Encyclopedia of Anxiety Disorders

Encyclopedia of Anxiety Disorders

Edited by **Peter Garner**

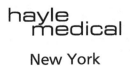

New York

Published by Hayle Medical,
30 West, 37th Street, Suite 612,
New York, NY 10018, USA
www.haylemedical.com

Encyclopedia of Anxiety Disorders
Edited by Peter Garner

International Standard Book Number: 978-1-63241-120-4 (Hardback)

Printed in the United States of America.

Contents

Preface

This book is a collection of contributions made by several clinical psychiatrists from across the globe, aimed at developing general research regarding anxiety and applying it in clinical contexts. It encompasses basic matters on clinical problems related to anxiety and novel therapeutic strategies applied. Substantial information regarding this field has been presented in this book.

This book has been the outcome of endless efforts put in by authors and researchers on various issues and topics within the field. The book is a comprehensive collection of significant researches that are addressed in a variety of chapters. It will surely enhance the knowledge of the field among readers across the globe.

It is indeed an immense pleasure to thank our researchers and authors for their efforts to submit their piece of writing before the deadlines. Finally in the end, I would like to thank my family and colleagues who have been a great source of inspiration and support.

Editor

Clinical Issues: Old Problems New Ideas

Social Anxiety, Beliefs About Expressing Emotions and Experiencing Positive Emotions

Jasminka Juretić and Ivanka Živčić-Bećirević

Additional information is available at the end of the chapter

1. Introduction

1.1. Social anxiety

Social anxiety refers to the excessive and persistent fear that a person will be embarrassed and/ or rejected by other people in one or more social or performance situations [1]. When a socially anxious person wants to present a desirable image of him/herself, a strong desire to accomplish it is accompanied by considerable uncertainty if he or she can really do it. Almost every person has to some extent felt socially anxious (feeling weird, blushing or stammer) in some social situations or situations in which he or she has been evaluated.

People differ in how often and with what intensity they feel socially anxious and show a certain degree of consistency in how anxious they are across social situations and over time [2]. Thus, some people are by nature strongly and more frequently socially anxious then other and we are considering this as a feature of the personality. Leary and Kowalski [2] find that, despite different results, there is little reason for assuming that social phobia/social anxiety disorder is qualitatively distinct from social anxiety as personality trait. Socially phobic persons experience a stronger intensity of anxiety in social situations, their attempts to escape unpleasant social contacts are more extreme and anxiety they are experiencing seriously affects their everyday life. A number of studies show that social anxiety is a continuum, from complete lack of social fear, through the usual forms of shyness and mild social anxiety, to social fears that significantly impair functioning and lead to social anxiety disorder [3]. When social situations become extremely unpleasant to a person and he or she starts to avoid them significantly impairing his/her quality of life, then we are talking of social anxiety disorder [1].

The fact that social phobia often precedes and/or occurs in comorbidity with other psychiatric disorders [4] and is often inadequately treated, stresses the need for further research and development of more efficient treatment [5, 6, 7]. When a person seeks professional help for many years after the social anxiety disorder has developed, it is possible that it has been primarily done because of symptoms related to other disorder/s.

Social anxiety disorder is a complex construct with which we try to describe a very heterogeneous group of people. It is important to distinguish people who are afraid of all or almost all social situations, from those who are afraid of only few of them. Likewise, it remains unclear whether the diagnostic subtypes are quantitatively different or reflect different qualitative entities of social phobia.

Studies have confirmed that at least two types of social anxiety should be distinguished: anxiety related to social interaction and anxiety related to some action performance. Anxiety related to social interaction consists of fears when meeting other people (e.g. initiating and maintaining conversation with other people, either in dyads or in groups), while performance anxiety relates to social evaluation concerns of doing something in front of other people (e.g. writing, playing an instrument, giving speeches) which the person would not be afraid doing if alone [8].

The role of cognitive processes and processes of focusing attention in the maintenance of social phobia are emphasized in contemporary theories [2, 9, 10]. According to these theories, extremely high standards of behavior in social environment maintain social phobia. These standards are characterized by negative thoughts, respectively statements of a person talking to him/herself and his/her assumption that other people see him/her as unsuitable, such as boring [9, 10]. In addition, socially anxious people consider beliefs and assumptions other people have about them as accurate and true. Consequences of these beliefs and assumptions are frequent negative self-statements, negative appraisal of their own behavior in social setting, increased self-focused attention on what has been done wrong in social interaction instead of focusing attention on those aspects which have been done well. Socially anxious people than become preoccupied with thoughts of how they would be evaluated by others and strongly shift attention to detailed monitoring and observation of themselves and impression they leave, including physiological symptoms of anxiety [9, 10, 11].

According to Clark and Wells [9, 11, 12, 13], when social phobics enter a feared situation, a set of assumptions (about themselves and their social world) is activated. If a person estimates situation as dangerous, so-called "anxiety program" is activated. The anxiety program includes physiological, cognitive, affective and behavioral changes that were designed to protect us from harm, but when the danger is largely overestimated this program loses its useful function. Anxiety symptoms, together with the strategies of coping with it, a person can misinterpret as sources of risk, which leads to an exacerbation of anxiety and a series of vicious circles that maintain social anxiety.

Several processes are important in development and maintenance of social anxiety [9]. One of the most important processes is the one concerning the self-focused attention. The shift in attentional focus happens to every social phobic – from perceiving the outside world to detailed monitoring and observation of oneself. The result is the construction of the self as a social object which helps creating an impression of how they appear to others. Onwards, entering feared situation, social phobics tend to use a wide range of safety behaviors they believe are helping them to prevent social disaster. Not only these behaviors are not helpful, they are also very harmful for social phobics. On one hand, safety behaviors can enhance feared behaviors and on the other, it prevents the person from perceiving any positive social feedback which might help in changing unrealistic beliefs. This means that unrealistic beliefs about feared behaviors or the consequences of these behaviors cannot be rejected. According to Clark and Wells, anticipatory and post event processing is very important; it contributes to the instability of self-image of social phobic person and in maintaining a high level of self-focused attention [11]. The basic feature of the anticipatory and post event processes is negativistic thinking concerning the extensive rumination about future failures or real or imagined past failures [14].

Besides importance of cognitive processes in developing and maintaining social anxiety disorder, it is also important to consider processes of emotion regulation. Many studies show that difficulties with emotion regulation are associated with psychopathology (e.g. 15, 16). It is necessary to explore the role of different ways of emotion regulation in development of specific disorders and to create models which integrate both cognitive and emotion regulation processes in development of psychopathology.

1.2. Emotion regulation

Through emotions we give other people information about our internal condition and behavioral intentions [17] and therefore they play an important role in interpersonal communication and our lives. They are manifested through specific cognitive, behavioral and physiological responses and are basis for adapting to new situations. If the person assess the situation as relevant to his or her goals and find it as an interesting one, then the emotions start to occur. Someone's goals may differ in many ways [18]. Goals may be enduring or temporary, conscious and complicated or unconscious and simple. They may be widely shared and understood or highly idiosyncratic. They may have a central role in understanding of ourselves or be peripheral. The base for developing an emotion is the meaning that a person gives to the situation. As the meaning changes over time, the emotion changes, too. Changes in emotional response can be triggered by situational changes or by the changes of significance that the situation has for the person [18].

Emotions occupy the whole body and include changes in the domains of subjective experience, behavior and physiological reactions. Impulses that encourage us to behave in certain ways and not act otherwise are associated with changes in the autonomic system and neuroendocrine changes. Those changes are followed by a particular behavior [18]. Because of a series of changes in various systems, emotions have imperative quality which means they can terminate the current activity and force a person to become aware of them. Also, when they occur, emotions often have to contend with other reactions that result from the same social context from which they have emerged. This is the most important fact for emotion regulation analysis because of the possibility to modulate emotions in many different ways.

Under certain circumstances, emotions have adaptive function; they have an evolutionary, a social and communicative and a decision making function [16] but they can also become a source of dysfunction and be maladaptive. It is a challenge to find the way how to regulate our own emotions in order to retain emotional useful features, and to limit their damaging aspect. Emotions can hurt us if they occur at the wrong time or with wrong intensity [18]. The ability to successfully regulate emotions is very important because those inappropriate emotional responses are involved in many forms of psychopathology or in somatic illness development.

A process model of emotion regulation supposes that specific strategies of emotion regulation can vary over a sequence of development of emotional responses [19- 21]. This conception of emotion regulation implies that emotion emerges with an evaluation of emotion cues that can be either external or internal. When a person pays attention to these cues and evaluate them in a certain way, the emotional cues trigger a coordinated set of response tendencies involving experiential, behavioral and physiological systems. Once these reactions occur, they can be modulated in different ways. As emotion develops over a certain period of time, emotion regulation strategies may differ by the point in the emotion-generative process at which they have their primary impact.

A process model of emotion regulation [19, 21- 23] highlights five families of emotion regulation strategies: situation selection, situation modification, attentional deployment, cognitive change and response modulation. Processes related to first four families are considered as *antecedent-focused* because they occur inclusive with appraisal based on which a complete emotional response will be created. In contrast, emotional regulation that is focused on response modulation is called *response-focused,* as it occurs after emotional response tendencies are activated (physiological, experiential and behavioral).

There are clear individual differences in preferred ways of emotional regulation which is important in predicting the behavior of other people [24]. It is shown that people who react better on life demands are the one able to recognize their own emotional states, to understand the meaning of emotions and use their informational value, as well as to adjust the expression of emotion and their own response in a way that fits the context of the situation. This set of abilities is often called emotional intelligence [25].

Suppression is one of the most widely studied emotion regulation strategies. It is a response-focused emotion regulation and refers to attempts of ignoring already generated emotions and avoiding their expression [21]. Suppression is a way to regulate emotions after cognitive reappraisal of emotional content, respectively it comes relatively late in the emotion-generative process after the behavioral tendencies have been initiated [19- 22]. Studies have shown that this way of emotion regulation is counterproductive because it actually leads to a paradoxical reinforcement of physiological arousal and unwanted affect itself [26]. Suppression of negative emotions brings no relief in sense of its subjective experience [22]. It also leads to decreased expression of both positive and negative emotions and is considered to interfere with relationships triggering unpleasant reactions in other people [20]. This emotional regulation strategy is associated with rare experience of positive emotions and their seldom expression [21, 24, 27].

Although suppression is generally considered to be a maladaptive emotion regulation strategy, it can be adaptive in situations where revealing emotions (e.g. anger or anxiety) should be restrained [28] or optimum distance between people should be maintained in order to facilitate a smooth social interaction [29].

1.3. Beliefs about expressing emotions

The way a person will regulate her or his emotion is strongly affected by beliefs she or he has about emotions [30]. If a person does not believe that efforts to regulate emotions will be successful, she or he will consider her/himself incompetent and uncertain and will invest a little effort and energy into implementing strategies of emotional regulation. In contrast, people who believe that emotions can be changed and controlled will be effective in regulating emotions using different adaptive strategies. Beliefs about emotions and emotional expression mediate the relation between experiencing emotions and there expression and thus have impact on emotion-generative process.

Negative reactivity to emotions refers to negative beliefs a person has about emotions, such as fearing consequences following emotion [25]. This construct applies to discomfort when experiencing emotions which leads to strong beliefs that emotional responses are dangerous and harmful for a person.

It has been assumed that socially anxious individuals may refrain from expressing their own emotions to avoid potential rejection. Refraining from expressing emotions offers less "material" for observation, which may cause rejection by others. Studies have shown that socially anxious people indicate a stronger suppression of their emotional experiences, they have lower capacity to monitor, differentiate and describe their own emotions and have more fears related to the experience of emotion and loss of control over them [31]. Spokas, Luterek and Heimberg [31] have found that beliefs about expressing emotions are significant mediators in the relationship between social anxiety and suppression of emotion, after controlling the effect of social phobics' ability to describe their own emotions to other people and their capacity to monitor them.

Tamir et al. [32] have confirmed that people who believe emotions are adaptable and changeable shape their own emotions by changing the evaluation of events that caused them. Regardless of the beliefs about emotions people have, they have an equal probability of masking their own feelings in certain situation. Those who believe in the malleability of emotions do not have fixed habit to use suppression as emotional regulation strategy.

1.4. Social anxiety, experiencing positive emotions and quality of life

Although inconsistent, positive emotions can have a lasting impact on our functioning through improvement of our well-being and relations with other people [33]. Research shows that induced positive emotions increase the personal feeling of unity with a close person and increase the confidence that we have in acquaintances. Likewise, the experience of positive emotions expands our attention and reflection in the field of personal and interpersonal functioning.

Other people and interaction with them are the source of positive events and emotions and therefore social activities and a sense of connection with other people are very important for our well-being [34]. There are also clear social benefits from sharing pleasant social events with other people, as they can be attributed to the relationship itself and thus reinforce social ties [35].

Social phobics are overly focused on the negative outcomes which interfere with their ability to recognize and respond to the potential rewards that come from the environment. It is expected that they experience high levels of negative affect and very low level of positive affect when anticipating participation, participating or constantly thinking about participating in social situation [36].

The current models of anxiety and depression (e.g., 37) generally assume that only depression is associated with deficits in positive emotions and events. Recent studies show that this deficit is also associated with social anxiety (e.g. 3, 36, 38). Socially anxious people have decreased positive affect and other positive psychological experiences (e.g., curiosity), even after controlling depressive symptoms, and have less frequent and less intense emotional response to positive social events [39]. They report about experiencing less frequent daily positive emotions and events than nonanxious people, and it could not be attributed to the conceptual overlap of social anxiety and other negative affective states [40]. The results have also shown that social phobics reported less positive events experienced during those days when they experienced higher levels of social anxiety and when tended to suppress emotions.

There is a strong evidence of correlation between social anxiety and reduced positive experi-ence [3]. Social anxiety explained an additional 4-5% of variance in positive experiences, after controlling for depression, which is important in understanding this relationship. In his meta-analysis a stable inverse relationship between social anxiety and positive affect has been found (r=-.36; 95% confidence limits (CI): -.31 to -.40) and it remains even after the variance attributed to depressive symptoms and disorders is removed.

It has been found that especially those aspects related to social interaction are related to low positive affect [8]. The significant and negative association of anxiety related to social interac-tion with all domains of positive psychological functioning, after controlling neuroticism, has been found [36], while anxiety and fear of being observed by others did not show significant association with these domains.

Social anxiety as a trait is negatively correlated with daily episodes of happiness, relaxation, and positive emotions in general and positively correlated with anger [41]. Results confirmed diminished experience of positive emotions and increased experience of anger in individuals with relatively high levels of social anxiety regardless of being alone or with other people. The authors believe that these two emotional experiences are potentially relevant to socially anxious people.

Socially anxious people express less positive emotions, overall pay less attention to their emotions and have more difficulty in describing their emotions than those with generalized anxiety disorder and control non-anxious group [42]. They express greater fear of anxiety, sadness, anger and even of positive emotions then control group. Insufficient attention to emotions or their frequent ignoring can contribute to difficulties that social phobics have in raising awareness and recognizing their own emotions and in understanding why they feel the way they do. Individuals who are able to recognize and use their emotions are better prepared to flexibly and adaptively respond to environmental requirements and appropriately regulate their affect [43].

Further studies of relationship between social anxiety and positive emotions are needed. It is well known that positive emotions induce more rapid recovery from adverse physiological effects of negative emotions, increase awareness during activity, efficacy and quality in decision making process and access to more creative and more flexible options in a particular situation [35]. Thus they have impact in life quality which has been found to be impaired in socially anxious people.

In order to understand better the relationship between social anxiety and experiencing positive and negative emotions and life satisfaction in general, the new model has been proposed and tested. Based on the model of social phobia [9], which emphasizes the role of cognitions, and process model of emotion regulation [20], especially the response modulation, proposed and tested model has included relationship between social anxiety (two dimensions: general fears and avoidance behaviors concerning social interactions and social evaluation concerns/anxiety related to being observed by others), beliefs about emotional expression, emotion suppression, positive and negative emotions and life satisfaction in general, controlling for depressive symptoms and neuroticism. It is assumed that the relationship between social anxiety and experiencing emotions and life satisfaction in general will be mediated by beliefs about expressing emotions and emotion suppression.

The further aim of the study was to test an interaction effect of social anxiety (with control of neuroticism and depression) and emotion suppression in explaining the frequency of experiencing positive and negative emotions.

2. Method

2.1. Participants

The sample consisted of 521 female students attending University of Rijeka and University of Pula, in Croatia. The average age of participants was 21.21 (SD = 2.5 years; range 18-37).

2.2. Instruments

To assess personality traits, The Big Five Inventory was used [44]. It provides a good coverage of all five personality traits (Extraversion, Agreeableness, Conscientiousness, Neuroticism and Openness), and has satisfactory psychometric properties. Inventory consists of 44 items, using five-point Likert-type format for answers scoring. For the purposes of this study only Neuroticism subscale was used (8 items). Cronbach-alpha for the present sample was .81.

Beck Depression Inventory-II [45] has been used to assess depressive symptoms. It is a 21-item self-report scale, using four-point Likert-type format (higher number meaning more severe depressive symptom). Cronbach-alpha in this sample was .90.

Anxiety in social interaction was assessed using Social Interaction Anxiety Scale [46] and fear of being observed and evaluated by others using Social Phobia Scale [46]. Both self-report scales consist of 20 items each, using five-point Likert-type format for scoring the answers. Cronbach-alpha for SIAS was .90 and for SPS .91.

Emotion Regulation Questionnaire [21] was used to assess emotional regulation strategies – reappraisal and suppression. For the purposes of this study only Suppression subscale was used. It consists of 4 items measuring the tendency to inhibit or conceal emotional expression that a person has experienced. Answers are scored by using seven-point Likert-type format. Internal reliability coefficient (Cronbach-alpha) for this subscale on the sample of participants of the present study was .74.

Attitudes Towards Emotional Expression Questionnaire [47] is constructed to measure negative beliefs and behaviors related to emotional expression and in the present study are used to assess beliefs about emotional expression. It is a 20-item self-report scale, using five-point Likert-type format for answers scoring. In the original form, the questionnaire consists of four factors: beliefs about meaning (sign of weakness), beliefs about expression (keep in control), beliefs about consequences (social rejection) and behavioral style (bottle up). The present study did not confirm these four subscales, but the authors recommended that subsequent research should focus on subscales as well as the overall scale. In the present study two factors were extracted, each of them with 10 items. The first factor is composed of items that are in the original questionnaire related to beliefs that expressing emotions is a sign of weakness, and beliefs that expressing emotions lead to social rejection. This factor is, therefore, called *the belief that expressing emotions leads to unpleasant consequences*. The second factor is composed of items that are in the original structure of the questionnaire related to the belief that it is important to have an expression of emotions under control and of items related to behavioral tendency to suppress the expression of emotion. This factor is called *the belief that emotions should not be expressed*. Cronbach-alpha for each subscale was .87.

To measure the subjective experience of emotion, Positive and Negative Affect Schedule – Expanded Form [48] has been used. This is a 20-item inventory that consists of 10 adjectives measuring positive affect (e.g. cheerful) and 10 adjectives measuring negative affect (e.g. irritable). Answers are scored by using five-point Likert-type format. Cronbach-alpha for positive affect subscale was .85 and for negative affect subscale .87.

In order to assess how a person is satisfied with her life, a Satisfaction with Life Scale [49] has been used. It is a 5-item self-report scale, using seven-point Likert-type format for answers scoring. Cronbach-alpha in the present sample was .86.

2.3. Procedure

Data were collected during classes in group format, anonymously. Goal of the study was briefly explained and students participated voluntarily. The students who were not willing to participate were allowed to leave the room.

3. Results

In order to determine the relationship between the variables involved in the study, correlation analyzes have been performed. Pearson's correlation coefficients are shown in Table 1.

	Fear of being evaluated by others	Belief – expressing emotions leads to unpleasant consequences	Belief – emotions should not be expressed	Suppression of emotions	Positive emotions	Negative emotions	Life satisfaction
Anxiety in social interactions	.74**	.45**	.29**	.28**	-.30**	.52**	-.40**
Fear of being evaluated by others		.41**	.21**	.18**	-.21**	.53**	-.38**
Belief – expressing emotions leads to unpleasant consequences			.64**	.48**	-.15**	.39**	-.31**
Belief – emotions should not be expressed				.75**	-.14**	.14**	-.18**
Suppression of emotions					-.15**	.12**	-19**
Positive emotions						-.17**	.43**
Negative emotions							-.43**

**p <.01

Table 1. Correlations between variables involved in the proposed model

According to results, if a young woman has a higher anxiety in social interactions, she will have increased fear of other people's evaluation. Socially anxious person will believe that emotions should not be expressed and that their expression leads to unpleasant consequences so will suppress emotions and will experience negative emotions more often. Such a female experiences positive emotions also less frequently and is less satisfied with her life. The belief that expressing emotions leads to unpleasant consequences and that emotions should not be expressed are highly positively correlated with each other, and are positively correlated with suppression of emotions and more frequent experience of negative emotions. Both beliefs are negatively correlated with life satisfaction and positive emotions. A female who uses a strategy of suppressing emotions as a way of emotion regulation, has lower life satisfaction and less frequently experiences positive but more often negative emotions. Frequent experience of positive emotions means less frequent experience of negative emotions and greater satisfaction with life, while often experiencing negative emotions means less satisfaction with life in general.

In order to determine the unique relationship between social anxiety and other variables in further analyzes, a common variance of social anxiety shared with neuroticism and depression is controlled. The aim was to eliminate the possibility that the potential negative effects of social anxiety, primarily in experiencing positive emotions, can be attributed to a common variance, or negative affectivity, which is shared by social anxiety, neuroticism and depression, and not to the uniqueness of social anxiety. Certain models suggest that neuroticism as a higher common vulnerability factor explains most of the covariance among the more specific constructs such as social anxiety, depression and anger [36]. It is considered that there are unique characteristics of high social anxiety that are not part of neuroticism. In order to control neuroticism and depression, regression analyzes were performed with standardized residuals calculated for both types of social fears. In regression analysis, the predictors included neuroticism and depression. Fear of social interaction was a criteria in the first analysis and a fear of being evaluated by others in the the second. After that the standardized values for both types of social fears were calculated. In this way we got two new variables, which were used for further analysis and in which negative affectivity related to neuroticism and depression is excluded, and only the part that is associated with a particular social fear has remained.

A variety of statistical analyzes were conducted in order to answer the research questions. The results were processed using the program LISREL 8 [50] and SPSS 15.0 for Windows.

3.1. Testing the model

The tested model included the relationship between both types of social fears, beliefs about expressing emotions, suppression of emotions and frequency of experiencing positive and negative emotions and life satisfaction.

The theoretical model is shown in Figure 1. Only significant direct and indirect effects are shown.

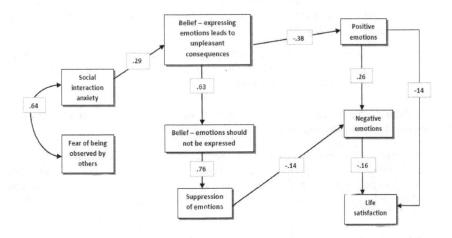

Figure 1. The model of relations between social anxiety, beliefs about the expression of emotions, suppression of emotions, experiencing positive and negative emotions and life satisfaction

Model fit indexes for this model are shown in Table 2.

	χ^2	degrees of freedom	χ^2/ degrees of freedom	RMSEA	GFI	NFI	CFI
Model	83.52***	19	4.39	0.09	0.96	0.93	0.95

***< p.001

Table 2. Fit indexes for theoretical model compared with empirical data

The indexes shown in Table 1. indicate that this model is acceptable. Chi-square index is significant, but it is affected by sample size and for large samples is generally significant. To reduce sensitivity of model chi-square to sample size, ratio chi-square and degrees of freedom have been calculated. This ratio indicates that the model is acceptable as well as RMSEA value. The values of GFI, NFI and CFI show that the model has a good fit with empirical data.

In this model, the fear of other people's evaluation does not have direct or indirect effects on remaining variables included in the model. Anxiety in social interactions has only a direct positive effect on the belief that the expression of emotions leads to unpleasant consequences (.29), while other effects of this variable, except the one mentioned, are mediated by the belief that emotions should not be expressed and by suppression of emotions. The belief that expressing emotions leads to unpleasant consequences have a direct, positive and strong effect on the belief that emotions should not be expressed (.63) and moderate, negative and direct effect on positive emotions (-.38). The belief that emotions should not be expressed has a direct, high and positive effect on the suppression of emotions (.76), which has a direct negative effect on negative emotions (-.14). Positive emotions have a direct positive effect on negative emotions (.26) and negative on life satisfaction (-.14). Negative emotions have a direct negative effect on life satisfaction (-.16).

According to obtained results it is evident that the effects of social anxiety on the experience of positive and negative emotions and life satisfaction are achieved indirectly through beliefs about emotional expression and suppression.

3.2. The contribution of interaction effect of social anxiety and suppression of emotions to the frequency of experiencing positive and negative emotions

In order to test whether there is an interaction effect of social anxiety (with control of neuroticism and depression) and suppression of emotions in explaining the variance of experiencing positive and negative emotions after determining the individual contributions of both types of social anxiety individually and suppression of emotions, hierarchical regression analyzes were conducted.

Four hierarchical regression analyzes were conducted. As the first step, anxiety in social interactions has been included in the first two analyzes, and the fear of other people's evaluation in the other two. In each of the hierarchical regression analyzes the suppression of emotions has been included in the second step. In the third step the interaction of anxiety in social interactions and suppression has been included in the first two analyzes, and interaction of fear of other people's evaluation and the suppression in the other two. For each analysis there were two criteria - positive and negative emotions.

Results are shown in Tables 3. and 4.

					positive emotions				
predictors	R^2	ΔR^2	F-change	β	predictors	R^2	ΔR^2	F-change	β
1.step anxiety in social interactions	.03	.03	12.72***	-.13**	1.step fear of being evaluated by others	.00	.00	1.21	-.03
2.step suppression of emotions	.05	.02	9.67**	-.15**	2.step suppression of emotions	.03	.03	13.86	-.17***
3.step anxiety in social interactions x suppression of emotions	.05	.00	.02	.00	3.step fear of being evaluated by others x suppression of emotions	.03	.00	.00	.00

** p<.01; *** p<.001

Table 3. Results of hierarchical regression analyzes for positive emotions as criteria

The results of hierarchical analysis which includes anxiety in social interactions show that included variables explain only 5% of the variance in frequency of experiencing positive emotions. Anxiety in social interactions explains 3% of the variance of criteria and suppression of emotions 2%, while the interaction of these two variables does not explain the frequency of experiencing positive emotions. Both anxiety in social interactions and suppression of emotions are negative predictors.

The results of hierarchical analysis which includes fear of being evaluated by others showed that only 3% of variance in frequency of experiencing positive emotions is explained, while suppression of emotions is the only significant and negative predictor.

					negative emotions				
predictors	R^2	ΔR^2	F-change	β	predictors	R^2	ΔR^2	F-change	β
1.step anxiety in social interactions	.04	.04	18.27***	.17***	1.step fear of being evaluated by others	.04	.04	21.65***	.20***
2.step suppression of emotions	.05	.01	3.51	.09	2.step suppression of emotions	.05	.01	4.83**	.10**
3.step anxiety in social interactions x suppression of emotions	.05	.00	.24	.02	3.step fear of being evaluated by others x suppression of emotions	.05	.00	.04	-.01

** p<.01; *** p<.001

Table 4. Results of hierarchical regression analyzes for negative emotions as criteria

The analysis with the anxiety someone is experiencing in social interactions, included in the first step, showed that only this variable is significant and positive predictor of the frequency of experiencing negative emotions and it explains 4% of the variance. Additional 1% of variance is explained by suppression of emotions as a strategy of emotional regulation, but as well as interaction included in the third step, it is not a significant predictor in the analysis.

The other conducted analysis showed that included variables explain only 5% of the variance in frequency of experiencing negative emotions. The fear of being evaluated by others and suppression of emotions are the only significant and positive predictors, while the interaction effect of these two variables is neither significant nor does it additionally explain the frequency of experiencing negative emotions.

4. Discussion

When presented model for the presumed relations was tested, only social anxiety that refers to the fear that a person experiences during encounters with other people (e.g. initiating and maintaining conversations either in dyads or in groups) was found significant. As previous studies revealed its role in experiencing positive emotions, it was expected for this aspect of social anxiety to be significant [3, 10, 35, 36, 38, 40]. The second type of social anxiety, the one related to fear of being observed and evaluated by others, has not been studied enough in previous research. Although it was expected that, as a social fear, it could have had some effects on other variables, it was not proven. There is a possibility that this kind of fear is not so important in comparison with anxiety felt during social interactions.

Anxiety in social interactions did not show the expected direct effects. In the first place there was no direct effect on the beliefs that emotions should not be expressed and on their suppression. Its relationship with these variables is only indirect through belief that expression of emotions leads to unpleasant consequences with high and positive effects. This kind of relationship would mean that the suppression of emotions in a socially anxious woman occurs when she has a strong belief that expressing emotions leads to unpleasant consequences, due to which the belief that emotions should therefore not be expressed will be activated, which will result in her scruple of expressing any emotion (emotional suppression). The importance of our beliefs in the process of emotion regulation is confirmed by these results. Cognitive model [9] assumes that when an individual finds him/herself in a particular social context, negative assumptions concerning the assessment of the situation as dangerous will be triggered. In this way a whole series of negative automatic thoughts about themselves and other people are triggered. The finding that the beliefs about expressing emotions have an indirect role in relation of social anxiety and suppressing emotions stresses the significant role of cognitions. It seems that the belief that expressing emotions leads to unpleasant consequences is "superior" to the belief that emotions should not be expressed. This result is not unusual because if someone believes that it is not good to express emotions, he or she must have a direct or an indirect experience that emotion expression has led to unpleasant outcome. Unpleasant consequences are related to the belief that expressing emotions is a sign of weakness, which means that the one expressing emotions will be perceived as weak by others. Evaluating someone as a weak person means a specific trait or flaw because it is expected that an adult must be able to effectively and appropriately regulate his or her own emotional expression. Those who can control emotions and know how not to express them are estimated as powerful, while those who aren't successful in it tend to be estimated as weak, possibly even less desirable as friends and partners.

Although someone's fear of being evaluated and perceived as weak is in the first place related to the aspect of emotion regulation, we might draw a parallel to research [7] which dealt with the fundamental fears that social phobics experience. One of the four dimensions of stimuli evaluation that elicit social fear refers to the fear of socially anxious individuals to be seen with some character flaws. Moscovitch [7] believes that this aspect can be represented with statements like "I'm boring", "I'm stupid", with activities in which there is a disclosure of personal information (e.g. talking one on one) and with those in which these features are being questioned (e.g. telling jokes). According to his model, social phobics are afraid that their features, in fact themselves, in the eyes of others might be seen as incomplete in comparison to other people. It carries certain consequences of which they are afraid. Unpleasant consequences are related to other people's negative evaluation and rejection, embarrassment, loss of social status and likewise, which is neither pleasant nor desirable. For the same reason, an individual will resort to a number of safety behaviors. Being afraid of ranking as socially undesirable person supports the belief that expressing emotions leads to unpleasant consequences which clearly leads to belief that it is better to be emotionally restrained and, ultimately, to emotional suppression. Since socially anxious people simultaneously feel desire to approach other people but are afraid of rejection, strategy of suppressing emotional expression and adherence to the belief that expressing emotions leads to unpleasant consequences seems, from their perspective, a wise strategy to maintain social status. This mode of emotion regulation is used with intention to reduce the likelihood of experiencing a single unpleasant consequence. It is actually a paradox since the suppression of emotions is counterproductive, as it does not reduce unwanted, unpleasant experience and even strengthen physiological arousal [20- 22, 24, 26, 27, 51].

Anxiety in social interactions has only indirect effects on positive and negative emotions. The effect on positive emotions is realized over the belief that expressing emotions leads to the unpleasant consequences. Its effect on negative emotions is achieved through the emotional suppression (with previous indirect role of beliefs about expressing emotions). If a woman believes that expressing emotions is not good because it will lead to unpleasant consequences, she rarely experiences positive emotions. When she decides to suppress her emotions, it leads to increased incidence of experiencing negative emotions.

However, there are results that differ from the expected. It is found that the more frequent experience of positive emotions also leads to increased incidence of experiencing negative emotions and to overall life satisfaction reduction. This result might be due to low negative correlation (-.17) between experiencing negative and positive emotions, which was not expected when the emotions are measured in this way. When measuring the experiencing of emotions in a way that the participants are asked to indicate how they usually feel, there should be no correlation between positive and negative emotions [52]. Increased emotionality of the participants (emotional reactivity) may be the reason for such result. Emotionality indicates individual's predominant intensity of emotional reactivity which includes a person's tendency to overreact even to weak stressors [53]. Emotional reactivity was found to be associated with high blood pressure [54]. People differ in emotional reactivity and those who are emotionally more reactive are lacking in control over thoughts related to the emotional content and therefore emotions themselves. It is possible that the participants in this study are prone to experience and to express positive emotions, which in turn has an effect on the more frequent experience of negative emotions. Generally speaking, it is possible that these women are more likely to experience positive and negative emotions. Some authors also suggest that people, who experience intense positive emotions, also experience intense negative emotions [55].

It is also uncommon to find that the emotional suppression leads to less often experience of negative emotions, which is not in accordance with paradoxical effect of this emotion regulation strategy [20-22; 24, 26, 27, 51]. It is possible that, despite the strong impact of the emotional expression beliefs, our participants do not come up with enough strong tendencies to inhibit or to conceal emotions (M = 3.05).

As expected, it has been confirmed that more frequent experience of negative emotions leads to reduced global life satisfaction [56]. According to the hierarchical model of happiness [57], subjective well-being is related to cognitive and emotional components that are interconnected. Experiencing positive and negative emotions is emotional component and global assessment of life satisfaction refers to a cognitive component. According to *bottom-up* theories (deductive theories) [58], life satisfaction and happiness are the result of an individual's total number of happy moments in his or her life. In line with this notion of subjective well-being, a person is happy when experiencing a lot of happy moments, so the measure of general life satisfaction is derived through the sum of satisfaction in different life areas. This would mean that if a person is satisfied with certain areas of her or his life (e.g. partnerships, finance, etc.) then she or he gives higher estimation of global life satisfaction.

The obtained result that the more frequent experience of negative emotions leads to a reduced life satisfaction is in line with the assumptions on the assessment of quality of life, but the finding that more frequent experience of positive emotions has the same effect, certainly is not. As already noted, there are data on the intense experience of both positive and negative emotions [55] which can be related to the higher frequency of experiencing both of them. It turns out that the frequency of experiencing both positive and negative emotions have unfavorable effects on global life satisfaction for our participants.

It can be concluded that this model has provided additional insight into understanding the relationship between social anxiety, beliefs about the expression of emotions, suppression of emotions, and the experiencing of positive and negative emotions and the global life satisfaction in women. The main contribution of this model is the result of the role that cognitions play in these relationships. Their role is reveled over the beliefs about expressing emotions to other variables that confirmed the mediating role of these beliefs in relation to social anxiety and suppression of emotions [31]. It has also been found that only aspect of social anxiety which refers to the anxiety experienced in social interactions has significant effects in these relations.

A further objective of this study was to examine whether there is an interactive effect of social anxiety (with control of neuroticism and depression) and suppression of emotions in explaining the frequency of experiencing positive and negative emotions after determining the individual contributions of each type of social anxiety and of emotion suppression. The starting point for setting this problem has been the assumption that severe social anxiety can become an even bigger problem if there are rigid tendencies in mastering and concealing emotional experiences [35]. The authors were primarily concerned with the relationship of one aspect of social anxiety, the one that refers to the anxiety experienced in social interactions, and experiencing positive emotions, so this paper aims to determine the contribution of other type of social fear (fear of other people's evaluation) in experiencing positive and negative emotions. Although the research is primarily focused on understanding the experience of positive emotions in socially anxious women, contribution of both types of social fears and the suppression of emotions and their interaction effect on negative emotions has been tested.

The results of the hierarchical regression analyzes reveled that the interaction effect of social anxiety and suppression of emotion was not significant in explaining the frequency of experiencing neither positive nor negative emotions. This result does not support the theory about the interactional effects of these two variables on the expression of positive emotions [35], although the authors themselves have failed to confirm the „joint vulnerability" model. The reason for this result may lie in the fact that women who participated in this study were low in social anxiety and suppression of emotion was not their main emotion regulation strategy (anxiety in social interactions M = 0.89, SD = 0.59; fear of other people's evaluation M = 0.73, SD = 0.61; suppression M = 3.05, SD = 1.22). It is possible that this result is a consequence of experiencing low frequency (or at least the reporting of it) of positive (M = 3.29, SD = 0.61) and negative emotions (M = 2.09, SD = 0.56), which again is the issue of emotional reactivity of the women involved in this research.

Only social fear related to anxiety experienced in social interactions was a significant predictor of the frequency of experiencing positive emotions. Expression of this type of fear contributes to less often experience of positive emotions. The results are consistent with findings about negative role of social anxiety in experiencing positive emotions (e.g. 3, 36). However, the role of anxiety in social interactions was confirmed, and the fear of other people's evaluation shows no significance in studying positive emotional experiences. Relationships with other people are very important for our welfare, and positive events and emotions are important for the development of such relations. Mastering fear of social interaction is important for the ability to develop relationships with other people and, to some extent, precedes fear of the other people's evaluation which could emerge after the contact. In this study, fear of other people's evaluation mostly includes evaluation of foreigners and people who are not emotionally important to us (which does not diminish the importance of this type of evaluation for socially anxious people). Women in this study are not diagnosed as socially anxious, so it is possible that this fear does not interfere with their relationships with other people as far as the fear of interaction with them do. The presence of other people is important for the frequency of experiencing positive emotional experiences, and if this fear is prevalent, the opportunity for such experiences is reduced.

Suppressing was found as a negative predictor of the frequency of experiencing positive emotions, which means that the use of this strategy of emotion regulation contributes to less often experience of positive emotions. The result is consistent with the finding that the suppression of emotions leads to decreased expression of both positive and negative emotions, thus interfering with relationships with other people [20] and that this strategy is associated with rare experiencing positive emotions and their seldom expression [21, 24, 27]. Suppression of emotions was significant predictor of experiencing negative emotions, but only in the analysis which included fear of other people's evaluation as a predictor. Selecting this emotion regulation strategy means more frequent experience of negative emotions. The result is consistent with previous studies that have found this mode of emotion regulation as counter-productive because it leads to paradoxical reinforcement of physiological arousal and unwanted affect itself [26], and the suppression of expressing negative emotions does not bring any relief in terms of the subjective experience of negative emotions [22].

Women who have expressed any of the two types of social fears experience more frequent negative emotions which is consistent with previous results. Anxiety disorders are associated with exaggerated and persistent negative emotions [59] and the relationship between social anxiety and frequent experience of negative emotions is confirmed in a number of studies (e.g. 3).

Results of this study showed that only anxiety in social interactions explains the experience of positive emotions with only 3% of the variance explained. In his meta-analysis Kashdan [3] also found that social anxiety explains 4-5% of the variance in positive experiences after controlling depression. Our study went a step further by controlling neuroticism as a personality trait, which would certainly „blur" independent contribution of social anxiety in explaining the experience of positive emotions. The data of this study provide significant contribution, showing that social anxiety has its own independent role in understanding the reduced experience of positive emotions, and that it cannot be attributed to effects of depression and neuroticism.

It was found that both types of social fears have a significant role for experiencing negative emotions and that each could explain 4% of the variance of frequency of experiencing negative emotions. This finding confirms and emphasizes the independent role of social anxiety in more frequent experiencing of negative emotions because effects of depression and neuroticism are controlled.

The results of this study should be considered within the context of its limitations. First, the study is based on participants' self-assessment. While this is the most common method of data collection, for this type of research it is important to use a clinical sample of socially anxious people who use different strategies of emotion regulation. In order to comprehend better this set of problem, experimental design would have been a better solution to answer the research questions. However, the results of previous studies have shown different ways of regulating emotion in the laboratory experiments and those implemented in everyday circumstances, so it would be better to implement this type of research in everyday circumstances of socially anxious individuals. Such research would better succeed to grasp impairment of social functioning in relation to emotional regulation strategies, as well as effects on close relationships.

Further limitation is the fact that only women participated in the study. Because of gender differences in the severity of social anxiety and ways of regulating emotions, future research should check the same model in a male sample and compare models for both sexes.

The sample included only those participants who agreed to participate in the study and who, on average, were not socially anxious. It is possible that some women who decided not to participate in the research were more socially anxious and their results would be valuable in the study of relationships of social anxiety and other variables. Research on a clinical sample of socially anxious women whose daily functioning is disrupted by disorder could be especially useful and might give different results.

Future research should focus on examining individual differences in emotional reactivity and sensitivity when studying the relationships that are examined here. As this study deals only with one of the strategies of emotion regulation - suppression, it would be important to test the model with reappraisal as emotion regulation strategy. This strategy has been found as adaptive and, as our data indicate the importance of cognitions in relationship between social anxiety and suppression of emotions, it would be important to see their relations when using this cognitive strategy of emotion regulation.

Considering that dimensions of social anxiety and emotion regulation are important for creating our relationships with others, future research might include assessment of quality of close relationships in the model. It was found that emotion regulation strategies have different effects on memory, and through the memory contents that are related to interpersonal relationships on the quality of close relationships [24, 60].

Practical contributions of this research are also worth mentioning. The results point out the importance that beliefs about emotions and their expression have on suppression of emotion, and experiencing emotions in general. Since these are dysfunctional beliefs that the expression of emotions leads to unpleasant consequences (to which a person does not want to be exposed), and due to which the belief that emotions should not be expressed is activated, the therapeutic work should focus on restructuring such beliefs about danger of emotions and their expression. On the other hand, the expression of emotions is important in interpersonal relationships. In development of quality close relationships it is necessary to mutually share emotional experiences which does not occur if someone perceives it as threatening. Therefore, it is important to teach socially anxious people about adaptive strategies of emotion regulation and to point out benefits, advantages and disadvantages of using different strategies. However, as the emotion regulation strategy is only a part of the entire system of self-regulation, it would be useful to check the person's capacities for self-regulation in general.

5. Conclusions

In conclusion, the results of this study have provided more insight into the complex relationship between social anxiety, emotional experiences and the quality of life in general. The mediation mechanisms that play a role in these relationships have been revealed by structural modeling, which has not been done in previous researches.

Author details

Jasminka Juretić and Ivanka Živčić-Bećirević

University of Rijeka, Faculty of Humanities and Social Sciences, Department of Psychology, Croatia

References

[1] American Psychiatric AssociationDiagnostic and statistical manual of mental disorders (4th ed.) text revision. Washington, DC: Am. Psychiatr. Assoc.; (2004).

[2] Leary, M. R, & Kowalski, R. M. Social Anxiety. New York: The Guilford Press; (1995).

[3] Kashdan, T. B. Social anxiety spectrum and diminished positive experiences: theoretical synthesis and meta-analysis. Clin Psychol Rev. (2007). , 27(3), 348-65.

[4] Brunello, N. den Boer JA, Judd LL, Kasper S, Kelsey JE, Lader M, Lecrubier Y, Lepine JP, Lydiard RB, Mendlewicz J, Montgomery SA, Racagni G, Stein MB, Wittchen HU. Social phobia: diagnosis and epidemiology, neurobiology and pharmacology, comorbidity and treatment. J Affect Disords. (2000). Oct; , 60(1), 61-74.

[5] Gilbert, P, Boxall, M, Cheung, M, & Irons, C. The relation of paranoid ideation and social anxiety in a mixed clinical population. Clin Psychol Psychother. (2005). Mar/ Apr; 12 (2), 124-33.

[6] Furmark, T, Tillfors, M, Every, P, Marteinsdottir, I, Gefvert, O, & Fredrikson, M. Social phobia in the general population: prevalence and sociodemographic profile. Soc Psychiatry Psychiatr Epidemiol. (1999). Aug; , 34(8), 416-24.

[7] Moscovitch, D. A. What is the core fear in social phobia? A new model to facilitate individualized case conceptualization and tretment. Cogn Behav Pract. (2009). , 16, 123-34.

[8] Hughes, A. A, Heimberg, R. G, Coles, M. E, Gibb, B. E, Liebowitz, M. R, & Schneier, F. R. Relations of the factors of the tripartite model of anxiety and depression to types of social anxiety. Behav Res Ther. (2006). Nov; , 44(11), 1629-41.

[9] Clark, D. M, & Wells, A. A cognitive model of social phobia. In: Heimberg RG, Liebowitz MR, Hope DA, Schneier FR, editors. Social phobia: diagnosis, assessment, and tretment. New York: The Guilford Press; (1995). , 69-94.

[10] Rapee, R. M, & Heimberg, R. G. A cognitive-behavioral model of anxiety in social phobia. Behav Res Ther. (1997). Aug; , 35(8), 741-56.

[11] Wells, A. Cognitive therapy of anxiety disorders: a practical manual and conceptual guide. Chichester: John Wiley & Sons Ltd; (1997).

[12] Clark, D. M. Panic disorder and social phobia. In: Clark DM., Fairburn CG, editors. Science and practice of cognitive behaviour therapy. New York: Oxford University Press; (1997).

[13] Clark, D. M. A cognitive perspective on social phobia. In: Crozier WR, Alden LE, editors. The essential handbook of social anxiety for clinicians. Chichester: John Wiley & Sons Ltd; (2005).

[14] Spurr, J. M, & Stopa, L. Self-focused attention in social phobia and social anxiety. Clin Psychol Rev.(2002). , 22, 947-75.

[15] Campbell-sills, L, & Barlow, D. H. Incorporating emotion regulation into conceptualizations and treatments of anxiety and mood disorders. In: Gross JJ, editor. Handbook of emotion regulation. New York: The Guilford Press; (2007). , 542-560.

[16] Amstadter, A. Emotion regulation and anxiety disorders. J Anxiety Disord. (2008). , 22(2), 211-221.

[17] Frijda, N. H. The Emotions. New York: The Press Syndicate of the University of Cambridge; (1986).

[18] Gross, J. J, & Thompson, R. A. Emotion regulation: conceptual foundations. In: Gross JJ, editor. Handbook of emotion regulation. New York: The Guilford Press; (2007). , 3-27.

[19] Gross, J. J. The emerging field of emotion regulation: an integrative review. Rev Gen Psychol. (1998). , 2, 271-99.

[20] Gross, J. J. Emotion regulation in adulthood: timing is everything. Curr Dir Psychol Sci. (2001). , 10, 214-19.

[21] Gross, J. J, & John, O. P. Individual differences in two emotion regulation processes: implications for affect, relationships, and well-being. J Pers Soc Psychol. (2003).

[22] Gross, J. J. Antecedent- and response-focused emotion regulation: divergent consequences for experience, expression, and physiology. J Pers Soc Psychol. (1998). , 74, 224-37.

[23] Gross, J. J. Emotion regulation. In: Lewis M, Haviland-Jones JM, Barrett LF, editors. Handbook of emotions. New York: The Guilford Press; (2008).

[24] Richards, J. M, & Gross, J. J. Emotion regulation and memory: the cognitive costs of keeping one's cool. J Pers Soc Psychol. (2000). Sep; , 79(3), 410-24.

[25] Mennin, D. S, Holaway, R, Fresco, D. M, Moore, M. T, & Heimberg, R. G. Delineating components of emotion and its dysregulation in anxiety and mood psychopathology. Behav Ther. (2007). , 38(3), 284-302.

[26] Hofmann, S. G, Heering, S, Sawyer, A. T, & Asnaani, A. How to handle anxiety: the effects of reappraisal, acceptance, and suppression strategies on anxious arousal. Behav Res Ther. (2009). May; , 47(5), 389-94.

[27] John, O. P, & Gross, J. J. Healthy and unhealthy emotion regulation: personality processes, individual differences, and life span development. J Pers. (2004). , 72, 1301-34.

[28] Butler, E. A, Egloff, B, Wilhelm, F. H, Smith, N. C, Erickson, E. A, & Gross, J. J. The social consequences of expressive suppression. Emotion. (2003). Mar; 3 (1), 48-67.

[29] Clark, M. S, & Taraban, C. Reactions to and willingness to express emotion in communal and exchange relationships. J Exp Soc Psychol. (1991). , 27, 324-36.

[30] John, O. P, & Gross, J. J. Individual differences in emotional regulation. In: Gross JJ, editor. Handbook of emotion regulation. New York: The Guilford Press; (2007). , 351-373.

[31] Spokas, M, Luterek, J. A, & Heimberg, R. G. Social anxiety and emotional suppression: the mediating role of beliefs. J Behav Ther Exp Psychiatry. (2009). Jun; , 40(2), 283-91.

[32] Tamir, M, John, O. P, Srivastava, S, & Gross, J. J. Implicit theories of emotion: affective and social outcomes across a major life transition. J Pers Soc Psychol. (2007). Apr; , 92(4), 731-44.

[33] Garland, E. L, Fredrickson, B, Kring, A. M, Johnson, D. P, Meyer, P. S, & Penn, D. L. Upward spirals of positive emotions counter downward spirals of negativity: insights from the broaden-and-build theory and affective neuroscience on the treatment of emotion dysfunctions and deficits in psychopathology. Clin Psychol Rev. (2010). Nov; , 30(7), 849-64.

[34] Langston, C. A. Capitalizing on and coping with daily life events: expressive responses to positive events. J Pers Soc Psychol. (1994). , 6, 1115-25.

[35] Kashdan, T. B, & Breen, W. E. Social anxiety and positive emotions: A prospective examination of a self-regulatory model with emotion suppression and expression tendencies as moderators. Behav Ther. (2008). , 39, 1-12.

[36] Kashdan, T. B. Social anxiety dimensions, neuroticism, and the contours of positive psychological functioning. Cognit Ther Res. (2002). , 26, 789-810.

[37] Clark, L. A, & Watson, D. Tripartite model of anxiety and depression: psychometric evidence and taxonomic implications. J Abnorm Psychol. (1991). Aug; , 100(3), 316-336.

[38] Kashdan, T. B. The neglected relationship between social interaction anxiety and hedonic deficits: differentiation from depressive symptoms. J Anxiety Disord. (2004). , 18(5), 719-30.

[39] Weeks, J. W, Jakatdar, T. A, & Heimberg, R. G. Comparing and contrasting fears of positive and negative evaluation as facets of social anxiety. J Soc Clin Psychol. (2010). , 29(1), 68-94.

[40] Kashdan, T. B, & Steger, M. Expanding the topography of social anxiety: an experience sampling assessment of positive emotions and events, and emotion suppression. Psychol Sci. (2006). , 17, 120-28.

[41] Kashdan, T. B, & Collins, R. L. Social anxiety and the experience of positive emotions and anger in everyday life: an ecological momentary assessment approach. Anxiety Stress Coping. (2010). May; , 23(3), 259-72.

[42] Turk, C. L, Heimberg, R. G, Luterek, J. A, Mennin, D. S, & Fresco, D. M. Delineating emotion regulation deficits in generalized anxiety disorder: a comparison with social anxiety disorder. Cognit Ther Res. (2005). , 29, 89-106.

[43] Feldman-barrett, L, Gross, J. J, Conner-christensen, T, & Benvenuto, M. Knowing what you're feeling and knowing what to do about it: mapping the relation between emotion differentiation and emotion regulation. Cogn Emot. (2001). , 15, 713-724.

[44] John, O. P, & Srivastava, S. The big five trait taxonomy: history, measurement, and theoretical perspectives. In: Pervin LA, John OP, editors. Handbook of personality: theory and research. New York: Guilford Press; (1999).

[45] Beck, A. T, Steer, R. A, & Brown, G. K. Beck depression inventory- second edition (BDI-II) manual. San Antonio: Harcourt Brace & Company; (1996).

[46] Mattick, R. P, & Clarke, J. C. Development and validation of measures of social phobia scrutiny fear and social interaction anxiety. Behav Res Ther. (1998). Apr; , 36(4), 455-70.

[47] Joseph, S, Williams, R, Irwing, P, & Cammock, T. The preliminary development of measure to assess attitudes towards emotional expression. Pers Individ Dif. (1994). , 16, 869-75.

[48] Watson, D, & Clark, L. A. The PANAS-X: Manual for the positive and negative affect schedule- expanded form. University of Iowa: Psychology Publications; (1994).

[49] Diener, E, Emmons, R. A, Larsen, R. J, & Griffin, S. The satisfaction with life scale. J Pers Assess. (1985). , 49, 71-5.

[50] Jöreskog, K, & Sörbom, D. LISREL 8.53. Scientific Software International, Inc., Chicago. (2002).

[51] Aldao, A, Nolen-hoeksema, S, & Schweizer, S. Emotion regulation strategies and psychopathology: a meta analysis. Clin Psychol Rev. (2010). , 30(2), 217-237.

[52] Diener, E, & Emmons, R. A. The independence of positive and negative affect. J Pers Soc Psychol. (1985). , 47, 1105-17.

[53] Rende, R. Emotion and behavior genetics. In: Lewis M, Haviland-Jones J, editors. Handbook of emotions. New York: Guilford Press; (2000). , 192-203.

[54] Melamed, S. Emotional reactivity and elevated blood pressure. Psychosom Med. (1987). May-Jun; , 49(3), 217-25.

[55] Magnus, K, Diener, E, Fujita, F, & Pavot, W. Extraversion and neuroticism as predictors of objective life events: A longitudinal analysis. J Pers Soc Psychol.(1993). Nov; , 65(5), 1046-53.

[56] Kuppens, P, Realo, A, & Diener, E. The role of positive and negative emotions in life satisfaction judgment across nations. J Pers Soc Psychol. (2008). Jul; , 95(1), 66-75.

[57] Diener, E, Scollon, C. N, & Lucas, R. E. The evolving concept of subjective well-being: the multifaced nature of happiness. Advances in Cell Aging and Gerontology. (2003). , 15, 187-219.

[58] Rijavec, M, Miljkovic, D, & Brdar, I. Pozitivna psihologija: znanstveno istraživanje ljudskih snaga i sreće. Zagreb, IEP-D2; (2008).

[59] Campbell-sills, L, Barlow, D. H, Brown, T. A, & Hofmann, S. G. Effects of suppression and acceptance on emotional responses on individuals with anxiety and mood disorders. Behav Res Ther. (2006). , 44(9), 1251-1263.

[60] Gross, J. J. Emotion regulation: Affective, cognitive, and social consequences. Psychophysiology. (2002). May; , 39(3), 281-91.

Chapter 2

Social Anxiety Disorder in Psychosis: A Critical Review

Maria Michail

Additional information is available at the end of the chapter

1. Introduction

Eugene Bleuler was one of the first to emphasize the importance of affect and its pronounced impact upon the course and outcome of psychosis. The famous *"Krapelian dichtocomy"* which supported the clear distinction between mood and psychotic illnesses on the basis of etiological origins, symptomatology, course and outcome was first challenged by Bleuler. Bleuler recognized the disorders of affect as one of the four primary symptoms (blunted *'Affect'*, loosening of *'Associations'*, *'Ambivalence'*, and *'Autism'*) of schizophrenia, as opposed to delusions and hallucinations which were perceived as secondary. Bleuler further postulated the incongruity between emotions and thought content in people with schizophrenia as well as their diminished or complete lack of emotional responsiveness. Bleuler's recognition of the importance of affective disturbances in schizophrenia has influenced current diagnostic definitions and criteria of schizophrenia.

The sharp distinction between affect and psychosis which has dominated both research and clinical practice during the nineteenth and twentieth century has gradually been abandoned. New evidence from epidemiological, familial and molecular genetic studies (Cardno et al, 2005; Craddock et al, 2005; Craddock & Owen, 2005) have come to light demonstrating the endemic nature of affective disturbances in psychosis. In a twin study by Cardno et al (2002), the authors identified significant overlap in risk factors between the schizophrenic, schizoaffective and manic syndromes. Specifically, considerable genetic correlations were reported between the schizophrenic and manic syndromes. This is in accordance with a review of genetic linkage studies of schizophrenia and affective disorders (Wildenauer et al, 1999) which supports the genetic overlap of the two syndromes. Furthermore, factor analytic studies of psychosis symptoms consistently point to a depression dimension in non-affective psychosis (Murray et al, 2005). Depression and social anxiety are each observed throughout the course (Koreen et al, 1993), including the prodromal phase (Hafner et al, 1999; Owens et al, 2005) and following symptomatic recovery. Post psychotic depression

(PPD) has been reported in 30-50% of individuals (McGlashan et al, 1976; Birchwood et al, 2000a) and social anxiety disorder (SaD) has been observed in up to one in three (Davidson et al, 1993; Cassano et al, 1999; Goodwin et al, 2003; Pallanti et al, 2004).

2. Social anxiety disorder

2.1. Definition

According to the DSM-IV (APA, 1994), social anxiety disorder (social phobia) is defined as "a marked and persistent fear of one or more social or performance situations in which the person is exposed to unfamiliar people or possible scrutiny by others. The individual fears that he or she will act in a way (or show anxiety symptoms) that will be humiliating or embarrassing". People with social anxiety desire to make a favourable impression during social encounters but at the same time doubt their ability to do so; they fear that they will be scrutinized and negatively evaluated due to perceived failed social performance. These fears lead people with social anxiety to avoid all or some social situations and in extreme cases this could lead to complete social isolation (Clark & Wells, 2005). Exposure to the feared situation is almost always accompanied by physical symptoms, for example, sweating, trembling, heart racing, which could develop (although not necessarily) to panic attacks.

Evidence regarding the distinction of social phobia into two subtypes, the non-generalized and generalized social phobia, is ambiguous; although the DSM-IV does acknowledge the presence of the latter. This encompasses a wider range of fears linked to interaction situations and therefore is not restricted to particular environmental circumstances (i.e. it is "free-floating"). It may include talking to others, asking questions, meeting new people, manifest in fear and avoidance of everyday situations (Wittchen et al, 1999). These kinds of social fears have been exclusively reported in approximately two-third of people with lifetime social phobia indicating that the generalized subtype might be more prevalent compared to the non-generalized one (Kessler et al, 1998). This, sometimes also called "specific" or "discrete", is mainly characterized by performance-type fears, the most common being that of speaking in public or performing in front of an audience (Schneier et al, 1992; Stein et al, 1996). It seems therefore that the generalized subtype reflects a more pervasive and debilitating form of the illness which is supported by evidence showing higher rates of comorbidity with mood and other anxiety disorders (Wittchen et al, 1999) and lower recovery rates, compared to the non-generalized, specific subtype (Kessler et al, 1998).

2.2. Epidemiology and course

One of the largest epidemiological investigations carried out in the United States, the National Comorbidity Survey (Kessler et al, 1994), has reported prevalence estimates of 12-month and lifetime social anxiety disorder as 7.1% and 12.1%, respectively. The lifetime prevalence of social anxiety in other western countries seems to range between 3.1% to 15.6 % (Favarelli et al, 2000; Furmark et al, 1999). The variation in prevalence rates among different epidemiological studies could be attributed to the application of different diagnostic criteria and instruments for the identification and assessment of social anxiety disorder.

Studies investigating the course of social anxiety have established the long-term morbidity of the illness (Chartiers et al, 1998; Yonkers et al, 2001). Social anxiety develops at an early age, usually during childhood or adolescence and once established, follows a stable, chronic course if treatment is not initiated (Chartiers et al, 1998; Yonkers et al, 2001). Recent findings show that social anxiety is also very prevalent in later life (Cairney et al, 2007). Findings regarding the sociodemographic characteristics of social anxiety disorder support that this is more prominent among the female population (Wittchen et al, 1999; Schneier et al, 1992; Davidson et al, 1993; Magee et al, 1996) although there have been studies (Stein et al, 2000) which have failed to confirm such gender differences. Moreover, higher incident rates have been consistently observed among unmarried individuals usually coming from a lower socioeconomic background, with poorer educational attainment and higher unemployment rates (Schneier et al, 1992; Davidson et al, 1993; Magee et al, 1996). The average duration of illness is approximately 29 years (Chartier et al, 1991; Keller et al, 2003) and the likelihood of a full remission or recovery is significantly lower compared to that of other anxiety disorder (Keller et al, 2003). In an eight year longitudinal study of 163 patients with social phobia, Yonkers et al (2001) found that only 38% and 32% of female and men respectively experienced a complete remission indicating the unremitting and persisting nature of the disorder. Additionally, such lower rates of recovery were found to be associated, particularly in women, with a history of suicide attempts, the presence of co-morbid disorders, the most prominent that of agoraphobia, avoidant personality disorder and alcohol abuse, and also with poor baseline functioning (Yonkers et al, 2001; Keller et al, 2003).

The highly impairing nature of the disorder is reflected in the marked disabilities affecting the majority of life domains. Deterioration of social functioning manifest in avoidance and withdrawal from social interactions, decrease in work productivity and interpersonal relations produce a significant decrease in quality of life (Wittchen et al, 2000). Despite the highly impairing nature of social anxiety only up to a half of patients seek and receive treatment during the course of the illness (Wittchen et al, 2000; Wang et al, 2005) and this is primarily in the form of pharmacological interventions.

3. Social anxiety in psychosis

Social anxiety is among the most prevalent and debilitating affective disturbances manifest in people with psychosis (Pallanti et al, 2004; Mazeh et al, 2009; Michail & Birchwood, 2009). In a recent study by Michail & Birchwood (2009), social anxiety was diagnosed in 25% of people with first-episode psychosis (FEP). In addition to the 25% with an ICD-10 diagnosis of SaD, there was also a further 11.6 % who reported clear social interaction difficulties and/or signs of avoidance not sufficient though to reach formal diagnostic criteria. Social anxiety is usually accompanied by high levels of depression (Michail & Birchwood, 2009; Birchwood et al, 2007) and leads to significant social disability (Voges & Addington, 2005), lower quality of life (Pallanti et al, 2004) and poorer prognosis as it raises the possibility of an early relapse (Gumley, 2007).

Despite the high prevalence and its debilitating nature, social anxiety has not been extensively investigated and the processes that underlie its emergence in psychosis remain unclear. The relationship between social anxiety and positive psychotic symptoms, particularly paranoia, is yet to be clarified. Particularly, it is not clear whether the development and maintenance of social anxiety in psychosis is simply driven by paranoia and persecutory beliefs.

4. Aim

This review aims to examine the prevalence and phenomenology of social anxiety disorder in psychosis and to investigate its relationship to positive psychotic symptoms and particularly paranoia and persecutory ideation.

5. Methods

A systematic search strategy was conducted and consisted of electronic searches of the following databases: PsycINFO, PubMed and Science Direct using the terms "anxiety AND psychosis", "anxiety AND schizophrenia", "social anxiety AND psychosis", "social anxiety AND schizophrenia", "social anxiety AND paranoia". For inclusion, studies had to meet the following criteria:

1. Published in an English language, peer-reviewed journal. This ensures a degree of quality assurance in the reviewing process

2. Published between 1990-2011

3. Participants with psychosis. This includes schizophrenia, schizoaffective disorder, schizophreniform, bipolar disorder and depression with psychotic features

4. Adult participants (≥16 years)

5. Diagnosis of social anxiety disorder (either ICD-10 or DSM-IV)

Following the electronic search, hand searches of identified literature were conducted in the form of citation chasing.

6. Results

Thirteen studies fulfilled the inclusion criteria of this review (Table 1): three studies (Cossof & Hafner, 1998; Tibbo et al, 2003; Braga et al, 2005) investigated the prevalence of anxiety disorders, (including social anxiety) in psychosis; six examined the prevalence of social anxiety disorder in psychosis (Penn et al, 1994; Pallanti et al, 2004; Voges & Addington, 2005; Birchwood et al, 2007; Mazeh et al, 2009; Michail & Birchwood et al, 2009), three studies (Lysaker & Ham-

mersley, 2006; Lysaker & Salyers; 2007; Romm et al, 2012) investigated the relationship of social anxiety with clinical psychotic symptoms and one review paper on anxiety disorders in
schizophrenia was also identified (Muller et al, 2004). Four studies recruited a first-episode
psychosis sample (Voges & Addington, 2005; Birchwood et al, 2007; Michail & Birchwood,
2009; Romm et al, 2012); three recruited in-patients with schizophrenia, schizoaffective or bipolar disorder (Cossof & Hafner, 1998; Penn et al, 1994; Mazeh et al, 2009) and three recruited
outpatients with schizophrenia (Tibbo et al, 2003; Braga et al, 2005; Pallanti et al, 2004).

6.1. Prevalence and phenomenology

Social anxiety appears to be among the most prevalent anxiety disorders in psychosis with
prevalence rates ranging between 17% to 36%. In samples with first-episode psychosis, prevalence rates range between 25%-32% based on formal diagnostic criteria (DSM-IV or ICD-10).
In a recent study by Michail & Birchwood (2009), social anxiety was diagnosed in 25% of people with first-episode psychosis. However, in addition to the 25% with formal SaD, there was
also a further 11.6 % who reported clear social interaction difficulties and/or signs of avoidance not sufficient though to reach formal diagnostic criteria (ICD-10). These *"borderline"* cases, though not satisfying formal criteria, were nevertheless reporting interpersonal difficulties
that may well warrant intervention at a clinical level. In studies with inpatient samples, the
prevalence of social anxiety ranged between 11%-43% among those with schizophrenia,
schizoaffective or bipolar disorder and in studies with outpatients with schizophrenia
17%-36% of them were diagnosed with social anxiety disorder or social phobia.

The highly impairing nature of social anxiety in psychosis has been consistently reported in
literature. In a study of outpatients with schizophrenia, Pallanti et al (2004) reported that
those diagnosed with comorbid social anxiety disorder had a higher rate of suicide attempts,
lower social adjustment and overall quality of life compared to those without social anxiety.
Braga et al (2005) also reported higher levels of global functional impairment and greater
limitations in the domains of work and social life in schizophrenic patients with comorbid
anxiety disorder compared to those without comorbid anxiety disorder. Previous findings
by Penn et al (1994) confirm the significant impact of social anxiety on social disability. Findings also show that those with schizophrenia and comorbid social anxiety have higher levels
of substance abuse compared to those with no comorbid social anxiety (Pallanti et al, 2004).

The phenomenology of social anxiety in psychosis has been thoroughly investigated by Michail & Birchwood (2009). In their study comparing the severity and phenomenology of social
anxiety in psychosis with that in non psychosis, the authors revealed a very similar clinical profile with regards to levels of social anxiety and social avoidance; the number and severity of autonomic anxiety symptoms and social evaluative concerns. What is more, social anxiety both in
people with psychosis and non psychosis occurred in the context of an equally high level of
other anxiety disorders underlying the similarity of the two groups. The presence of social
anxiety in people with psychosis was also accompanied by marked levels of depression; approximately 31% of FEP people exhibited moderate to severe levels of post-psychotic depression. This is in line with findings from previous studies (Voges & Addington, 2005; Birchwood
et al, 2007) and confirmed by Romm et al (2012) who found that high levels of social anxiety in
people with first-episode psychosis were accompanied by high levels of depression.

Study	Participants	Aim	Key results
Penn et al. (1994)	38 in-patients with a diagnosis of schizophrenia or schizoaffective disorder according to the SCID-P	Investigate the relationship between social anxiety and positive and negative symptoms in schizophrenia	Behavioural indices of social anxiety (e.g. slower speech rated, less fluent speech, global social anxiety) were associated with negative symptoms. Self-report measures of social anxiety and related fears (e.g. fear of being negatively evaluated, fear of walking alone in the streets, fear of talking to people in authority) were associated with positive symptomatology. Such fears may be related to certain aspects of the illness e.g. paranoia, persecutory ideation whereas behavioural manifestations of social anxiety may reflect a deficit in social skills prominent in negative symptom
Cossof & Hafner (1998)	100 consecutive in-patients diagnosed with schizophrenia, schizoaffective disorder or bipolar disorder(based on the SCID)	Determine the prevalence of anxiety disorders in treated psychiatric inpatients with a DSM-IV diagnosis of schizophrenia, schizoaffective or bipolar disorder	43% of inpatients with schizophrenia were also diagnosed with a comorbid anxiety disorder (based on the SCID): 17% social phobia (SP), 12% generalized anxiety disorder (GAD), 13% obsessive-compulsive disorder (OCD)
Tibbo et al (2003)	30 outpatients with a diagnosis of DSM-IV schizophrenia (based on the MINI)	Determine the prevalence of anxiety disorders (as assessed by the MINI) controlling for anxiety symptoms related to delusions and hallucinations	16.7% prevalence of GAD 13.3% prevalence of SP 3.3% prevalence of panic disorder with/without agoraphobia 16.7% prevalence of agoraphobia without panic, excluding individuals whose anxiety symptoms were related to delusions or hallucinations
Muller et al (2004)	A review of the literature on comorbid anxiety disorders in schizophrenia	Review the epidemiology, phenomenology, and neurobiologic underpinnings of comorbid anxiety symptoms and disorders in schizophrenia, and address treatment strategies	Anxiety disorders are very prevalent in schizophrenia. The mechanisms that underpin this comorbidity require further investigation. Randomized controlled trials of pharmacotherapy and psychotherapy are necessary to establish the best way of managing this comorbidity
Pallanti et al (2004)	80 outpatients with schizophrenia (based on the SCID for DSM-IV) and 27 outpatients with primary diagnosis of social anxiety disorder	Prevalence and severity of social anxiety in schizophrenia Compare the severity and phenomenology of social anxiety in those with schizophrenia and those with social anxiety as primary diagnosis (no schizophrenia)	36.3% of people with schizophrenia were diagnosed with social anxiety based on the Liebowitz Social Anxiety Scale (LSES). The severity of social anxiety and avoidance in this group was as elevated in those with social anxiety without schizophrenia People with social anxiety and schizophrenia had a higher rate of suicide attempts, lower social adjustment and overall quality of life compared to those with schizophrenia only No differences in positive and negative symptoms (as assessed by the SAPS and SANS) between patients with schizophrenia and social anxiety and those with schizophrenia only

Study	Participants	Aim	Key results
Voges & Addington (2005)	60 patients with first-episode psychosis (FEP)	Examine the relationship between social anxiety and social functioning and determine whether those with psychosis have any maladaptive or irrational beliefs regarding social situations	32% of patients with FEP were diagnosed with social anxiety disorder (SCID-I for DSM-IV) Higher levels of social anxiety, as assessed by the Social Phobia and Anxiety Inventory (SPAI) were related to depression and negative symptoms but not positive symptoms. Social anxiety was associated with greater negative self-statements, and the lack of social anxiety with higher levels of positive self-statements. The authors suggest that negative self-statements may be prominent in the development and maintenance of social anxiety in first-episode patients
Braga et al (2005)	53 outpatients with a DSM-IV diagnosis of schizophrenia	Describe the prevalence of comorbid lifetime anxiety disorders in outpatients with schizophrenia and to compare the subjective quality of life of patients with and without comorbid anxiety disorders	Prevalences of anxiety comorbidity (based on SCID-IV) were: social phobia (17%), OCD (15.1%), GAD (9.4%), anxiety disorder Not Otherwise Specified (7.5%), panic disorder (5.7%), specific phobia (5.7%), Post-traumatic stress disorder (PTSD) (3.8%), and agoraphobia (1.9%) Higher levels of global functional impairment, more severe limitations in the domains of work and social life in schizophrenic patients with comorbid anxiety disorder compared to those without comorbid anxiety disorder
Birchwood et al (2007)	79 participants with first-episode psychosis	1. Examine the rate and severity of social anxiety in FEP 2. investigate the relationship of social anxiety with positive and negative symptoms 3. investigate the relationship between social anxiety and shame of psychosis	29% prevalence of social anxiety in FEP (based on the SIAS/SPS) No relationship between delusions, hallucinations and suspiciousness/ persecution and social anxiety (based on the positive scale of PANSS). Also, no relationship between negative symptoms and social anxiety and avoidance Greater levels of shame attached to their diagnosis and feelings of being down-ranked and rejected in the socially anxious psychotic group compared to the non socially anxious psychotic group
Mazeh et al (2009)	117 inpatients with a SCID-P for DSM-IV diagnosis of schizophrenia	Investigate the prevalence and correlates of social phobia in patients with schizophrenia	11% were diagnosed with comorbid social phobia (based on the SCID-P) Schizophrenic patients with comorbid social phobia had higher (although not statistically significant) level of PANSS total score compare to those without social phobia The "fear" component of social phobia (as measured by the Leibowitz Social Anxiety Scale, LSAS) was related to positive psychotic symptoms Avoidance (as measured by LSAS) was associated with negative symptoms

Study	Participants	Aim	Key results
Michail & Birchwood (2009)	80 participants with FEP	Determine the phenomenology of psychotic SaD and how this is different to non-psychotic SaD Investigate whether psychotic SaD is linked to the nature and severity of psychotic symptoms and particularly paranoia	25% of FEPs received an ICD-10 diagnosis of social anxiety based on the SCAN (WHO, 1999). Equally elevated levels of social anxiety (SIAS), avoidance (SPS), depression (CDSS) and autonomic anxiety symptoms in the psychotic and non psychotic socially anxious group No relationship between positive symptoms including suspiciousness/persecution (PANSS) and social anxiety (SIAS/SPS) in the FEP group. However, a subgroup of socially anxious psychotic people reported higher levels of persecutory threat (Details of Threat Questionnaire) compared to psychotic people without social anxiety.
Romm et al (2012)	144 participants with FEP (based on SCID-I for DSM-IV)	Investigate whether SaD in psychosis is associated with poorer premorbid functioning, higher levels of psychotic symptoms and reduced QoL	50% of FEPs suffered from severe social anxiety (LSAS). Social anxiety was associated with greater levels of depression, poorer premorbid functioning and reduced QoL. No relationship between social anxiety and positive psychotic symptoms was reported.
Lysaker & Salyers (2007)	128 participants with schizophrenia & schizoaffective disorder (based on SCID for DSM-IV)	Investigate the relationship between anxiety (as measured by the Multidimensional Anxiety Questionnaire) and psychotic symptoms (as measured by the PANSS)	Higher levels of anxiety were associated with greater hallucinations, withdrawal, depression, hopelessness, better insight and poorer function.
Lysaker & Hammersley (2006)	71 participants with schizophrenia & schizoaffective disroder	Examine the possible roots of social anxiety in schizophrenia by investigating its relationship to delusions and flexibility of abstract thought	Participants classified as having both significant delusions (based on the PANSS) and impairments in flexibility of abstract thought had significantly higher levels of social anxiety (based on the LSAS) compared to those with only one or neither of these difficulties

Table 1. Studies investigating social anxiety in people with psychosis

6.2. The relationship between social anxiety and positive psychotic symptoms

The relationship between social anxiety and positive psychotic symptoms, particularly paranoia, has attracted considerable attention; however, the processes that underlie this relationship are yet to be clarified. Ten studies identified in this review examined the relationship of
social anxiety with positive symptoms (Penn et al, 1994; Tibbo et al, 2003; Pallanti et al, 2004;
Voges & Addington, 2005; Birchwood et al, 2007; Mazeh et al, 2009; Michail & Birchwood,
2009; Lysaker & Hammersley, 2006; Lysaker & Salyers, 2007; Romm et al, 2012). Four studies
(Penn et al, 1994; Mazeh et al, 2009; Lysaker & Hammersley, 2006; Lysaker & Salyers, 2007)
reported a link between social anxiety and positive symptoms. Penn et al (1994) showed that
self-report measures of social anxiety and related fears (e.g. fear of being negatively evaluated, fear of walking alone in the streets, fear of talking to people in authority) were associated
with positive symptomatology. The authors suggested that such fears may be related to cer-

tain aspects of the illness e.g. paranoia, persecutory ideation whereas behavioural manifestations of social anxiety (e.g. slower speech rated, less fluent speech, global social anxiety) may reflect a deficit in social skills prominent in negative symptoms. This was also supported by Mazeh et al (2009) who found the "fear" component of social phobia in schizophrenic patients (as measured by the Leibowitz Social Anxiety Scale, LSAS) to be related to positive psychotic symptoms. Lysaker & Hammersley (2006) and Lysaker & Salyers (2007) found that in people with schizophrenia severe social anxiety was accompanied by severe levels of delusions and greater levels of hallucinations, respectively.

Five studies (Pallanti et al, 2004; Voges & Addington, 2005; Birchwood et al, 2007; Michail & Birchwood, 2009, Romm et al, 2012) reported no differences in severity levels of positive symptoms (including paranoia) between those with schizophrenia and comorbid SaD vs no SaD, suggesting that SaD may be unrelated to clinical psychotic symptoms. In a study of young people with first-episode psychosis, Michail & Birchwood (2009) conducted a thorough investigation of the relationship between positive symptoms and social anxiety. The authors compared levels of positive symptoms, including suspiciousness and persecution, as measured by the PANSS (Positive and Negative Symptom Scale) between people with psychosis and social anxiety (FEP/SaD) and those with psychosis only (FEP/no SaD). Findings revealed no differences in PANSS positive symptoms between psychotic individuals with vs. without social anxiety; including no relationship between PANSS suspiciousness/persecution and social anxiety in the whole FEP (with and without SaD) sample. Furthermore, the level of PANSS suspiciousness/persecution did not affect the severity of social anxiety within the FEP/SaD group itself. These findings confirm previous studies reporting no link between positive symptoms (similarly assessed using the PANSS) and social anxiety (Pallanti et al, 2004; Voges & Addington, 2005) which suggests that the presence of social anxiety in psychosis is not simply driven by clinical paranoia and persecutory threat. It is important to mention though findings in the Michail & Birchwood (2009) study also revealed a subgroup of socially anxious psychotic people (45%) which reported significantly more persecutory threat and anticipated harm as measured by the Details of Threat Questionnaire (Freeman et al, 2001) compared to psychotic people without social anxiety. When investigating further the inter-relationship between social anxiety and persecutory threat within this sub-group no link between level of social anxiety and persecutory threat was revealed. This is of particular interest as it suggests that even among those individuals with psychosis and social anxiety, social anxiety is not necessarily contaminated by ongoing persecutory beliefs.

7. Discussion

Social anxiety is among the most commonly reported and disabling of the co-morbidities in people with psychosis. It is characterized by a highly impairing nature which is evident by its impact on social functioning and social disability. Despite its elevated prevalence and severity in psychosis, social anxiety remains under-recognized and under-treated. One of the reasons for this could be that the exact relationship between social anxiety and psychotic symptoms is yet to be determined and the available empirical findings are inconclusive. Although theoretical models and empirical evidence consistently point towards a link between general anxiety and positive symptoms of psychosis, predominantly paranoia and persecutory delusions (Freeman et al, 2001), social anxiety appears to have a distinct quality and its relationship to paranoia and persecutory thinking is not straightforward.

Three pathways have been proposed for the understanding of the ontogeny of social anxiety in psychosis (Michail & Birchwood, 2009; 2011) and they are summarized here:

a.   social anxiety predates the onset of paranoia and helps maintain persecutory beliefs

This suggests that symptoms of social anxiety, avoidance and withdrawal develop in the early or prodrome phase. This is confirmed by studies showing how social withdrawal and socio-emotional dysfunction in people identified as being at risk for developing psychosis are highly predictive predicting of psychosis (Johnstone et al, 2005; Miller et al, 2002; Yung et al, 2004). The development of paranoia and persecutory ideation follows the onset of social anxiety which serves the function of maintaining or strengthening persecution ideation. The work by Freeman et al (2005a; 2005b) has shown how common social anxieties, for example, fear of rejection, interpersonal sensitivity and negative beliefs about the self are amongst the most commonly reported types of suspiciousness (2005a) and form the basis upon which ideas of reference and more severe levels of paranoid thinking are established. Furthermore, these anxieties and social evaluative concerns were found to predict paranoid thinking in a non-clinical sample (2005b).

b.   social anxiety and paranoia develop concurrently in the early phase of psychosis and
      follow a similar course

This pathway suggests that for a sub-group of individuals, social anxiety and paranoia may develop at the same time and follow a similar course. According to Freeman et al (2001), social anxiety and paranoia are underlined by common fears and concerns which refer to the anticipation of *threat* and danger which drives behaviours of avoidance and withdrawal from social interactions. It is expected therefore that for this sub-group of people, addressing paranoid concerns and ideas of persecution, would inevitably lead to the remission of symptoms of social anxiety and avoidance.

c.   social anxiety may develop for some people as a consequence of paranoid beliefs

The third pathway suggests that for a sub-sample of people with psychosis, symptoms of social anxiety and avoidance may develop as a direct consequence of their paranoid ideation. Persecutory beliefs and perceived threat regarding other people's intentions to cause harm can lead to elevated social anxiety and apprehension during social encounters. As a way of protecting or "saving" oneself from such social threats, individuals may engage in safety behaviours by isolating themselves from the social world and actively avoiding all social interactions.

Following the findings of a thorough investigation into the psychological processes that underlie the emergence and maintenance of social anxiety in psychosis (Michail & Birchwood, 2012), a fourth potential pathway is provided here:

d. social anxiety as a response to the shame and social stigma attached to a diagnosis of mental illness

In a recent study by Michail & Birchwood (2012), the authors examined the relationship between shame cognitions, shame proneness and perceived loss of social status in people with first-episode psychosis and social anxiety disorder. Findings showed that psychotic individuals with social anxiety expressed high levels of shame proneness which was accompanied by perceived loss of social status. They also reported significantly greater negative appraisals arising from a stigmatizing illness, including shame and fear of rejection, compared to their counterparts without social anxiety. These findings were consistent with those of earlier studies (Birchwood et al, 2007, Gumley et al, 2004) reporting that dysfunctional appraisals held by socially anxious psychotic people were characterized by shamefulness, humiliation and perceived rejection by others.

The authors proposed that individuals with psychosis are characterized by an established vulnerability to shame linked to early developmental anomalies. This shame proneness is likely to be catalysed by the stigma attached to the diagnosis of mental illness and there is evidence to suggest that psychosis is indeed considered as a highly stigmatized condition (Thornicroft et al, 2009). As with any type of *social stigma*, this can affect the social identity of the individual by suggesting qualities that deviate from the norm and are socially discrediting (Goffman, 1963). Individuals with psychosis are aware of the social stereotypes surrounding mental illness and some may even accept and endorse these (Hayward & Bright, 1997; Angermeyer et al, 2003). This internalization of stigma or *self-stigma* leads to increased shamefulness -particularly when individuals agree with the stigma and the associated negative responses (Corrigan & Watson, 2002a; 2002b)- and fear of the illness being revealed to others due to the consequences of this discovery (e.g. social exclusion, marginalization). Hence, the authors suggested that people with psychosis will attempt to conceal their stigmatized identity to prevent or minimise this threat by promoting behaviours of submissiveness or by avoiding and withdrawing from social interactions.

8. Clinical implications

There is lack of evidence on the clinical effectiveness and cost effectiveness of psychological interventions for the treatment of affective dysregulation and associated distress in psychosis. Cognitive behaviour therapy (CBT) is recommended for people with psychosis (NICE, 2009); however, its focus and evaluation has primarily revolved around the reduction of psychotic symptoms, and not for comorbid depression and social anxiety. Furthermore, psychological interventions such as CBT for the treatment of affective disorders in non-psychotic populations are proposed for the management of affective dysfunction when this is comorbid in psychosis (Halperin et al, 2000; Kingsep et al, 2003). This could be challenging as such treatments in order to be effective, would need to adapt to the specific nature of symptoms and difficulties experienced by people with psychosis (Tarrier, 2005). The findings of the recent study by Michail & Birchwood (2012) suggest that the "conventional" CBT for social anxiety in psychosis could be considerably enhanced with an additional focus on shame cognitions linked to psychosis and accompanying concealment behaviours which are suggested to form part of the safety behaviour repertoire of socially anxious psychotic individuals. A randomised controlled trial testing the effectiveness of a CBT intervention in targeting shameful cognitions while reducing or eliminating concealment linked behaviours could be effective in psychosis.

Author details

Maria Michail

Address all correspondence to: maria.michail@nottingham.ac.uk

School of Nursing, Midwifery & Physiotherapy, University of Nottingham, UK

References

[1] American Psychiatric Association(1994). Diagnostic and statistical manual of mental health disorders (4th ed). Washington DC

[2] Angermeyer, M. C., & Matschinger, H. (2003). The stigma of mental illness: effects of labeling on public attitudes towards people with mental disorder. *Acta Psychiatrica Scandinavica*, 108, 304-309.

[3] Birchwood, M., Iqbal, Z., Chadwick, P., & Trower, P. Cognitive Approach to Depression and Suicidal Thinking in Psychosis I. Ontogeny of post-psychotic depression. British Journal of Psychiatry (2000a). , 177, 516-521.

[4] Cairney, J., Mc Cabe, L., Veldhuizen, S., Corna, L., Streiner, D., & Herrmann, N. (2007). Epidemiology of social phobia in later life. Am J Geriatr Psychiatry, 15 (3), 224-233

[5] Cardno, A., G., , Rijsdijl, F. V., Sham, P. C., et al. (2002). A twin study of genetic relationships between psychotic symptoms. American Journal of Psychiatry, , 159, 539-545.

[6] Cassano, G. B., Pini, S., Saettoni, M., & Dell'Oso, L. (1999). Multiple Anxiety Disorder Comorbidity in Patients with Mood Spectrum Disorders with Psychotic Features. American Journal of Psychology, , 156, 474-476.

[7] Chartier MJ, Hazen AL, Stein MB. (1998). Lifetime patterns of social phobia: a retrospective study of the course of social phobia in a nonclinical population. *Depression and Anxiety*, 113 EOF-21 EOF.

[8]   Clark, D., & Wells, . (1995). A Cognitive Model of Social Phobia. In Heimberg, Liebo-
      witz (eds.), Social Phobia. New York, Guildford Press

[9]   Corrigan PW, Watson CA(2002a). The paradox of self-stigma and mental illness.
      Clinical Psychology and Science Practice , 9, 35-53.

[10] Corrigan PW, Watson CA(2002b). Understanding the impact of stigma on people
      with mental illness. World Psychiatry , 1, 16-20.

[11] Craddock, N., O'Donovan, M. C., & Owen, M. J. (2005). Genetics of schizophrenia
      and bipolar disorder: dissecting of psychosis. Journal of Medical Genetics, , 42,
      193-204.

[12] Craddock, N., & Owen, M. J. (2005). The beginning of the end of the Kraepelian di-
      chotomy. British Journal of Psychiatry, , 186, 364-366.

[13] Davidson, J., Hughes, D., George, L., & Blazer, D. (1993). The Epidemiology of Social
      Phobia: Findings from the Duke Epidemiological Catchment Area Study. *Psychologi-
      cal Medicine*, 23, 709-718.

[14] Favarelli, C., Zucchi, T., Viviani, B., Salmoria, R., Perone, A., Paionni, A., Scarpato,
      A., Vigliaturo, D., Rosi, S., Dadamo, D., Bartolozzi, D., Cecchi, C., & Abrardi, L.
      (2000). Epidemiology of Social Phobia: A Clinical Approach. European Psychiatry, ,
      15, 17-24.

[15] Freeman, D., Garety, P. A., & Kuipers, E. (2001). Persecutory delusions: Developing
      the understanding of belief maintenance and emotional distress. *Psychological Medi-
      cine*, 31, 1293-1306.

[16] Freeman, D., Garety, P. A., Bebbington, P., Slater, M., Kuipers, E., Fowler, D., Green,
      C., Jordan, J., Ray, K., & Dunn, G. (2005a). The psychology of persecutory ideation. II.
      A virtual reality exp. erimental study. Journal of Nervous Mental Disorders, , 193,
      309-315.

[17] Freeman, D., Garety, P. A., Bebbington, P. E., Smith, B., Rollinson, R., Fowler, D.,
      Kuipers, E., Ray, K., & Dunn, G. (2005b). Psychological investigation of the structure
      of paranoia in a non-clinical population. Br J Psychiatry, , 186, 427-435.

[18] Furmark, T., Tillfors, M., Everz-O, P., Marteinsdottir, I., Gefrert, O., & Fredrikson, M.
      (1999). Social Phobia in the General Population: Prevalence and Sociodemographic
      Profile. *Social Psychiatry and Psychiatric Epidemiology*, 34, 416-424.

[19] Goodwin, D. R., Amador, F. X., Malaspina, D., Yale, A. S., Goetz, R. R., & Gorman,
      M. J. (2003). Anxiety and Substance Use Comorbidity among Inpatients with Schizo-
      phrenia. *Schizophrenia Research*, 61, 89-95.

[20] Gumley, A., O'Grady, M., Power, K., & Schwannauer, M. (2004). Negative Beliefs
      about Self and Illness: A Comparison of Individuals with Psychosis with and without
      Comorbid Social Anxiety Disorde. r. Aust ranlian and New Zealand Journal of Psy-
      chiatry, , 38, 960-964.

[21] Gumley et al(2007). Staying well after psychosis: a cognitive interpersonal approach to emotional recovery after relapse preventi. on. Tidsskrift for Norsk Psykologforening, 44 (5), 667-676

[22] Hafner, H., Loffler, W., Mauer, K., Hambrecht, M., & an der, Heiden. W. (1999). Depression, Negative Symptoms, Social Stagnation and Social Decline in the Early Course of Schizophrenia. Acta Psychiatrica Scandinavica,, 100, 105-118.

[23] Halperin, S., Nathan, P., Drummond, P., & Castle, D. (2000). A cognitive-behavioural, group-based intervention for social anxiety in schizophrenia. Australian and New Zealand Journal of PsychiatryHayward, P. & Bright, J. (1997) Stigma and mental illness: a review and critique. Journal of Mental Health, 6, 345-354, 34, 809-813.

[24] Johnstone, C. E., Ebmeier, P. K., Miller, P., Owens, G. C. D., & Lawrie, M. S. (2005). Predicting Schizophrenia: Findings from the Edinburgh High-Risk Study. British Journal of Psychiatry, , 186, 18-25.

[25] Keller, B. (2003). The lifelong course of social anxiety disorder: a clinical perspective. *Acta Psychiatrica Scandinavica*, 108, 85-94.

[26] Kessler, R., Murray, B., & Berglund, M. (1998). Social Phobia Subtypes in the National Comorbidity Survey. American Journal of Psychiatry,, 155, 613-619.

[27] Kessler, R. C., Mc Gonagle, K. A., Zhao, S., Nelson, C. B., Hughes, M., Eshleman, S., Wittchen-U, H., & Kendler, K. S. (1994). Lifetime and 12-month prevalence of DSM-III-R psychiatric disorders in the United States: results from the National Comorbidity Survey. *Archives of General Psychiatry*, 51, 8-19.

[28] Kingsep, P., Nathan, P., & Castle, D. (2003). Cognitive behavioural group treatment for social anxiety in schizophrenia. *Schizophrenia Research*, 63, 121-129.

[29] Koreen, A., Siris, S., Chakos, M., Alvir, J., Mayerhoff, D., & Lieberman, J. (1993). Depression in First-Episode Schizophrenia. American Journal of Psychology, , 150, 1643-1648.

[30] Magee, W. J., Eaton, W. W., Wittchen, H. U., Mc Gonagle, K. A., & Kessler, R. C. (1996). Agoraphobia, simple phobia, and social phobia in the National Comorbidity Survey. Archives of General Psychiatry, , 53, 159-168.

[31] Mazeh et al(2009). Co-morbid social phobia in schizophrenia. International Journal of psychiatry, , 55, 198-202.

[32] Mc Glashan, T., & Carpenter, W. (1976). An Investigation of the Post-psychotic Depressive Symptom. American Journal of Psychology, 133 (1), 14-19

[33] Michail, M., & Birchwood, M. (2009). Social anxiety disorder in first-episode psychosis: Incidence, phenomenology and relationship with paranoia. *British Journal of Psychiatry*, 195, 234-241.

[34] Michail, M., & Birchwood, M. (2011). Understanding the role of emotion in psychosis: social anxiety disorder in first-episode psychosis.. In: RITSNER, M., ed., Hand-

book of Schizophrenia Spectrum Disorders: Phenotypic and Endophenotypic Presentations 1st. 2nd. Springer. , 89-110.

[35] Michail, M., & Birchwood, M. (2012). Social anxiety disorder and shame cognitions in psychosis. Psychological Medicinee-pub), 1 EOF-10 EOF.

[36] Miller, P., Byrne, M., Hodges, A., Lawrie, M. S., Owens, G. C. D., & Johnstone, C. E. (2002). Schizotypal Components in People at High-Risk of Developing Schizophrenia: Early Findings from the Edinburgh High-Risk Study. British Journal of Psychiatry, , 180, 179-18.

[37] Murray, V., Mc Kee, I., Miller, P. M., Young, D., Muir, W. J., Pelosi, A. J., & Blackwood, D. H. (2005). Dimensions and classes of psychosis in a population cohort: a four-class, four-dimension model of schizophrenia and affective psychoses. Psychological Medicine, , 35, 499-510.

[38] Owens, C., Miller, P., Lawrie, S., & Johnstone, E. C. (2005). Pathogenesis of schizophrenia: a psychopathological perspective. British Journal of Psychiatry, , 186, 386-393.

[39] Pallanti Stefano, Quercioli Leonardo, Hollander Eric.(2004). Social Anxiety in Outpatients with Schizophrenia. A Relevant Cause of Disability. American Journal of Psychology, , 161, 53-58.

[40] Romm, K., Melle, I., Thoresen, C., Andreassen, O., & Rossberg, J. (2012). Severe social anxiety in early psychosis is associated with poor premorbid functioning, depression and reduced quality of life. Comprehensive Psychiatry, 434 EOF-440 EOF.

[41] Schneier, F., Johnson, J., Horing, C., Liebowitz, A., Weissman, M., & (2002, . (2002). Social Phobia Comorbidity and Morbidity in an Epidemiological Sample. Archives of General Psychiatry, , 49, 282-288.

[42] Stein, M. B., Walker, J. R., Forde, D. R., & (1996, . (1996). Public speaking fears in a community sample: Prevalence, impact on functioning, and diagnostic classification, Archives of General Psychiatry, 53, 169-174.

[43] Stein, M., Torgrud, J. L., & Walker, R. J. (2000). Social Phobia Subtypes, Symptoms and Severity. Arch Gen Ps. ychiatry, , 57, 1046-105.

[44] Tarrier, N. (2005). Co-morbidity and associated clinical problems in schizophrenia: Their nature and implications for comprehensive cognitive-behavioural treatment. Behaviour Change, 125 EOF-142 EOF.

[45] Thornicroft, G., Brohan, E., Rose, D., Sartorius, N., & Leese, M. (2009). Global pattern of experienced and anticipated discrimination against people with schizophrenia: a cross-sectional survey. The Lancet, 373, 408-415.

[46] Voges, M., & Addington, J. (2005). Association between social anxiety and social functioning in first-episode psychosis. Schizophrenia Research, , 76, 287-291.

[47] Wang, P. S., Lane, M., Olfson, M., et al. (2005). Twelve month use of mental health services in the US: Results from the National Comorbidity Survey Replication (NCS-R). Archives of General Psychiatry, , 62, 629-640.

[48] Wildenauer, D. B., Schwab, S. G., Maier, W., & Detera-Wadleigh, S. D. (1999). Do schizophrenia and affective disorder share susceptibility genes? Schizophrenia Research , 39, 107-11.

[49] Wittchen-U, H., Stein, M., & Kessler, R. (1999). Social Fears and Social Phobia in a Community Sample of Adolescents and Young Adults: Prevalence, Risk Factors and Comorbidity. *Psychological Medicine*, 29, 309-323.

[50] Wittchen, H. U., Fuetsch, M., Sonntag, H., Muller, N., & Liebowitz, M. (2000). Disability and quality of life in pure and comorbid social phobia. Findings from a controlled study. European Psychiatry, , 15, 46-58.

[51] Yonkers, K. A., Dyck, I. R., & Keller, M. B. (2001). An eight-year longitudinal comparison of clinical course and characteristics of social phobia among men and women,. Psychiatric Services, 52 (5), , 637 EOF-43 EOF.

[52] Yung, R. A., Phillips, J. L., Yven, P. H., & Mc Gorry, P. (2004). Risk Factors for Psychosis in an Ultra-High Risk Group: Psychopathology and clinical features. *Schizophrenia Research*, 67, 131-152.

Chapter 3

Anxiety Syndromes and Their Correlates in Children and Adolescents: A Two-Year- Follow-Up Study at Primary Health Care in Mexico City

Jorge Javier Caraveo-Anduaga,
Alejandra Soriano Rodríguez and Jose Erazo Pérez

Additional information is available at the end of the chapter

1. Introduction

Anxiety disorders are among psychiatric conditions the earliest to manifest, with a median age at onset of 15 years, using retrospective information (WHO ICPE, 2000). As a group, anxiety disorders are frequent and persistent in childhood and adolescence. The prevalence of anxiety disorders in nonrefered children 4-6 years old has been estimated in 6.1% (Briggs-Gowan et al., 2000), and studies on older children and adolescents have reported lifetime prevalence ranging from 8.3% to 27.0% (Costello et al., 2005). Separation anxiety disorder (SA), specific phobias (SP) and generalized anxiety disorder (GA) are the most common. Left untreated, anxiety disorders tend to have a chronic and unremitting course (Yonkers et al., 2003; Ramsawh et al, 2009) and also increase the risk for adult psychiatric disorders (Pine et al., 1998; Costello et al., 2011).

In primary care settings studies have shown that approximately 9% to 15% (Benjamin et al., 1990; Costello, 1989) of 7- to 11-year-olds meet the criteria for an anxiety disorder, and at least 17% in pediatric patients (Chavira et al., 2004). Most contact with GPs is for physical health problems; only 2–5% of child and adolescent consultations involve presentations with emotional or behavioural problems (Giel et al., 1981). Pediatric anxiety disorders often feature somatic complaints such as abdominal pain, chest pain or discomfort, headaches, nausea, or vomiting, and are often comorbid with medical conditions such as asthma and other atopic disorders (Ramsawh et al., 2010). However, children and adolescents with mood and anxiety disorders in primary care and pediatric settings are underrecognized, not commonly treated onsite, and less likely than youths with behavioral disorders to be referred to specialized mental health settings (Wren et al., 2003, 2005).

Mental health presentations may also relate to educational or social issues and other risk factors for functioning and development rather than to diagnosable disorders per se. In children, anxiety disorders can be associated with school absenteeism or school refusal, poor academic performance, or grades that are lower than would be expected based on the child's abilities (Mazzone et al, 2007). It is the concerns of parents that typically alert the primary care clinician to psychosocial issues (Dulcan et al., 1990), but parents are often either unaware of their child's internalizing symptoms or do not see a need for services (Wu et al., 1999; Caraveo et al., 2002).

2. Mental health surveillance for children and adolescents: A pilot study at a primary care center in Mexico City

2.1. Background

Having identified that children's and adolescent's mental health problems are frequent and unrecognized conditions in Mexico City (Caraveo et al, 2002) and that an epidemiological study on the general population showed evidence about the familial risk for developing psychopathology acoss three generations (Caraveo et. al., 2005), a pilot study aimed on the surveillance of children's and adolescent's mental health at primary care level was launched. The initiative was conceived as a potential action-research oriented project for the enhancement of the role of primary care in the preventive actions that are needed for mental health care. Primary care has great potential as a source of education, triage, and frontline intervention. However, this role requires simple and efficient methods and tools to accurately identify, in collaboration with the family, the child's core areas of difficulty (Wren et al., 2005).

Eventually, the information to be gathered by this program may contribute to a better understanding of the natural history of different psychiatric syndromes and disorders such as attention deficit and hyperactivity disorder, affective disorders, anxiety disorders and other neuro-psychiatric conditions. All of these produce varying degrees of handicap and may create a risk for other disorders such as alcohol and drug abuse (Merikangas et al., 1998; Hofstra et al. 2000), hence the importance of their surveillance, early detection and care.

As a first step in the development of this pilot study, the concurrent validity and efficiency of the Brief Screening and Diagnostic Questionnaire (CBTD for its initials in Spanish) was evaluated. The CBTD was built based on our previous experience using the Report Questionnaire for Children, RQC (Caraveo et al., 1995) adding 17 items to explore symptoms frequently reported as motives for seeking attention at the out-patient mental health services. The aim was to include cardinal symptoms that could lead to identify probable specific syndromes and disorders, based on the parent's report. The instrument was tested and further developed using information gathered from a general population sample. Internal consistency showed a Cronbach's alpha of 0.81 with a 0.75-0.85 range by age groups; cluster and factor analyses identified eight groups of symptoms that correlate with the most frequent syndromes seen in children and adolescents (Caraveo, 2006). Logistic regression analyses were then performed between cardinal symptoms for different diagnoses and the rest of the items from the questionnaire, and statistically significant associations were evaluated clinically and compared to psychiatric syndromes as defined by the DSM-IV (APA,1994) and the ICD-10 (WHO, 1993) classifications. Based on these results, algorithms for probable psychiatric syndromes, including subclinical forms, were created (Caraveo, 2007a) and the concurrent validity between some of them and the psychiatric diagnoses of children who received care at two out-patient mental health services showed a fair agreement (Yule's Y: 0.43- 0.55; Caraveo, 2007b). However, as psychiatric diagnoses did not follow a structured clinical interview, there was the need to confirm these results using a standardized evaluation and on primary health attendants in order to evaluate the screening instrument adequacy for establishing a surveillance of mental health in childhood and adolescence.

Results showed an overall Sensitivity of 68%, Specificity of 82%, Positive Predictive Value (PPV) of 88% and a Negative Predictive Value (NPV) of 57%. When two or more CBTD syndromes are present the PPV is almost 100%. Concurrent validity showed a fair agreement for most of the CBTD syndromes as compared to DSM-IV diagnoses (Caraveo et al., 2011).

Once established the validity and efficiency of CBTD as the basic tool for screening purposes, an impairment measurement was considered as a priority for the surveillance pilot study, along with the obtention of psychiatric antecedents in both parents. Also, as besides genetic predisposition a variety of mechanisms have been postulated as being responsible for intergenerational continuity of psychopathology such as impairments in parenting and dysfunctional family relationships (Malcarne et al., 2010), and because along the field work of the surveillance study, these issues were frequently reported by the population, they were subsequently assessed during the two-year follow-up.

As this chapter is focused on anxiety disorders in children and adolescents, we will review research on these aspects as related to anxious children and adolescents.

2.1.1. Familial antecedents

Findings from family studies, either using a "top-down" design where the children of parents with anxiety disorders are evaluated or a "bottom-up" design which ascertain the parents of children with anxiety disorders, have clearly establish the cross-generation transmission of anxiety from parents to children (Klein & Pine, 2002). A detailed revision of the literature has been presented in a previous work (Caraveo-Anduaga, 2011).

An epidemiological study on the general population of Mexico City investigated the presence of psychopathology across three generations (Caraveo et al., 2005). Anxiety syndromes, as defined in the Brief Screening and Diagnostic Questionnaire (CBTD) showed a familial transmission pathway that is consistent with results from studies on Caucasian populations in developed countries (Klein & Pine, 2002), suggesting that familial risk for developing anxiety disorders is a fact, thus not limited by ethnicity or culture, but mediated by socio-economic conditions (Caraveo-Anduaga, 2011).

Results showed that comorbid anxiety disorders in grandparents seem to interact with anxiety-only as well as with anxiety comorbid disorders in parents, determining a robust morbid risk for the generalized anxiety screening syndrome in descendants, while the familial anxiety risk across generations for the anxiety with inhibition syndrome is less pronounced.

Results considering only the adult proband's information showed that parent's history of anxiety-only as well as comorbid anxiety-depression were significantly associated with both screening anxiety syndromes in their offspring. Male children developed more generalized anxiety as compared to females, and the relationship with spouse was inversely associated with the presence of the syndrome of anxiety with inhibition in the descendant. Additionally, household higher income showed a significant association with the presence of the generalized anxiety syndrome in the children, and poor adult proband's own health perception was associated with both anxiety syndromes in their offspring (Caraveo-Anduaga, 2011).

A limitation of the study was that as the principal objective of the survey was focused on adult population, only one adult was selected at each household, and so familial risk across generations, was based on information about only one parent.

2.1.2. Functional impairment

Functional impairment describes the impact of psychopathology on the life of the child with respect to daily life activities (Üstun & Chatterji, 1997); it refers to ways in which symptoms interfere with and reduce adequate performance of important and desired aspects of the child's life (Rapee et al., 2012). Most common conceptualisations indicate three areas of impairment within family, school and social domains. Ezpeleta et al. (2001) identified three dimensions: interference with parents, peers and education.

Different authors have shown the importance of including impairment indicators in the diagnostic definitions in order to reduce the prevalence rates of the disorders in epidemiological studies (Bird et al., 1988; Roberts, et al., 1997; Shaffer, et al, 1996; Simonoff et al., 1997). The knowledge of the degree of impairment is also necessary for the proper identification of those persons affected by a psychological disorder or in need of psychological help.

Measures of functional impairment besides being an aid in case definitions in epidemiological studies and in nosology are useful for studies of treatment effectiveness, planning services, service eligibility determination, evaluating and planning of programs, but, mainly, they are used as outcome indicators (Ezpeleta et al., 2006).

Available instruments of level of functioning could be classified either as one-dimensional or multidimensional. For the definition of impairment three primary measurement strategies have been identified (Bird et al., 2000): a) measures that incorporate the symptoms and their correlates into the definition of disorder, b) specific impairment measures associated with each diagnosis, and c) global omnibus impairment measures.

Goals for assessment of functional impairment should help to decide what the best strategy is. If the goal is to decide if a child needs intervention or not, a global strategy could be used, but if the objective is to plan the areas of intervention, then a decomposed instrument could be more appropriate.

Anxiety disorders are especially susceptible to impairment thresholds; however, the importance of impairment is uncertain in early diagnoses. Moreover, anxiety symptoms that are not impairing in early childhood may become so as development and life-experiences continues (Malcarne et al., 2010). Thus, knowledge of the degree of impairment is a necessary component for the surveillance of anxiety and other children's mental health disorders at the primary care level.

Kashani & Orvaschel (1990) in a community sample of 210 children and adolescents found that children diagnosed with anxiety disorder demonstrated greater impairment on both the physical and cognitive measures on self-competence, temperamental flexibility, and levels of self-esteem than non-clinic controls. Research on the psychosocial implications of anxiety indicates the disabling consequences affecting schooling and academic functioning, peer relationships, autonomous activities, self-esteem, family functioning and overall psychosocial impairment (Strauss et al, 1988; Bell-Dolan & Brazeal, 1993; Kendall et al., 1992; Wittchen, Nelson & Lachner, 1998; Essau et al., 2000).

Manassis and Hood (1998) determined the correlates of anxiety disorders that were predictive of impairment. They concluded that predictors were different depending on disorder. The impairment for generalized anxiety disorder was mainly determined by psychosocial adversity, but in the case of phobia, it was determined by mothers' ratings of conduct problems of the child, the depressive symptoms reported by the child, the maternal phobic anxiety, and the development difficulties suffered by the child.

Whiteside (2009) found that the greatest impairment report from both the child and parents was associated with obsessive compulsive disorder and social anxiety disorder, followed by separation anxiety disorder, and then generalized anxiety disorder. Thus, level of impairment seems to be associated with the type of anxiety disorder. However, literature suggests that there are many shared risk or associated factors for psychiatric morbidity and functional impairment in children (Wille N, et al, 2008).

2.1.3. Child-rearing and parenting practices

Darling and Steinberg (1993) defined child-rearing style as 'a constellation of attitudes toward the child that are communicated to the child and create an emotional climate in which the parent's behaviours are expressed'; it describes the quality of the parent-child relationship, whereas parenting practices describes the content and frequency of specific parenting behaviour (Stevenson-Hinde, 1998).

In the literature on child-rearing style, the term 'care' is interchangeably used with warmth, acceptance, nurturance, affection, responsiveness or supportiveness on the one end of the dimension and rejection, hostility or criticism on the other.

Ever since the seminal paper of Bell and Chapman (1986) about the child's influence on parental behaviour, parenting is no longer considered to be a purely parental characteristic affecting the child, but rather an interactional phenomenon in which parent and child participate and reciprocally influence one another.

Relationship may be reciprocal, that is, anxious child influences the parental style exhibited and vice versa (Samerof & Emde, 1989; Thomasgard & Metz, 1993; Bögels and Brechman-Toussaint, 2006).

Behavioural genetic research (Rowe & Plomin, 1981; Plomin & Daniels, 1987) has shown that environmental factors that all children in a family share may have a different influence than those that are unique. Child-rearing style is often considered to belong to the shared environment, but when the contribution of the child to parenting style is taken into consideration, it should rather be regarded as part of the nonshared environment. When differences in parenting behaviour regarding different children within the same family are very outspoken, this is called parental differential treatment (Lindhout, 2008).

Anxiety disorders could be conceptualized, considering the multi factorial aetiological view of the phenomenom, as a self-perpetuating cycle of elevated biological responses to stress, debilitated cognition and avoidance of stressful circumstances reinforced by environmental factor including a parenting style, which interferes with children's attempts at solving their own problems, and instead emphasizes threat in situations, and encourages children's avoidance behavior. The exposure to traumatic or aversive situations also increases the risk of children developing anxious responses (Webster, 2002).

Studies have shown that parents of anxious children behave in ways that increase the chance that their child behaves in an anxious manner. High levels of maternal control and anxiety, and maternal rejection and depression (Rapee, 1997) as well as less accepting, aversiveness, intrusiveness, overinvolved, over protective and more controlling parenting styles have been found associated with anxiety disorders in children (Siqueland et al., 1996; Hudson & Rapee, 2001; Wood et al., 2003; Moore et al., 2004; McLeod et al., 2007; Hudson et al., 2008).

2.1.4. Family style of solving problems and domestic violence

Family relationships are viewed as critical factors influencing a child's social and emotional development (Hannan & Luster, 1991; Levitt, 1991). A number of broad classes of dysfunction such as psychosocial stress, poverty, parental marital discord, parental psychopathology, maltreatment, and parental emotional unavailability, have been associated with both internalizing and externalizing problems (Gotlib & Avison, 1993).

Exposure to conflict has been shown to influence children directly. Witnessing adult anger is physiologically and affectively stressful for children, and exposure to conflict has been shown to influence children indirectly through its effect on parenting and parents' psychological wellbeing. Some researchers have shown that the effects of parental conflict can be more harmful to children than parental absence through death or divorce (Emery, 1982; Jekielek, 1998; Mechanic & Hansell, 1989; Peterson & Zill, 1986). Marital fighting has been found to be more predictive of children's functioning than divorce (Cummings, 1994; Jekielek, 1998). More specifically, the quality of the marital relationship in early life has been found to predict future anxiety in the child (Bögels & Brechman-Toussaint, 2006).

In children exposed to chronic violence, increasing sensitization has been reported. Hennessy et al. (1994) found that children exposed to violence, in comparison to peers, were more fearful and emotionally reactive to videotaped scenes of anger between adults. Sensitization may be related to hypervigilance, the tendency to anxiously scan the environment for possible threat that is one of the hallmarks of posttraumatic stress.

Also, deficits in emotion regulation have been observed in children exposed to uncontrolled anger and distress in the very figures they would turn to for soothing and solace (Graham-Bermann & Levendosky, 1998).

Exposure to violence at home is recognized as a form of child maltreatment. Witnessing domestic abuse, especially when it is perpetrated against the mother, in itself is a traumatic experience. Although children growing up in violent homes do not consistently show cognitive deficits, they often display academic problems. Distractibility and inattention in school may occur as a result of the trauma that is associated with exposure ot violence. Research suggest that children exposed to domestic violence show a range of emotional and behavioral problems including insecure attachment in younger children and both externalizing and internalizing problems in the school years (Wenar & Kerig, 2006).

Some children experience negative effects in the short term, others have both short and longer term effects, and still others seem to experience no effects related to witnessing violence. Children's age and sex, as well as severity, intensity and chronicity of the violence are variables that play a role in the outcome of the exposure. In a longitudinal study of a sample of 155 children followed from birth through adolescence, Yates et al. (2003) found that exposure to violence in the home was an independent predictor of externalizing problems in boys and internalizing problems in girls. A study in Canada reported that children aged 4 to 7 years old who witnessed violence at home showed more overt aggression two and four years later. For boys the experience was also linked to indirect aggression, and for girls, with anxiety (Moss, 2003).

2.2. Objective

This chapter will focus on testing whether the basic issues included for the surveillance of mental health in childhood and adolescence are somehow significantly associated with the presence of anxiety syndromes in children an adolescents attended at a primary care setting and followed along a two-year period.

The specific goals for this report are:

1. Confirm familial associations between parental psychiatric history and anxiety CBTD screening syndromes in their offspring.

2. Determine if a higher score on the scale for the assessment of impairment is associated with anxiety CBTD screening syndromes in children and adolescents.

3. Determine if a higher score on the scales examining child-rearing and parental practices are associated with anxiety CBTD screening syndromes in children and adolescents.

4. Determine if a higher score on the scale for the assessment of a potential dysfunctional environment at home is associated with anxiety CBTD screening syndromes in children and adolescents.

5. Evaluate the morbid risk of these variables for the development of anxiety CBTD screening syndromes.

2.3. Method

All consecutive children and adolescents aged 4 to 16 years attended during a six-month period at a primary care health center (PCHC) were included for this study. Children and adolescents already in treatment at the mental health service were excluded. Informed consent was obtained from the parents of the minors at the beginning of the study. At the initial interview, socio demographic data was obtained and parents responded the Brief Screening and Diagnostic Questionnaire (CBTD). Whenever a probable case was detected, parents were advised to seek help from the mental health service at the PCHC or at another facility. The cohort was followed for two years (2005-2007); at each consecutive evaluation a follow-up version of the CBTD was used and complementary information was gathered at different points of time as will be explained.

2.3.1. Instruments

1. The Brief Screening and Diagnostic Questionnaire (CBTD for its initials in Spanish) is a 27-item questionnaire answered by the parents of the child exploring symptoms frequently reported as motives for seeking attention at the outpatient mental health services. Presence of the symptom requires that each item has to be reported as "frequently" presented. The internal consistency of the questionnaire showed a Cronbach's alpha of 0.81, range: 0.76 to 0.85 (Caraveo, 2006). Diagnostic algorithms in order to define probable DSM-IV disorders in children were created based on data from the general population epidemiological study (Caraveo, 2007a). The generalized anxiety screening syndrome was defined as follows: Key symptom: a positive response to the question: Does the child gets scared or nervous for no good reason?, and at least two of the following: can't seat still, irritable, sleep problems, and frequent nightmares. The anxiety with inhibition screening syndrome was defined as follows: Key symptom: a positive response to the question: Is the child excessively dependent or attached to adults?; and at least two positive answers on the following: aloof, frequent headaches, afraid of school, physical complains without a medical problem, sleep problems, low weight, overweight, do not work at school, and backward compared to other children. Concurrent validity of the two screening anxiety syndromes, generalized anxiety and anxiety with inhibition, as compared to DSM-IV anxiety diagnoses using the E-MiniKid standardized interview (Sheehan et al., 1998; 2000) showed Kappa agreement to be 0.53 and 0.68 respectively, and using Yule's Y coefficient results were 0.65 and 0.92 respectively.

Receiver Operating Characteristic Curves (ROC) analyses showed Area under the Curve (AUC) to be 0.82 and 0.78 respectively (Caraveo-Anduaga et al., 2011).

2. Psychiatric parental antecedents about anxiety, affective and substance-use disorders were obtained following the Family-history research criteria (Andreasen et al., 1977; 1986; Kendler et al., 1997) as was used in the general population study (Caraveo-Anduaga, 2011).

3. Functional impairment in children and adolescents was measured using the Brief Imparment Scale (BIS) (Bird et al., 2005) which is a 23-item questionnaire that has three sub-scales exploring interpersonal relationships, work/school performance and self-attitudes. Each question is responded in Likert scale with 4 options: 0= never or no problem; 1= some problems; 2= several problems; 3= serious problems. The internal consistency of the BIS in our population showed a Cronbach's alpha of 0.87.

4. The Parent Practices Inventory (PPI) (Bauermeister et al. 1995 as presented in Barkley R., Murphy K. & Bauermeister J., 1998) is a 37-item questionnaire exploring child rearing as well as disciplinary practices. Two dimensions were identified: a positive one that considers approval, acceptance, positive motivation and affection as predominant practices, while the negative dimension includes inconsistency, cohersion and negative affect. Each question is evaluated in a 4-point Likert scale: 0= never or almost never; 1= rarely; 2= frequently; 3= very frequently. The internal consistency of the PPI in our population showed a Cronbach's alpha of 0.87.

5. The style of solving problems at home was explored with a 7-item scale adapted from answers used by Kessler in the National Comorbity Study. In the present study they were asked as follows: All persons solve their conflicts in different manners. How often do you and your spouse/partner display the following conducts when there is a conlict? Insults or swores; become furious; sulk or refuse to talk; stomp out of the room; say something to spite; threaten to hit; smash or kick something in anger. Each item is responded in a 4-point Likert scale: 0= never; 1= rarely; 2= sometimes; 3= always. The internal consistency of this scale in our population showed a Cronbach's alpha of 0.98. If some kind of physical violence was reported on the previous scale, it was asked if the child have witnessed the episodes.

2.3.2. Procedure

Field work started on May of 2005 and in an intensive way, children and adolescents aged 4 to 16 years attending the general health clinicians at the PHC were assessed. During the vacation period, months of July and August, attendance during the morning turn was numerous but after that, it was parctically reduced to the afternoon turn. Moreover, new elegible subjects became fewer, so that in December it was decided to end the incorporation phase of the study and start preparing the first follow-up evaluation.

Besides the clinical evaluation using the CBTD in a follow-up version, information about familial psychiatric antecedents of both parents, (that was initiated during the last two months of the incorporation phase), as well as the assessment of impairment in the child using the BIS were sistematically obtained. It is important to note that even tough follow-up evaluations were cost-free and that reminder of appointments were made, the participation of the study population was scarse as shown in Table 1. In order to deal with this, telephone interviews were carried out by the child psychiatrists working in the project under the supervision of the principal researcher (JC).

For the second follow-up, assessments started on July 2007; based on the previous field clinical work, it was decided to incorporate measures of parental child-rearing practices and of domestic violence. Also, besides clinical follow-up appointments at the PHC, and telephone interviews, it was decided to have home-interviews. For this purpose, psychologists with experience in community studies were trained in the use of all the instruments, and a computarized program was created in order to facilitate the assessments, control, and management of the information. This strategy probed to be more efficient as a higher participation of the study population was accomplished; altough losses were considerable as shown in Table 1. At each follow-up interview, we look for that preferably the informant would be the same person as in the initial assessment.

2.3.3. Analyses

Longitudinal morbid risk in terms of the odds ratio was calculated using the random effects logistic regression analysis as our interest was in the individual development over time of dichotomous outcome variables (Twisk, 2003), for this chapter the two screening anxiety syndromes in children and adolescents.

Bivariate analyses between anxiety syndromes and each independent variable were performed. Scores of the different scales used in the study were converted into dummy variables using quartiles, where higher scores indicated major problems.As each independent variable of interest and its corresponding measure was incorporated at different times along the study period, the number of observations are somehow different in each analysis.

Multivariate analysis including all variables was performed in terms of the odds ratio using the random effects logistic regression analysis. It was assumed that child-rearing practices as well as the style of solving problems at home were the same during the two-year period.

2.4. Results

A total cohort of 846 consecutive children and adolescents patients attended at the PHC was initially evaluated. Girls represented 55% and boys 45%, with a mean age of 9 years (s.d. 3.5). On 87% the informant was the child's mother. For 60% of the cohort at least one follow-up was completed, and in 21%two follow-up interviews were done (Table 1).

Children/ Adolescents	Initial Evaluation		1 year follow-up		2 year follow-up	
N	%	n	%	n	%	
Interviewed	846	100	298	35.2	454	53.7
Not interviewed	-	-	548	64.8	392	46.3

Table 1. Interviewed population

The total prevalence of the anxiety screening syndromes at the initial interview was 29.4% (95%CI: 26.4, 32.5) for the generalized anxiety syndrome, and 31.2% (95%CI: 26.4, 35.9) for the anxiety with inhibition syndrome. Both anxiety syndromes were slightly more frequently reported in boys than in girls. In adolescents anxiety syndromes were more frequent among girls. Prevalence of both anxicty syndromes tended to be somehow similar to the initial prevalence at the one-year follow-up, but they both considerably dimisnished at the two-year follow-up; prevalence of anxiety with inhibition decreased to be less than a half of the initial prevalence (Table 2).

2.4.1. Is the morbid risk higher for developing anxiety syndromes in the offspring when anxiety parental psychiatric antecedents are present as compared to when they are not?

The analysis of the association between specific types of pychiatric parental antecedents and the two anxiety syndromes in the offspring shows that parental antecedents of anxiety-only, and comorbid anxiety with depression, as well as with substance abuse are significantly associated with both types of anxiety syndromes in the offspring. Parental antecedents of depression are associated with generalized anxiety syndrome in the offspring, but the odds ratio is considerably lower; and parental antecedents of substance abuse alone, are not significantly associated with neither anxiety syndromes in the offspring (Table 3).

2.4.2. Does a higher impairment score is significantly associated with each anxiety syndrome? If so, is it different for each anxiety disorder?

For this analysis, 741 observations were included; 187 correspond to observations on subjects presenting generalized anxiety, 25.5%, and 135 presenting anxiety with inhibition, 18.2%.

For the next tables, on the second column, the proportions of observations with each anxiety syndrome as related to scores on the BIS are presented. The odds ratio in tables represent the longitudinal strenght of the association between those observed subjects with anxiety syndromes within the corresponding quartile of the impairment scale as compared to observed subjects with anxiety syndromes within the first quartile.

Initial assessment	4 – 5	6 – 8	9 – 12	13 – 16	TOTAL (95%CI)	
Boys	(n= 88)	(n= 99)	(n= 128)	(n= 66)	(N= 381)	
Generalized anxiety	29.5	34.3	36.0	22.7	31.5 (26.8, 36.2)	
Anxiety with inhibition	43.2	38.4	28.0	18.2	33.3 (26.0, 40.6)	
Girls	(n= 87)	(n= 112)	(n= 157)	(n= 109)	(N= 465)	
Generalized anxiety	20.7	29.5	26.7	33.0	27.7 (23.6, 31.8)	
Anxiety with inhibition	27.6	39.3	22.9	30.3	29.4 (23.2, 35.7)	
1 year follow-up						
Boys	(n= 15)	(n= 30)	(n= 54)	(n= 34)	(N= 133)	
Generalized anxiety	53.3	30.0	40.7	17.6	33.8 (25.7, 42.0)	
Anxiety with inhibition	40.0	36.7	24.1	11.8	25.6 (18.1, 33.1)	
Girls	(n= 18)	(n= 45)	(n= 56)	(n= 46)	(N= 165)	
Generalized anxiety	27.8	20.0	30.3	32.6	27.9 (21.0, 34.8)	
Anxiety with inhibition	38.9	20.0	25.0	15.2	22.4 (16.0, 28.9)	
2 year follow-up						
Boys	(n= 9)	(n= 54)	(n= 51)	(n= 69)	(N= 183)	
Generalized anxiety	11.1	22.6	34.7	17.7	23.2 (16.9, 29.4)	
Anxiety with inhibition	11.1	28.3	14.3	10.6	16.9 (11.4, 22.5)	
Girls	(n= 38)	(n= 60)	(n= 92)	(n= 81)	(N= 271)	
Generalized anxiety	0.0	15.5	32.3	21.2	20.7 (15.8, 25.6)	
Anxiety with inhibition	0.0	17.2	16.7	11.2	12.8 (8.7, 16.8)	

Table 2. Prevalence of anxiety syndromes at the initial assessment and follow-ups

Nearly half of the observations on children and adolescents with any screening anxiety syndrome are reported as having considerable impairment and with strong longitudinal morbid risk in terms of the odds ratio. Another one fith of the observations on children and adolescents with any screening anxiety syndrome shows moderate impairment as well as moderate longitudinal morbid risk. Notably, one quarter of the observations on children and adolescents presenting anxiety with inhibition also shows some impairment with moderate longitudinal morbid risk (Table 4).

Anxiety Syndromes and Their Correlates in Children and Adolescents: A Two-Year-Follow-Up Study at Primary Health Care in Mexico City

55

Antecedents	Generalized anxiety OR (95% CI)	P	Anxiety with inhibition OR (95% CI)	P
Anxiety	9.4 (2.8, 31.8)	.000	8.7 (2.3, 33.2)	.001
Depression	3.9 (1.1, 14.2)	.040	2.6 (0.8, 7.9)	.093
Substance abuse	1.0 (0.2, 5.7)	.979	1.9 (0.3, 10.4)	.464
Anxiety depression	6.5 (2.4, 17.8)	.000	4.4 (1.6, 11.9)	.004
Anxiety, depression Substance abuse	21.7 (6.7, 70.6)	.000	5.2 (1.9, 14.5)	.002

No.obs: 1003; No. gps 433; Wald chi2=33.03; gl=5; p= 0.0000;Wald chi2=17.18;gl=5; p= 0.0042

Table 3. Specific parental antecedents and anxiety syndromes in the offspring

BIS total score	Generalized anxiety %	OR (95% CI)	P	Anxiety with inhibition %	OR (95% CI)	P
0-4	13.9	1.0	.	10.4	1.0	
5-8	18.1	2.0 (0.8, 4.9)	.149	25.9	4.7 (1.7, 12.8)	.003
9-12	22.5	5.5 (2.0, 14.6)	.001	17.8	5.0 (1.6, 15.2)	.005
13-48	45.5	19.1 (6.6, 55.1)	.000	45.9	20.6 (6.5, 65.9)	.000

No.obs: 741; No. gps.540; Wald chi2=34.75;gl=3; p= 0.0000;Wald chi2=26.97;gl=3; p= 0.0000

Table 4. BIS impairment total score and anxiety syndromes

Further analyses on the different sub-scales of the BIS show that interpersonal relationships are significantly impaired in all of the observations of anxious children and adolescents as compared to those observed in the first quartil (Table 5).

Interpersonal Sub-scale score	Generalized anxiety %	OR (95% CI)	P	Anxiety with inhibition %	OR (95% CI)	P
0	11.8	1.0		12.6	1.0	
1-2	32.1	4.3 (1.7, 10.7)	.002	37.8	4.5 (1.7, 11.6)	.002
3	12.8	11.7 (3.4, 40.5)	.000	12.6	10.6 (2.7, 41.2)	.001
4-20	43.3	17.2 (6.1, 48.7)	.000	37.0	10.0 (3.3, 30.4)	.000

No.obs: 741; No. gps.540; Wald chi2=31.0;gl=3; p= 0.0000;Wald chi2=18.00;gl=3; p= 0.0004

Table 5. BIS interpersonal relationships sub-scale and anxiety syndromes

Seventy percent of the observations on anxious children and adolescents show moderate to severe impairment on the school/work sub-scale of the BIS as compared to those observed in the first quartile (Table 6).

School/work Sub-scale score	Generalized anxiety %	OR (95% CI)	P	Anxiety with inhibition %	OR (95% CI)	P
0-1	20.3	1.0		17.8	1.0	
2	9.1	0.8 (0.3, 2.3)	.725	10.4	1.0 (0.3, 2.8)	.992
3-5	34.2	3.7 (1.6, 8.4)	.002	34.8	3.4 (1.4, 8.2)	.006
6-21	36.4	14.7 (5.5, 39.4)	.000	37.0	14.7 (4.9, 43.9)	.000

No.obs: 741; No. gps.540; Wald chi2=32.26;gl=3; p= 0.0000;Wald chi2=25.17;gl=3; p= 0.0000

Table 6. BIS work/school performance sub-scale and anxiety syndromes

Finally, on the self attitudes sub-scale, 85% of all the observations on children and adolescents presenting anxiety with inhibition show different degrees of impairment that are significantly diferent from those in the first quartile, as compared to 60% of the observations on children and adolescents with generalized anxiety syndrome (Table 7).

Self-attitudes Sub-scale score	Generalized anxiety %	OR (95% CI)	P	Anxiety with inhibition %	OR (95% CI)	P
0-1	22.5	1.0		14.1	1.0	
2-3	20.3	1.0 (0.4, 2.4)	.978	25.2	3.5 (1.4, 9.2)	.010
4-5	22.5	3.7 (1.3, 10.4)	.012	28.9	7.5 (2.7, 21.1)	.000
6-18	34.7	8.1 (3.0, 22.0)	.000	31.8	8.5 (3.1, 23.6)	.000

No.obs: 741; No. gps.540; Wald chi2=21.31;gl=3; p= 0.0001;Wald chi2=19.77;gl=3; p= 0.0002

Table 7. BIS self-attitudes sub-scale and anxiety syndromes

2.4.3. Does the exposure to a more outrageous family environment is significantly associated with each anxiety syndrome? If so, is it different for each anxiety disorder?

Bivariate analyses between anxiety syndromes and the score on the style of solving problems at home scale (SSPHS) do not show a significant association with either anxiety syndrome in children and adolescents; however, a higher score on the SSPHS was close to be significantly associated with generalized anxiety (Table 8).

SSPHS score	Generalized anxiety %	OR (95% CI)	P	Anxiety with inhibition %	OR (95% CI)	P
7-8	27.5	1.0		26.4	1.0	
9-11	25.0	1.2 (0.3, 6.1)	.784	24.0	1.2 (0.4, 3.3)	.790
12-15	13.7	0.2 (0.05, 1.2)	.089	16.3	0.7 (0.2, 2.1)	.526
16-28	33.8	3.4 (0.9, 11.9)	.060	33.3	2.3 (0.8, 6.6)	.129

No.obs: 794; No. gps.321; Wald chi2=12.75;gl=3; p= 0.0052;Wald chi2=4.42;gl=3; p= 0.22

Table 8. More outrageous family environment and anxiety syndromes

Having witnessed physical violence at home was found significantly associated with gener-alized anxiety syndrome in children and adolescents, OR= 2.6. (95% CI: 1.2, 5.9), but not for anxiety with inhibition, OR= 1.3 (95% CI: 0.6, 2.6).

2.4.4. Does the exposure to a parental's less positive reinforcement rearing practice is significantly associated with each anxiety syndrome? If so, is it different for each anxiety disorder?

Bivariate analyses show that a higher score on parental's less positive reinforcement rearing practice is only associated with observations on children and adolescents with generalized anxiety as compared to those in the first quartile (Table 9).

Less positive reinforcement sub-scale score	Generalized anxiety %	OR (95% CI)	P	Anxiety with inhibition %	OR (95% CI)	P
0-17	25.7	1.0		29.1	1.0	
18-23	17.2	0.7 (0.3, 2.0)	.507	21.2	0.7 (0.3, 1.7)	.490
24-28	25.6	2.4 (0.8, 6.7)	.103	17.3	0.7 (0.3, 1.8)	.463
29-51	31.5	2.9 (1.1, 7.9)	.033	32.4	1.6 (0.7, 3.8)	.244

No.obs: 1088; No. gps.444; Wald chi2=9.71;gl=3; p= 0.0212;Wald chi2=4.27;gl=3; p= 0.2336

Table 9. Less positive reinforcement practices and anxiety syndromes

2.4.5. Does the exposure to a parental's more negative reinforcement rearing practice is significantly associated with each anxiety syndrome? If so, is it different for each anxiety disorder?

Bivariate analyses show that exposure to a parental's higher negative reinforcement is sig-nificantly associated with roughly one third of the observations on children and adolescents with either anxiety syndromes. However, the strenght of the association is higher on the offspring with general anxiety (Table 10).

Negative reinforcement Sub-scale score	Generalized anxiety %	OR (95% CI)	P	Anxiety with inhibition %	OR (95% CI)	P
1-5	25.3	1.0		23.5	1.0	
6-8	14.2	0.4 (0.2, 1.2)	.112	18.4	0.9 (0.4, 2.4)	.918
9-12	22.0	1.5 (0.5, 4.3)	.442	24.6	1.8 (0.7, 4.4)	.186
13-37	38.5	5.6 (2.2, 14.3)	.000	33.5	2.8 (1.2, 6.8)	.018

No.obs: 1088; No. gps.444; Wald chi2=25.41;gl=3; p= 0.0000;Wald chi2=7.84;gl=3; p= 0.0494

Table 10. High negative reinforcement practices and anxiety syndromes

Multivariable analysis using the random effects logistic regression shows that for both anxiety syndromes in children and adolescents parental psychiatric antecedents and a higher score on the BIS are the only two predictive variables significantly associated with the outcome. The contribution of parental psychiatric antecedents in terms of the odds ratio is considerably higher for generalized anxiety than for anxiety with inhibition, and impairment is higher in this latter syndrome than in generalized anxiety (Table 11).

	Generalized anxiety	P	Anxiety with inhibition	P
No. of Familial antecedents	4.7 (1.8, 11.9)	.001	1.9 (1.1, 3.4)	.024
Less positive reinforcement	1.3 (0.7, 2.4)	.365	0.7 (0.5, 1.2)	.177
Higher negative reinforcement	1.2 (0.6, 2.2)	.626	1.3 (0.8, 2.2)	.311
Conflict resolution	1.4 (0.8, 2.6)	.248	1.0 (0.6, 1.6)	.980
Witnessed agression	0.6 (0.1, 2.5)	.455	0.8 (0.2, 2.6)	.662
Impairment	1.9 (1.2, 3.3)	.011	2.5 (1.4, 4.2)	.001
Sex female	0.7 (0.2, 3.0)	.684	1.1 (0.4, 3.4)	.835
Age	1.1 (0.9, 1.3)	.264	0.9 (0.8, 1.1)	.315

No.obs: 454; No. gps.:307; Wald chi2=17.90;gl=8; p= 0.0220;Wald chi2=18.32;gl=7; p= 0.0189

Table 11. Predictor variables and anxiety syndromes

2.5. Discussion

This study has shown that variables included for the surveillance of mental health problems in children and adolescents at a primary care setting, probed to be useful and complementary for the study of anxiety syndromes as defined in the CBTD. Furthermore, results are consistent with findings reported in the literature on child's anxiety disorders as previously reviewed, although none to our knowledge have attempted to collect them as a whole in a primary care setting and evaluate their risk contribution for anxiety disorders in children and adolescents.

Results obtained on the association between specific parental's psychiatric antecedents and the two anxiety syndromes replicated our previous findings in general population (Caraveo-Anduaga,2011) in that anxiety parental's psychiatric antecedents either alone or comorbid with depression and substance abuse are significantly associated with the development of anxiety syndromes in their offspring.

The odds ratios in the present study are higher than most of the crude odds ratios found on the general population study. For example, the strength of the association between parental's antecedents of anxiety-only and general anxiety syndrome in the offspring was OR= 5.7 (95% CI: 2.1, 15.9) in the general population, while in the present study is OR=9.4 (2.8, 31.8). An explanation for such differences is that regression coefficients calculated with logistic GEE analysis, as in the general population study, always will be lower than the coefficients calculated with a logistic random coefficient analysis as in the present study (Twisk, 2003).

One currently key issue is the extent to which diagnostic thresholds defining mental disorders represent unique entities that lead to functional impairment (Rapee et al., 2012). Results showed that, as expected, higher scores on the BIS were significantly associated with CBTD's anxiety screening syndromes. For most observations on children and adolescents with the generalized anxiety syndrome, 68%, significant risk impairment was found, mainly on interpersonal relationships and work/school performance. Also, for 90% of the observations on children and adolescents reporting anxiety with inhibition, significant risk impairment is associated, and for this syndrome mainly on interpersonal relationships and self-attitudes. These findings are consistent with other reports in the literature, as previously reviewed (see 2.1.2) and contribution of this study is to have documented its presence and relevance in a primary care setting.

Moreover, it is important to highlight that in the present study only frequency of each symtom on the CBTD determined its rating for presence and persistance, so that impairment measurement was obtained irrespective of symptoms and syndromes. The significant association between the measurement of functional impairment and the CBTD's screening anxiety syndromes not only enhance the accuracy and usefulness of these later, but also, impairments identified with the BIS, may become targets for specific interventions and eventually used as outcome indicators as signaled by Ezpeleta et al. (2006).

The exposure to a more outrageous family environment as evaluated by the SSPHS was not significantly associated with any anxiety syndrome in the offspring. However, having witnessed aggression at home was found associated only with generalized anxiety in children and adolescents. As reviewed, exposure to violence has been found as an independent pre-dictor of different problems in boys as compared with girls (Yates et al., 2003; Moss, 2003). Further analysis is needed to bring more light about this issue.

Roughly, one third of the observations on children and adolescents reporting any screening anxiety syndrome have been exposed to more adverse child-rearing and parental practices, as measured by the two sub-sacles of the PPI. A less positive reinforcement rearing practice seems to be a risk only for generalized anxiety syndrome, while higher negative reinforce-ment is for both anxiety syndromes; however, the strenght of the association in terms of the odds ratio is higher for children and adolescents with generalized anxiety. Thus, generalized anxiety syndrome in children and adolescents is associated with more adverse child-rearing and parental practices than children and adolescents presenting anxiety with inhibition. As disscussed for impairment, results from the PPI sub-scales not only showed differences in their association with the two screening anxiety syndromes, but also the information is im-portant for planning interventions.

Finally, among the variables included in the study, it is important to distinguish nonmodifi-able risk factors from those that could be modifiable (Opler et al., 2010). Results evaluating the morbid risk of all independent variables on anxiety showed that familial psychiatric an-tecedent, mainly anxiety, is the major nonmodifiable risk factor for both anxiety syndromes, although slightly higher for generalized anxiety than for anxiety with inhibition syndrome. Impairment, which is the second mayor contributor, is actually a consequence of the psycho-pathology, so it seems that once an anxiety syndrome is detected, efforts should be directed toward the other modifiable risk factors such as rearing and parenting practices in order to prevent further impairment; diminishes suffering and modify maladjustment.

3. Conclusion

The present report has confirmed that anxiety disorders in children and adolescents attend-ing a primary care center in Mexico City are frequent, persistent and represent a great part of the unmet treatment needs of children's mental health. In order to tackle this problem and enhace the role of primary care in the preventive actions that are needed, results from this pilot surveillance program on child's mental health have developed and adapted simple and efficient tools that identified child's core areas of difficulty associated with the two screening anxiety syndromes. Future work should be focused on acceptable and relatively simple interventions that, as part of a step-care strategy, could modify risk factors such as rearing and parenting practices, evaluating the impact on impairment measures.

Acknowledgment

This is study was funded by The National Council of Science and Technology (CONACYT) award 2003-C01-60.We would like to thank: M Psic. Jorge L. López Jimenez; Dr. Julio López

Hernández; Dra. Aurora Contreras Garza; Psic. Arlette Reyes Mejía; Enf. Nayely Meneses Zamudio; Psic. Blanca T. Rodríguez Gavia; Dra. Cynthia Rincón González; Psic. Araceli Aguilar Abrego; Psic. Brenda Jiménez Ramos; Psic. Alejandra Guerrero Carillo; Psic. Denisse Meza Mercado & Psic. Sergio Bernabé Castellanos, for their collaboration and participation in this study.

Author details

Jorge Javier Caraveo-Anduaga, Alejandra Soriano Rodríguez and Jose Erazo Pérez

Instituto Nacional de Psiquiatría "Ramón de la Fuente Muñiz", México

References

[1] American Psychiatric Association. (1994) *Diagnostic and statistical manual of mental disorders*, (Fourth edition), American Psychiatric Association, ISBN 0-89042-062-9, Washington D.C.

[2] Andreasen, N. C.; Endicott, J.; Spitzer, R. L. & Winokur, G. (1977) The family history method using diagnostic criteria. *Archives of General Psychiatry*, 34, pp. 1229-1235, ISSN: 0003-990X.

[3] Barkley, R. A.; Murphy, K. R. & Bauermeister, J. J. (1998) *Attention-Deficit Hyperactivity Disorder. A clinical Workbook*, (Second edition), The Guilford Press, ISBN 1-57230-301-8, New York, NY.

[4] Bell-Dolan, D. & Brazeal, T. J. (1993) Separation anxiety disorder, overanxious disorder, and school refusal. *Child and Adolescent Psychiatric Clinics of North America*, 2, pp. 563-580, ISSN 1056-4993.

[5] Bell, R. Q. & Chapman, M. (1986) Child effects in studies using experimental or brief longitudinal approaches to socialization. *Developmental Psychology*, 22, pp. 595-603, ISSN 0012-1649.

[6] Benjamin, R. S.; Costello, E. J. & Warren, M. (1990) Anxiety disorders in a pediatric sample. *Journal of Anxiety Disorders*, 4, pp. 293-316, ISSN 0887-6185.

[7] Bird, H. R.; Canino, G.; Rubio-Stipec, M.; Gould, M. S.; Ribera, J.; Sesman, M.; Woodbury, M.; Huertas-Goldman, S.; Pagan, A.; Sanchez-Lacay, A. et al. (1988) Estimates of the prevalence of childhood maladjustment in a community survey in Puerto Rico: The use of combined measures. *Archives of General Psychiatry*, 45, pp. 1120-1126, ISSN 0003-990X.

[8] Bird, H. R.; Davies, M.; Fisher, P.; Narrow, W.; Jensen, P.; Hoven, C.; Cohen, P. & Duncan, M. K. (2000) How specific is specific impairment? *Journal of the American Academy of Child and Adolescent Psychiatry*, 39, pp. 1182-1189, ISSN 0890-8567.

[9] Bird, H. R.; Canino, G. J.; Davies, M.; Ramírez, R.; Chávez, L.; Duarte, C. & Shen, S. (2005) The Brief Impairment Scale (BIS): A Multidimensional Scale of Functional Impairment for Children and Adolescents. *Journal of the American Academy of Child & Adolescent Psychiatry*, 44, pp. 699-707, ISSN 0890-8567.

[10] Bögels, S. M. & Brechman-Toussaint, L. (2006) Family issues in child anxiety: Attachment, family functioning, parental rearing and beliefs. *Clinical Psychology Review*, 26, pp. 834-856, ISSN 0272-7358.

[11] Briggs-Gowan, M. J.; Horwitz, S. M.; Schwab-Stone, M. E.; Leventhal, J. M. & Leaf, P. J. (2000) Mental health in pediatric settings: distribution of disorders and factors related to service use. *Journal of the American Academy of Child and Adolescent Psychiatry*, 39, pp. 841-849, ISSN 0890-8567.

[12] Caraveo-A, J.; Medina-Mora, M. E.; Villatoro, J., and López-Lugo, E. K. & Martínez-Vélez A. (1995) Detección de problemas de salud mental en la infancia. *Salud Pública De México*, 37, pp. 446-451, ISSN 0036-3634.

[13] Caraveo-Anduaga, J. J.; Colmenares, E. & Martínez, N. A. (2002) Síntomas percepción y demanda de atención en salud mental en niños y adolescentes de la Ciudad de México. *Salud Pública De México*, 44, pp. 492-498, ISSN 0036-3634.

[14] Caraveo-Anduaga, J. J.; Nicolini, S. H.; Villa, R. A. & Wagner, E. F. (2005) Psicopatología en familiares de tres generaciones: un estudio epidemiológico en la Ciudad de México. *Salud Pública De México*, 47, pp. 20-26, ISSN 0036-3634.

[15] Caraveo-Anduaga, J. J. (2006) Cuestionario Breve de tamizaje y diagnóstico de problemas de salud mental en niños y adolescentes, CBTD: confiabilidad, estandarización y validez de construcción. *Salud Mental*, 29, pp. 65-72, ISSN 0185-3325.

[16] Caraveo-Anduaga, J. J. (2007a) Cuestionario Breve de tamizaje y diagnóstico de problemas de salud mental en niños y adolescentes: algoritmos para síndromes y su prevalencia en la Ciudad de México. *Salud Mental*, 30, pp. 48-55, ISSN 0185-3325.

[17] Caraveo-Anduaga, J. J. (2007b) Validez del Cuestionario Breve de Tamizaje y Diagnóstico (CBTD) para niños y adolescentes en escenarios clínicos. *Salud Mental*, 30, pp. 42-49, ISSN 0185-3325.

[18] Caraveo-Anduaga, J. J. (2011) Intergeneration Familial Risk and Psychosocial Correlates for Anxiety Syndromes in Children and Adolescents in a Developing Country, In: *Anxiety and Related Disorders*, Á. Szirmal, (Ed.), 49-68, InTech, ISBN 978-953-307-254-8, Croatia.

[19] Caraveo-Anduaga, J. J.; López, J. J. L.; Soriano, R. A.; López, H. J. L.; Contreras, G. A. & Reyes, M. A. (2011) Eficiencia y validez concurrente del CBTD para la vigilancia de

la salud mental de niños y adolescentes en un centro de atención primaria de México. *Revista De Investigación Clínica*, 63, pp. 590-600, ISSN 0034-8376.

[20] Chavira, D. A.; Stein, M. B.; Bailey, K. & Stein, M. T. (2004) Child anxiety in primary care: prevalent but untreated. *Depression and Anxiety*, 20, pp. 155-164, ISSN 1091-4269.

[21] Costello, E. J. (1989) Child psychiatric disorders and their correlates: a primary care pediatric sample. *Journal of the American Academy of Child & Adolescent Psychiatry*, 28, pp. 851-855, ISSN: 0890-8567.

[22] Costello, E. J.; Egger, H. C. & Angold, A. (2005) The developmental epidemiology of anxiety disorders: Phenomenology, prevalence and comorbidity. *Child and Adolescent Psychiatric Clinics of North America*, 14, pp. 631-648, ISSN 1056-4993.

[23] Costello, E. J.; Copeland, W. & Angold, A. (2011) Trends in psychopathology across the adolescent years: what changes when children become adolescents, and when adolescents become adults? *Journal of Child Psychology and Psychiatry and Allied Disciplines*, 52, pp. 1015-1025, ISSN 0021-9630.

[24] Cummings, E. M. (1994) Marital conflict and children's functioning. *Social Development*, 3, pp. 16-36, ISSN 0961-205X.

[25] Darling, N. & Steinberg, L. (1993) Parenting style as context: an integrative model. *Psychological Bulletin*, 113, pp. 487-496, ISSN 0033-2909.

[26] Dulcan, M. K.; Costello, E. J.; Costello, A. J.; Edelbrock, C.; Brent, D. & Janiszewski, S. (1990) The pediatrician as gatekeeper to mental health care for children: do parents' concerns open the gate? *Journal of the American Academy of Child & Adolescent Psychiatry*, 29, pp. 453-458, ISSN 0890-8567.

[27] Emery. R. E. (1982) Interparental conflict and the children of discord and divorce. *Psychological Bulletin*, 3, pp. 310-330, ISSN 0033-2909.

[28] Essau, C. A.; Conradt, J. & Petermann, F. (2000) Frequency, comorbidity, and psychosocial impairment of anxiety disorders in German adolescents. *Journal of Anxiety Disorders*, 14, pp. 263-279, ISSN 0887-6185.

[29] Ezpeleta, L.; Granero, R.; De La Osa, N.; Doménech, J. M. & Bonillo, A. (2006) Assessment of functional impairment in spanish children. *Applied Psychology*, 55, pp. 130-143, ISSN 0269-994X.

[30] Ezpeleta, L.; Keeler, G.; Alaatin, E.; Costello, E. J. & Angold, A. (2001) Epidemiology of psychiatric disability in childhood and adolescence. *Journal of Child Psychology and Psychiatry*, 42, pp. 901-914, ISSN 0021-9630.

[31] Giel, R.; de Arango, M. V.; Climent, C. E.; Harding, T. W.; Ibrahim, H. H.; Ladrido-Ignacio, L.; Murthy, R. S.; Salazar, M. C.; Wig, N. N. & Younis, Y. O. (1981) Childhood mental disorders in primary health care: results of observations in four developing countries. A report from the WHO collaborative Study on Strategies for Extending Mental Health Care. *Pediatrics*, 68, pp. 677-683, ISSN 0031-4005.

[32] Gotlib, I. H. & Avison W. R. (1993) Children at risk for psychopathology, In: *Basic issues in psychology*, C. G. Costello, (Ed.), 271-319, The Guilford Press, ISBN 0-8986-2139-9, New York, NY.

[33] Graham-Bermann, S. A. & Levendosky, A. A. (1998) The social functioning of preschool-age children whose mothers are emotionally and physically abused. *Journal of Emotional Abuse*, 1, pp. 59-84, ISSN: 1092-6798.

[34] Hannan, K. & Luster, T. (1991) Influence of parent, child and contextual factors on the quality of the home environment. *Infant Mental Health Journal*, 12, 17-30, ISSN 0163-9641.

[35] Hennessy, K. D.; Rabideau, G. J.; Cicchetti, D. & Cummings, E. M. (1994) Responses of Physically Abused and Nonabused Children to Different Forms of Interadult Anger. *Child Development*, 65, pp. 815-828, ISSN 0009-3920.

[36] Hofstra, M. B.; Van der Ende, J. & Verhulst, F C. (2000) Continuity and Change of Psychopathology From Childhood Into Adulthood: A 14-Year Follow-up Study. *Journal of the American Academy of Child and Adolescent Psychiatry*, 39, pp. 850-858, ISSN 0890-8567.

[37] Hudson, J. L.; Comer, J. S. & Kendall, P. C. (2008) Parental responses to positive and negative emotions in anxious and nonanxious children. *Journal of Clinical Child and Adolescent Psychology*, 37, pp. 303-313. ISSN 1537-4416.

[38] Hudson, J. L. & Rapee, M. R. (2001) Parent-child interactions and anxiety disorders: an observational study. *Behaviour Research and Therapy*, 39, pp. 1411-1427, ISSN 0005-7967.

[39] Jekielek, S. M. (1998) Parental conflict, marital disruption and children's emotional well-being. *Social Forces*, 76, pp. 905-935, ISSN 0037-7732.

[40] Kashani, J. H. & Orvashel, H. A. (1990) A community study of anxiety in children and adolescents. *American Journal of Psychiatry*, 147, pp. 313-318, ISSN 0002-953X.

[41] Kendall, P. C.; Kortlander, E.; Chansky, T. E. & Brady, E. U. (1992) Comorbidity of anxiety and depression in youth: Treatment implications. *Journal of Consulting and Clinical Psychology*, 60, pp. 869-880, ISSN 0022-006X.

[42] Kendler, K.; Davis, C. G. & Kessler, R. C. (1997) The familial aggregation of common psychiatric and substance use disorders in the National Comorbidity Survey: a family history study. *British Journal of Psychiatry*, 170, PP. 541-548, ISSN 0007-1250.

[43] Klein, R. G. & Pine D. S. (2002) Anxiety disorders, In: *Child and Adolescent Psychiatry: Modern Approaches*, M. Rutter & E. Taylor, (Eds.), 486-509, BlackWell, ISBN 0-632-05361-5, Oxford, UK.

[44] Levitt, M. J. (1991) Attachment and close relationships: A life-span perspective, In: *Intersections with attachment*, J. L. Gewirtz & W. M. Kurtines, (Eds.), 183-205, Lawrence Erlbaum Associates, ISBN 0-8058-0176-6, Hillsdale, NJ.

[45] Lindhout, I. E. (2008) *Childhood anxiety disorders - a family perspective*, University of Amsterdam (UvA) [UvA-DARE], ISBN 978-90-8559-382-9, Rotterdam, The Netherlands.

[46] Malcarne, V. L.; Hansdottir, I. & Merz, E. L. (2010) Vulnerability to anxiety disorders in childhood and adolescence, In: *Vulnerability to Psychopathology. Risk across the Lifespan*, R. E. Ingram & J. M. Price, (Eds.), 357-362, The Guilford Press, ISBN 978-1-60623-347-4, New York, NY.

[47] Manassis, K. & Hood, J. (1998) Individual and familial predictors of impairment in childhood anxiety disorders. *Journal of the American Academy of Child and Adolescent Psychiatry*, 37, pp. 428-434, ISSN 0890-8567.

[48] Mazzone, L.; Ducci, F.; Scoto, M. C.; Passaniti, E. D.; Arrigo, V. G. & Vitiello, B. (2007) The role of anxiety symptoms in school performance in a community sample of children and adolescents. *BMC Public Health*, 7, p. 347-352, ISSN 1471-2458.

[49] McLeod, B. D.; Wood, J. J. & Weisz, J. R. (2007) Examining the association between parenting and childhood anxiety: a meta-analysis. *Clinical Psychology Review*, 27, pp. 155-172. ISSN 0272-7358.

[50] Mechanich, D. & Hansell, S. (1989) Divorce, family, conflict and adolescents well-being. *Journal of Health and Social Behavior*, 30, pp. 105-116. ISSN 0022-1465.

[51] Merikangas, K. R.; Mehta, R. L.; Molnar, B. E.; Walters, E. E.; Swendsen, J. D.; Aguilar-Gaxiola, S.; Bijl, R.; Borges, G.; Caraveo-Anduaga, J. J.; Dewit, D. J.; Kolody, B.; Vega, W. A.; Wittchen, H-U. & Kessler, R. C. (1998) Comorbidity of substance use disorders with mood and anxiety disorders: results of the International Consortium in Psychiatric Epidemiology. *Addictive Behaviors*, 23, pp. 893-907, ISSN 0306-4603.

[52] Moore, P. S.; Whaley, S. E. & Sigman, M. (2004) Interactions between mothers and children: Impacts of maternal and child anxiety. *Journal of Abnormal Psychology*, 113, pp. 471-476, ISSN 0021-843X.

[53] Moss, K. (2003) Witnessing violence aggression and anxiety in young children. *Supplement to Health Reports*, 14, pp. 53-66, ISSN 0033-3506.

[54] Opler, M.; Sodhi, D.; Zaveri, D. & Madhusoodanan, S. (2010) Primary psychiatric prevention in children and adolescents. *Annals of Clinical Psychiatry*, 22, pp. 220-234, ISSN 1040-1237.

[55] Peterson, J. I. & Zill, U. (1986) Marital disruption, Parent-child relationships, and Behavior Problems in Children. *Journal of Marriage and Family*, 48, pp. 295-307, ISSN 0022-2445.

[56] Pine, D. S.; Cohen, P.; Gurley, D.; Brook, J. & Ma, Y. J. (1998) The risk for early-adulthood anxiety and depressive disorders in adolescents with anxiety and depressive disorders. *Archives of General Psychiatry*, 55, pp. 56-64, ISSN 0003-990X.

[57] Plomin, R. & Daniels, D. (1987) Why are children in the same family so different from one another? *Behavioral and Brain Sciences*, 10, pp. 1-16, ISSN 0140-525X.

[58] Ramsawh, H. J.; Raffa, S. D.; Edelen, M. O.; Rende, R. & Keller, M. B. (2009) Anxiety in middle adulthood: effects of age and time on the 14-year course of panic disorder, social phobia and generalized anxiety disorder. *Psychological Medicine*, 39, pp. 615-624, ISSN 0033-2917.

[59] Ramsawh, H. J.; Chavira, D. A.; & Stern, M. B. (2010) Burden of Anxiety Disorders in Pediatric Medical Settings. *Archives of Pediatrics and Adolescent Medicine*, 164, pp. 965-972, ISSN 1072-4710.

[60] Rapee, R. M. (1997) The potential role of childrearing practices in the development of anxiety and depression. *Clinical Psychology Review*, 17, pp. 47-67, ISSN 0272-7358.

[61] Rappe, R. M.; Bögels, S. M.; van der Sluis, C. M. & Craske, M. G. (2012) Conceptualizing functional impairment in children and adolescents. *The Journal of Child Psychology and Psychiatry*, 53, pp. 454-468, ISSN 0021-9630.

[62] Roberts, R. E.; Roberts, C. R. & Chen, Y. R. (1997) Ethnocultural differences in prevalence of adolescent depression. *American Journal of Community Psychology*, 25, pp. 95-110, ISSN 0091-0562.

[63] Rowe, D. C. & Plomin, R. (1981) The importance of nonshared (E1) environmental influences in behavioral development. *Developmental Psychology*, 17, pp. 517-531, ISSN 0012-1649.

[64] Sameroff, A. J. & Emde, R. N. (Eds.). (1989) *Relationship Disturbances in Early Childhood. A Developmental Approach*, (First edition), Basic Books, ISBN 0-46506-897-9, New York, NY.

[65] Sheehan, D. V.; Lecrubier, Y.; Sheehan, K. H.; Amorim, P.; Janavs, J.; Weiller, E.; Hergueta, T.; Baker, R.; Dunbar, G. C. (1998) The Mini-International Neuropsychiatric Interview (M.I.N.I.): the development and validation of a structured diagnostic psychiatric interview for DSM-IV and ICD-10. *Journal of Clinical Psychiatry*, 59(suppl 20), pp. 22-33, ISSN 0160-6689.

[66] Sheehan, D. V.; Lecrubier, Y.; Shytle, D.; Milo, K.; Hergueta, T.; Colón-Soto, M.; Díaz, V. & Soto, O. (2000) Mini International Neuropsychiatric Interview for children and adolescents [M.I.N.I. KID]. Version 1.2.5 Medical Outcome Systems, Inc.

[67] Shaffer, D.; Fisher, P.; Dulcan, M. K. & Davies, M. (1996) The NIMH Diagnostic Interview Schedule for Children Version 2.3 (DISC-2.3): Description, acceptability, prevalence rates, and performance in the MECA study. *Journal of the American Academy of Child and Adolescent Psychiatry*, 35, pp. 865-877, ISSN 0890-8567.

[68] Simonoff, E.; Pickles, A.; Meyer, J. M.; Silberg, J. L.; Maes, H. H.; Loeber, R.; Rutter, M.; Hewitt, J. K. & Eaves, L. J. (1997) The Virginia Twin Study of Adolescent Behavioral Development: Influence of age, sex, and impairment on rates of disorder. *Archives of General Psychiatry*, 54, pp. 801-808, ISSN 0003-990X.

[69] Siqueland. L.; Kendall, P. C. & Steinberg, L. (1996) Anxiety in children: Perceived family environments and observed family interaction. *Journal of Clinical Child Psychology*, 25, pp. 225-237, ISSN 0047-228X.

[70] Stevenson-Hinde, J. (1998) Parenting in different cultures: time to focus. *Developmental Psychology*, 34, pp. 698-700, ISSN 0012-1649.

[71] Strauss, C. C.; Lahey, B. B.; Frick, P.; Frame, C. L. & Hynd, G. W. (1988) Peer social status of children with anxiety disorders. *Journal of Consulting and Clinical Psychology*, 56, pp. 137-141, ISSN 0022-006X.

[72] Thomasgard, M. & Metz, W. P. (1993) Parental overprotection revisited. *Child Psychiatry and Human Development*, 24, pp. 67-80, ISSN 0009-398X.

[73] Twisk, J. W. R. (2003) *Applied longitudinal data analysis for epidemiology*, (First edition), Cambridge University Press, ISBN 0-521-52580-2, Cambridge, UK.

[74] Üstun, B. & Chatterji, S. (1997) Measuring functioning and disability-a common framework. *International Journal of Methods in Psychiatric Research*, 7, pp. 79-83, ISSN 1049-8931.

[75] Webster, H. M. (2003) Thesis, Ph D: *An Ecological Approach to the Prevention of Anxiety Disorders during Childhood*, In: National Library of Australia, Access: 1 agosto 2012, Available from: <http://trove.nla.gov.au/work/28495437?versionId=34606732>

[76] Wenar, C. & Kerig P. (2006) Risk in the Family Context: Child Maltreatment and Domestic Violence, In: *Developmental Psychopathology From Infancy through Adolescence*, C. Wenar & P. Kerig, (Eds.), 431-464, McGraw-Hill, ISBN: 0-072-82019-5, New York, NY.

[77] Whiteside, S. P. (2009) Adapting the Sheehan Disability Scale to assess child and adolescent impairment related to childhood anxiety disorders. *Journal of Clinical Child and Adolescent Psychology*, 38, pp. 721-730, ISSN 1537-4416.

[78] WHO-ICPE. (2000) Cross-national comparisons of the prevalences and correlates of mental disorders. *Bulletin of The World Health Organization*, 78, pp. 413-426, ISSN 0042-9686.

[79] Wille, N.; Bettge, S.; Wittchen, H. U. & Ravens-Sieberer, U. (2008) How impaired are children and adolescents by mental health problems? Results from the BELLA study. *European Child and Adolescent Psychiatry*, 17(Suppl. 1), pp. 42-51, ISSN 1018-8827.

[80] Wittchen, H. U.; Nelson, C. B. & Lachner, G. (1998) Prevalence of mental disorders and psychosocial impairments in adolescents and young adults. *Psychological Medicine*, 28, pp. 109-126, ISSN 0033-2917.

[81] Wood, J. J.; McLeod, B. D.; Sigman, M.; Hwang, W. C. & Chu, B. C. (2003) Parenting and childhood anxiety: theory, empirical findings, and future directions. *Journal of Child Psychology and Psychiatry*, 44, pp. 134-151, ISSN 0021-9630.

[82] World Health Oragnization. (1993) *The ICD-10 Classification of Mental and Behavioural Disorders: Diagnostic criteria for research*, MEDITOR, ISBN 84-87548-13-X, Madrid, España.

[83] Wren, F. J.; Scholle, S. H.; Heo, J. & Comer, D. M. (2003) Pediatric mood and anxiety syndromes in primary care: who gets identified? *The International Journal of Psychiatry in Medicine*, 33, pp. 1-16, ISSN 0091-2174.

[84] Wren, F. J.; Scholle, S. H.; Heo, J. & Comer, D. M. (2005) How do primary care clinicians manage pediatric mood and anxiety syndromes. *The International Journal of Psychiatry in Medicine*, 35, pp. 1-12 ISSN 0091-2174.

[85] Wu, P.; Hoven, C. W.; Bird, H. R.; Moore, R. E.; Cohen, P.; Alegria, M.; Dulcan, M. K.; Goodman, S. H.; Horwitz, S. M.; Lichtman, J. H.; Narrow, W. E.; Rae, D. S.; Regier, D. A. & Roper, M. T. (1999) Depressive and disruptive disorders and mental health service utilization in children and adolescents. *Journal of the American Academy of Child & Adolescent Psychiatry*, 38, pp. 1081-1092, ISSN 0890-8567.

[86] Yates, T. M.; Egeland, B. & Sroufe, L. A. (2003) Rethinking resilience: a developmental process perspective, In: *Resilience and Vulnerabilities: Adaptation in the Context of Childhood Adversities*, S. S. Luthar, (Ed.), Cambridge University Press, ISBN 0-521-80701-8, New York, NY.

[87] Yonkers, K. A.; Bruce, S. E.; Dyck, I. R. & Keller, M. B. (2003) Chronicity, relapse, and illness: course of panic disorder, social phobia, and generalized anxiety disorder: findings in men and women from 8 years of follow-up. *Depression and Anxiety*, 17, pp. 173-179, ISSN 1091-4269.

Chapter 4

Co-Morbid Anxiety and Physical Disorders: A Possible Common Link with Joint Hypermobility Syndrome

Guillem Pailhez and Antonio Bulbena

Additional information is available at the end of the chapter

1. Introduction

As we stated in a previous book chapter titled "Somatic conditions intrinsic to anxiety disorders" [1], Johann Christian August Heinroth (1773-1843) was the person who introduced for the first time the term 'psychosomatic' into medical literature. The psychosomatic approach offers an overall or holistic "body and mind" perception that can be often useful for prevention purposes. Unfortunately, up to the present day Heinroth's contributions to the development of medicine and psychosomatics have been little acknowledged. Possibly, the current medical tendency towards specialisation makes it difficult to embody such paradigms in current psychiatric and medical nosology.

In this sense, the group of anxiety disorders have been included alternatively among the somatic and among the mental conditions when, in fact, anxiety disorders include both strong somatic and mental dimensions which need to be dealt with. The study of somatic conditions linked to anxiety disorders provide insights into the biology of these mental disorders that may result in a greater understanding of its aetiology, treatment, and prevention. In this second chapter we shall review, up to the last findings, the comorbidity of anxiety and physical disorders linked to joint hypermobility syndrome (JHS). This relationship is one of the strongest available evidences of the somatic components of anxiety disorders.

2. Anxiety disorders do relate to some somatic conditions

Patients with anxiety disorders often complain of somatic features, especially cardiac (tachycardia, chest pain), gastrointestinal (epigastric pain), and neurological complaints (headaches, dizziness, or presyncope), in emergencies and primary services [2-4]. This clinical phenomenon helped to deepen into the study of differential diagnoses: are they symptoms of the primary anxiety disorder or are they symptoms of a comorbid physical illness? [5-7]. Besides, more recent research suggests a strong association between anxiety disorders and somatic conditions, although some authors emphasize the huge amount of published research about somatic conditions and depression in contrast to the few studies about the same relationship with anxiety disorders [8-10]. Furthermore, results from the National Comorbidity Survey-Replication (NCS-R) showed that various anxiety disorders had equal or greater association than depression with four chronic physical disorders (hypertension, arthritis, asthma, and ulcers) [11].

The more recent review articles about this relationship are organized according to medical illness specifically associated to anxiety disorders in several descriptive and analytic studies with clinical samples [2,3,9,12,13]. These reviews often include the following somatic conditions: irritable bowel syndrome, asthma, cardiovascular disease, cancer, chronic pain, vestibular and thyroid dysfunction, chronic obstructive pulmonary disease, and mitral valve prolapse. Some of the main general conclusions of these reviews are the following: 1) emerging evidence about the bi-directional relationship between anxiety disorders and medical illness suggests that they may be as important as depression [9]; 2) such associations provide important clues for understanding the neurobiology of anxiety disorders [2]; and 3) such associations are greater for panic disorder [12,3], worsening its identification, presentation and treatment [13].

Along this way, there are four studies relying on clinical samples that have shown higher rates of somatic conditions among patients with anxiety disorders (table 1). The first one was published in 1994. Rogers et al. examined the prevalence and characteristics of medical illness in 711 patients with present or past index anxiety disorders [14]. Patients were assessed using structured diagnostic interviews and the Medical History Form II. The rates of medical illness for all subjects were later compared with data extracted from an epidemiological sample. Results showed that patients with panic disorder had more reported medical problems than the general population, in particular, more ulcer disease, angina, and thyroid disease.

In 2003, Härter et al. studied the associations between anxiety disorders and medical illnesses in a total of 262 probands (169 cases with an anxiety disorder and 93 controls with no evidence of an anxiety disorder according to DSM-III-R criteria) [8]. Diagnoses were obtained based on direct interview (SADS) or family history information, and lifetime history of numerous medical illnesses was obtained. Results showed that patients with a lifetime anxiety disorder reported higher rates of several medical illnesses than did persons without anxiety. After controlling for the effects of gender, comorbid substance abuse/dependence and/or depression, significant associations were found between anxiety disorders and cardiac disorders (OR = 4.6), hypertension (OR = 2.4), gastrointestinal problems (OR = 2.4), genitourinary disorders (OR = 3.5), and migraine (OR = 5.0). A similar pattern was observed for probands with panic or generalized anxiety disorder.

In 2005, Sareen et al. examined the relationship between anxiety disorders and a wide range of physical conditions in a nationally representative sample. Data came from the

National Comorbidity Survey (N=5,877). Physical disorders were assessed based on a list of several conditions shown to respondents. Results showed that anxiety disorders were positively associated with physical conditions even after adjusting for mood disorders, substance-use disorders, and sociodemographics. Among specific anxiety disorders, panic disorder and agoraphobia were more likely to be associated with cardiovascular disease and bone and joint diseases [10].

In 2008, in a case-control study carried out by our group [15] using retrospective data extracted from clinical records, patients with anxiety disorders showed higher risk of medical illnesses than patients without anxiety disorders. The aim of the study was to investigate the comorbidity between anxiety disorders and somatic conditions in three groups: patients with anxiety disorders (n=130) including panic disorder with/without agoraphobia and agoraphobia without panic attacks, patients from a primary care unit without any psychiatric disorder (n=150), and patients from a psychiatric service without anxiety disorders (n=130). Multivariate statistical logistic regression analysis showed that patients with anxiety disorders presented 4.2-fold increase in the risk of cephalea, 3.9 of cardiopathy, 3.8 of osteomuscular disorder and 2-fold increase in the risk of digestive diseases.

	Type	N	Data assessment	Main associations
Rogers et al. 1994 [14]	D	711	Structured diagnostic interview	Ulcer disease, angina & thyroid disease
Härter et al. 2003 [8]	CC	262	Direct interview & medical records	Cardiac disorders, hypertension, digestive problems, genitourinary disorders & migraine
Sareen et al. 2005 [10]	E	5877	List of several conditions	Cardiac disorders & bone and joint diseases
Pascual et al. 2008 [15]	CC	410	Medical records	Cephalea, cardiac disorders, bone and joint diseases & digestive problems

Table 1. Relationship between medical conditions and anxiety disorders. Basic features of studies reviewed. D, descriptive study; CC, case–control study; E, epidemiological study.

3. Measuring medical conditions in anxiety patients

Despite the significant prognostic and therapeutic implications derived from the comorbidity between mental disorders and medical conditions, there is a lack of measuring instruments designed to quantify the physical health and disease in psychiatric population. Obviously, the use of these instruments in clinical settings is virtually absent. In this sense, our team developed, for over a decade, the Spanish version of the Cumulative Illness Rating Scale [16] designed for the assessment of medical conditions in general. The issues chosen for this instrument to assess illness severity were related to life-risk, functional disability and the need for treatment. Our group is now actively working on a variation of this scale, specially designed to detect medical conditions, including some functional diseases, on anxiety and depressive patients. Some of these functional diseases assessed are atopy and allergies, tensional headache and migraine, fibromyalgia, irritable bowel syndrome, dysfagia and dyspepsia, interstitial cystitis, sexual dysfunction, temporo-mandibular joint disorder, and chronic fatigue syndrome.

There are various hypotheses on how anxiety disorders and medical conditions may be related [14]. Medical illness may sometimes directly trigger the development of anxiety symptoms (e.g., cardiomyopathy or anxiety as a psychological reaction towards an illness), or mimic anxiety symptoms (e.g. pheochromocytoma). Conversely, anxiety disorders may sometimes directly trigger the development of somatic symptoms (e.g., angina in cardiovascular disease), mimic symptoms of a medical illness (leading to high costly procedures or inadequate treatment), or may contribute to the onset or exacerbation of certain somatic conditions (e.g., hypertension or gastric ulcer).

However, there is evidence that some medical conditions that are often comorbid with anxiety disorders could share a common genetic etiology [17-19]. For example, Talati et al. studied probands with diagnosis and family history of panic disorder (n=219), social anxiety disorder (n=199), or both (n=173), and 102 control subjects with no personal/family history of anxiety. Subjects were blindly interviewed with a diagnostic instrument and medical history was obtained via medical checklist and the family history screen [20]. They found that panic or social anxiety patients and their first-degree relatives were more likely to have interstitial cystitis, mitral valve prolapse and headaches, and this was hypothesized to be linked to a common genetic susceptibility. According to this hypothesis, several studies have shown a noticeable association between anxiety disorders (particularly panic/phobic cluster) and the joint hypermobility syndrome (JHS) [21-23]. This association has allowed a wider "body and mind" comprehension of anxiety disorders and has provided new clues in order to measure medical conditions in these patients.

4. Anxiety disorders and the role of collagen tissue

JHS is an inherited connective tissue disorder associated with a generalized collagen laxity and characterized by an increase of active or passive joint mobility. The condition was not described for the first time until fifty years ago by Rotés, when it was properly identified and associated to pathology of the musculoskeletal system [24]. In 1973, after an epidemiological study by Beighton et al., the syndrome gained general interest in the rheumatological field and began to be studied in a broader way, as a separate entity [25] (see Fig.1).

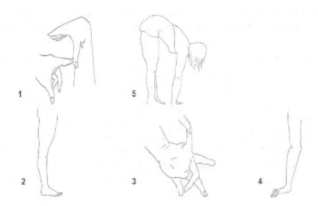

Figure 1. Joint Hypermobility criteria [25]1.Passive apposition of the thumbs to the flexor aspects of the forearm (one point for each thumb). 2. Hyperextension of the knee beyond 10° (one point for each knee). 3. Passive dorsiflexion of the little fingers beyond 90° (one point for each hand). 4. Hyperextension of the elbows beyond 10° (one point for each elbow). 5. Forward flexion of the trunk with knees fully extended so that the palms of the hands rest flat on the floor (one point).

In 1992, the Hospital del Mar criteria (table 2) compiled all the items included in the most clinically used criteria. This new scale showed consistent indicators of reliability, internal consistency and predictive validity, and provided evidence for using different scores according to age and gender [26].

Upper extremities
Passive apposition of the thumb to the flexor aspect of the forearm at a distance of less than 21 mm.
The passive dorsiflexion of the fifth finger is 90° or more.
The active hyperextension of the elbow is 10° or more.
External rotation of the shoulder up to more than 85°.
Lower extremities. Supine position
The passive hip abduction can be taken to an angle of 85° or more.
Hypermobility of the rotula.
Hypermobility of the ankle and foot.
Dorsal flexion of the toe of 90° or more.
Lower extremities. Prone position
Hyperflexion of the knee.
Ecchymoses.

Table 2. Hospital del Mar criteria for JHS [26]. Male patients scoring 4 or more are considered cases; female patients are considered cases with scores 5 or over.

JHS has an estimated prevalence in the general population ranging between 10% – 15%, it is more frequent among females (3:1) and is one of the hereditary disorders of the connective tissue, which include other conditions such as Ehlers-Danlos syndrome, Marfan syndrome and ostogenesisimperfecta [27]. Clinical features in JHS can be articular or extra-articular and are always related to the connective tissue. Among the best known articular features of JHS are arthralgia, lumbalgia, soft-tissue rheumatism (e.g., epicondilytis, tenosynovitis, bursitis), recurrent dislocations, childhood scoliosis, or rheumatoid arthritis [28,29]. Among the best-known extra-articular features of JHS are hernias, varicose veins, "easy bruising", keloids, uterine or rectal prolapse, spontaneous pneumothorax, fibromyalgia, dysautonomia and some other conditions also linked to panic disorder as asthma, mitral valve prolapse, thyroid dysfunction or irritable bowel syndrome [29,30]. Therefore, most of the conditions linked to anxiety disorders can be explained as clinical features of JHS. Unfortunately, the relationship between anxiety disorders and JHS is often neglected.

The clinical relationship between anxiety disorders and JHS was found 50 years ago. In 1957, the rheumatologist J. RotésQuerol pointed out for the first time the remarkable degree of nervous tension suffered by patients with hypermobility [24]. To a certain extent, there are some indirect references about the relationship between "hypotonia" and anxiety/phobias in the classical psychosomatic literature [31]. On the other hand, Carlsson and Rundgren in 1980 [32] found a higher score in hypermobility among alcoholic patients than among controls. Although not mentioned, the percentage of anxiety patients among the case group might have been high.

Empirical history of the clinical relationship between anxiety disorders and JHS starts in the case-control study conducted by our group in 1993, with rheumatologic outpatients affected by JHS [21]. Diagnoses of panic disorder, agoraphobia and simple phobia were significantly more frequent among hypermobile patients. There were no significant differences in the diagnoses of generalized anxiety disorder, dysthymia, or major depressive disorder. Around 70% of rheumatological patients with JHS had some kind of anxiety disorder. However, this only occurred in 22% of controls, a usual figure in chronic patient samples. Cases were 10 times more likely to suffer from anxiety than controls. Specifically, agoraphobia and panic disorders were, respectively, 5 and 7 times more likely (table 3).

	% JHS	% Non-JHS	Age-Sex Adjust. Odds Ratio	95 % C. I.
Any Anxiety D.	69,3	22,0	10.69	4.80-23.81
Panic D.	34.2	6.8	6.96	2.31-20.91
Panic & Agora.	24.6	5.1	6.40	1.82-22.43
Simple Phobia	29.8	8.5	5.77	2.05-16.24
Agoraphobia	37.7	11.9	5.08	2.06-12.49
General.Anx.	10.5	5.1	2.49	0.65-9.45
Major Depress.	14.9	3.4	4.51	0.99-20.56
Dysthymic D.	7.9	5.1	2.15	0.53-8.65

Table 3. Lifetime psychiatric disorders in JHS cases (n=114) and non-JHS controls (n=59) seen at an outpatient rheumatological unit [21].

For a subsequent second study, conducted to support this hypermobility-anxiety association, outpatients with new diagnoses of panic disorder and/or agoraphobia were examined, as well as non-anxious psychiatric and non-psychiatric outpatients as control groups [33]. Results showed that JHS was present in almost 70% of anxiety cases, versus slightly over 10% of controls. This meant that cases with panic disorders and/or agoraphobia were 17 times more likely to suffer from JHS. Conclusions were valid for women [OR=23.7; CI95% 10.6-52.9] (figure 2), but also for men [OR=10.5; CI95% 3.0-36.3] (figure 3).

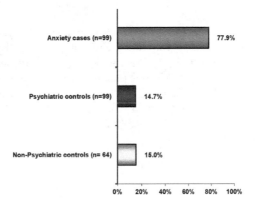

Figure 2. Women frequencies of JHS diagnoses in anxiety cases (n=99), psychiatric (n=99) and non-psychiatric controls (n=64) [33].

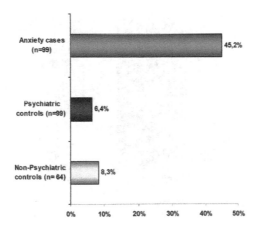

Figure 3. Men frequencies of JHS diagnoses in anxiety cases (n=99), psychiatric (n=99) and non-psychiatric controls (n=64) [33].

Later on, it was suggested that this association needed to be studied in the general population. To that end, a two-phase cross-sectional epidemiological study was carried out in a ru-
ral town in order to establish lifetime risk for anxiety and affective disorders in subjects with
JHS. A sample of 1,300 individuals were examined at baseline and over 500 were subsequently subjected to follow-up in a two-stage epidemiological study. Hypermobile patients
were eight times more likely to suffer from panic disorder (OR 8.2, CI 95% 3.4 to 19.7), eight
times more likely to suffer from social phobia (OR 7.8; CI 95% 2.4 to 24.8) and six times more
likely to suffer from agoraphobia (OR 5.9; CI 95% 3 to 11.7) than non-JHS patients. Results
were valid for both genders. No differences were found for other anxiety disorders or mood
disorders [22].

In the same sample of general population it was also reported that hypermobiles had significantly higher scores in fear and phobia scales, reinforcing the hypothesis that intensity of
fears is greater in subjects with JHS [34]. We assessed fear intensity and frequency using a
modified version of the Fear Survey Schedule (FSS-III). When we compared the groups with
and without joint hypermobility, the mean total scores for both genders were significantly
higher for the hypermobile group (figure 4). These results showed that the association of
JHS and phobic anxiety is sustained for intense fears and might represent a susceptibility
factor for these anxiety conditions.

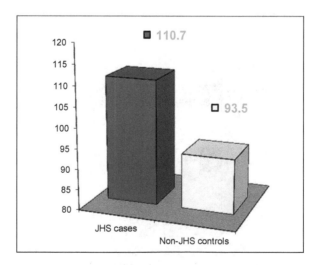

Figure 4. Mean total scores of the Fear Survey Schedule (FSS-III) in JHS cases (n=182) and non-JHS controls (n=1,123) [34].

The same design was replicated in 2011 in a sample of 150 nonclinical students [35]. Severe fears and daily consumption of cigarettes, alcohol, coffee, and chocolate were compared with the hypermobility scores. We found significant differences when comparing severe fears between the groups with and without hypermobility (7.6 vs. 11; p = 0.001). The frequency of chocolate intake was also significantly higher among subjects with joint hypermobility (31.2% vs. 51.2%; p = 0.038). There were no significant differences regarding cigarette (19.5% vs. 19.3%), alcohol (36.6% vs. 34.9%), and coffee (46.3% vs. 35.8%) consumption. Therefore, these patterns of consumption may be interpreted as self-treatment attempts of subsyndromal anxiety in hypermobile subjects (figure 5).

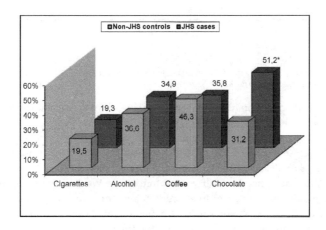

Figure 5. Frequencies of daily consumption of cigarettes, alcohol, coffee, and chocolate in JHS cases (n=41) and non-JHS controls (n=109) [35]. *p = 0.038

In 2004, our group also assessed a non-clinical sample of subjects working in the same company (N=526) [36]. Subjects with JHS had significantly higher scores in STAI trait anxiety [female average: 16.5 vs. 11, p<0.001] [male average: 13 vs. 11, p<0.03]. STAI state anxiety scores were also higher among hypermobile subjects, although not significantly (figure 6).

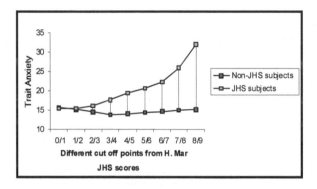

Figure 6. STAI trait anxiety scores (range: 0-60) in 203 women with or without joint hypermobility according to all possible cutoff scores on the Hospital del Mar hypermobility criteria [36].

In 2005, we studied schizophrenic outpatients (N=124) with the hypothesis that anxiety disorders mediated by JHS were not symptoms, but an independent comorbid entity in schizophrenic patients [37,38]. Joint Hypermobility was noticeably more likely among panic disorder/phobia-clustered schizophrenic patients, than among the non-comorbid group (OR = 9.35; IC = 95% [3.85-22.73]; p<0.0001). The cluster panic disorder/phobia had higher scores in fear scales and schizophrenia positive symptom scales. We are now performing a voxel-based morphometric study in order to examine brain structure, comparing magnetic resonance images of 20 schizophrenic-anxious patients and 20 schizophrenic patients. The preliminary results indicated gray matter volume differences in the schizophrenic-anxiety group in the dorsolateral prefrontal cortex related to the interaction between both conditions. Our findings suggest that the schizophrenic-anxiety group is characterised by specific neural abnormalities that cannot be explained by the presence of schizophrenia or anxiety, but by their conjunction, and this might result in a certain symptomatology [39].

After several significant cross-sectional studies we sought to conduct a prospective incidence analysis that assesses whether JHS could be a risk factor in developing anxiety conditions [23].

The main objective was to determine the cumulative incidence of anxiety disorders in a cohort of young subjects recruited from the general population who had not developed any type of anxiety condition up to then; consequently we planned a scheduled 15-year follow-up covering subjects from late adolescence to adulthood. The total population sample was 1,305 subjects, and in order to observe the development of anxiety disorders during the 15-

year study period, only the lower age segment (at that time subjects aged between 16 and 20) included in the town's municipal registry was invited to participate. We sought to describe the occurrence of new cases of anxiety disorders during the study period, therefore the exclusion criterion for the study was having already had an anxiety disorder at baseline examination. At baseline, 158 subjects were screened for participation in the study, and after the 15-year follow-up the final sample comprised 137 subjects (86.7% retention rate). Results showed that cumulative incidence of panic/agoraphobia at follow-up was significantly higher for the JHS group (41.4%) than for the control group (1.9%) with relative risk of 22.3 (CI 95% 4.6-108.7), p<0.0001, (NNT 3, CI 95% 2.9-2.3). Incidence of social phobia and simple phobia was also significantly higher for the JHS group at (RR=6.52; CI 95% 1.7-24.2) p<0.001 and (RR=3.31; CI 95% 1.1-9.6) p=0.02, respectively (table 4). Moreover, anxiolytic drug use was nearly fourfold higher among JHS subjects compared to non-JHS.

Recent work from another Spanish group [40] has shown again a high prevalence of JHS (61.8%) among panic subjects compared with 10.9% in the healthy control group and 9% in the psychiatric control group. Interestingly these authors found an intermediate figure among subjects suffering from fibromyalgia (25.4%). A paper from a Turkish group [41], albeit declaring no significant association, also found JHS in 59.5% of panic disorder patients with mitral valve prolapse, in 42.9% of patients without mitral valve prolapse but also in 52.6% of control subjects. Gülsün et al. [42], studying subjects with thorax deformities, found that the anxiety level of males with thorax deformity and JHS is higher than males with thorax deformity without JHS. And finally, Baeza-Velasco [43] also found high prevalence of social anxiety and joint hypermobility among subjects of high stature.

Total Sample	JHS Status						
	JHS present		JHS absent		RR	95% CI	P
n = 137	n = 29		n = 108				
	n	%	n	%			
Anxiety Disorders							
Panic/Agoraphobia	12	41.4	2	1.9	22.3	(4.6 to 108.7)	0.0001***
Social Phobia	7	24.1	4	3.7	6.5	(1.7 to 24.2)	0.001*
Simple Phobia	8	27.6	9	8.3	3.3	(1.1 to 9.6)	0.02*
GAD	7	24.1	9	8.3	2.9	(0.97 to 8.62)	0.14 ns
Other Disorders							
Depression/Dysthymia	7	24.1	7	6.48	3.7	(1.2 to 11.7)	0.15 ns

JHS, Joint Hypermobility Syndrome according to Beighton criteria assessed at baseline. GAD, Generalized Anxiety Disorder Statistical significance: * p<0.05, ** p<0.001, *** p<0.0001, ns: non significant

Table 4. Incident cases and relative risk after 15 years of follow-up according to JHS status [23].

	Type	Popul.	N groups	Sex	Age	JHS ass.	Association tendencies
Bulbena et al., 1993 [21]	CC	Spain	114 JHS 59 CTL	Matched	Matched	Beighton	JHS cases: 5 x Aph and 7 x PD
Martin-Santos et al., 1998 [33]	CC	Spain	99 PD &APh 99 Psychiatric CTL 64 Medical CTL	Matched	Matched	Beighton	PD cases: 17 x JHS
Benjamin et al., 2001 [52]	CC	Israel	101 PD 39 Healthy CTL	35 / 65 64 / 36	39.3 (11) 23.4 (3)	Beighton	No statistically significant relationship
Bulbena et al., 2004 [22]	E	Spain	1305 subjects	45.7 / 54.3	43.4 (18.3)	Beighton	JHS cases: 6 x Aph, 8 x SPh and 8 x PD
Gulpek et al., 2004 [41]	CC	Turkey	42 PD & MVP 35 PD 38 MVP CTL	Matched	Matched	Beighton	No statistically significant relationship
Bulbena et al., 2004 [36]	D	Spain	526 subjects	61.4 / 38.6	25.4 (3)	H. Mar	JHS cases: higher scores in STAI trait anxiety
Bulbena et al., 2005 & 2007 [37,38]	D	Spain	124 SCHZ	54 / 46	33.6 (10)	Beighton & H. Mar	Schizophrenic & PD cases: 9 x JHS and higher positive symptoms
Bulbena et al., 2006 [34]	D	Spain	1305 subjects	45.7 / 54.3	43.4 (18.3)	Beighton	JHS cases: higher scores in fear and phobia scales
Gülsün et al., 2007 [42]	CC	Turkey	52 thorax deformity 40 CTL	Males	21.9 (1.3)	Beighton	JHS cases: higher scores in HAM-A
Baeza-Velasco &Bulbena 2009 [43]	D	Several countries	158 high stature	46.8 / 53.2	25.7 (8.1)	Hakim & Grahame	JHS cases: higher scores in LSAS
García-Campayo et al., 2010 [40]	CC	Spain	55 PD 55 Psychiatric CTL 55 Fibromyalgia 55 Healthy CTL	Matched	Matched	Beighton	PD cases: 13 x JHS
Pailhez et al., 2011 [35]	D	Spain	150 subjects	44 / 56	16.4 (0.6)	Hakim & Grahame	JHS cases: higher scores in fear and phobia scales
Bulbena et al., 2011 [23]	C	Spain	137 subjects	53.3 / 46.7	31.9 (2.4)	Beighton & H. Mar	JHS cases: 22 x PD, 6.5 x SPh and 3.3 x Ph

Table 5. Relationship between JHS and anxiety disorders. Basic features of studies reviewed. D, descriptive study; CC, case–control study; C, cohort study; E, epidemiological study; CTL, controls; PD, Panic disorder; Aph, Agoraphobia; MVP, Mitral valve prolapse; SCHZ, Schizophrenia; SPh, Social phobia; Ph, Specific phobia. Sex expressed in percentage (%) male/female. Age expressed in mean (SD).

5. Weather, medical conditions and panic attacks

The relationship between meteorological variables and human behaviour has been subject of conjecture since Hippocrates. This interaction has been held more in popular belief than in scientific verification. However, since mid 1900s it has been more thoroughly studied, and we are now in a better position to test popular beliefs regarding this connection. Numerous studies in different fields have been carried out in an attempt to assess this relationship and its implications. Studies about meteorological variables and stroke onset [44], myocardial infarction [45] and arthritic pain [46] have shown significant results. Moreover, subjective experience from patients, such as variations in pain thresholds and mood swings when the weather changes, points towards this association and paves the road towards further research.

There are few studies designed to specifically assess the association between meteorological variables and clearly defined psychiatric disorders. Our group has studied this relationship with anxiety disorders [47]. Anxiety disorders are a clinically heterogeneous group that should be evaluated by differentiating panic and non-panic anxiety states due to the different clinical features present in each. Panic disorder has been associated with JHS, which is not seen in generalized anxiety disorder. Due to this association, the physical variables tend to be more relevant. This evidence has partly motivated the need to assess the association of meteorological variables with anxiety disorders and panic attacks separately and specifically.

All psychiatric emergencies attended at a general hospital in Barcelona (Spain) during 2002 with anxiety as main complaint were classified as panic or non-panic anxiety according to strict independent and retrospective criteria. Both groups were assessed and compared with meteorological data (wind speed and direction, daily rainfall, temperature, humidity and solar radiation). Seasons and weekend days were also included as independent variables. Episodes of panic were three times more common with the *poniente* wind (hot wind), twice less often with rainfall, and one and a half times more common in autumn than in other seasons (table 6). These three trends (hot wind, rainfall, and autumn) were accumulative for panic episodes in a logistic regression formula. Significant reduction of episodes on weekends was found only for non-panic episodes. Panic attacks, unlike other anxiety episodes, in a psychiatric emergency department in Barcelona seem to show significant meteorotropism.

	Any Anxiety Days			Panic Anxiety Days			Non-panic Anxiety Days		
Variables	OR	(95%CI)		OR	(95%CI)		OR	(95%CI)	
Poniente Wind	1.23	0.66	2.36	3.32	1.76	6.34	0.60	0.30	1.15
Saturday-Sunday	0.69	0.43	1.09	0.92	0.55	1.52	0.55	0.34	0.89
Autumn	1.63	0.99	2.72	1.67	1.00	2.77	1.40	0.86	2.27
Rain	0.78	0.49	1.26	0.55	0.31	0.93	0.94	0.58	1.51
Whole Model p	0.11			0.0003			0.035		

Table 6. Odds ratio for days with anxiety (all, panic and non panic), through logistic regression models [47].

On the whole, the results show a higher meteorological sensitivity in patients suffering from panic disorder. In these patients, warm wind increases the risk by three, rain onset reduces it to one-half, and autumn increases it by one and a half. This is not observed in non-panic anxiety, where meteorological effects were not found to be significant.

6. Perspectives

There is enough evidence showing that comorbidity of anxiety disorders and some medical conditions share a similar physiopathological mechanism mediated by the clinical features of JHS. Having arrived at this point, it might be relevant to remind the high association of JHS and the so called dysautonomia. In this way, significant research by Gazit and colleagues [48] found that symptoms related to anxiety such as palpitations, light-headedness, nausea, shortness of breath, hyperventilation, tremulousness, chest discomfort, fatigue, etc., were significantly more common among patients with JHS. Moreover, they found that orthostatic hypotension, postural orthostatic tachycardia syndrome and uncategorized orthostatic intolerance were present in 78% of the studied patients with JHS compared to 10% of control subjects. Thus, they suggested that dysautonomia could be an extra-articular related feature of JHS. It is plausible that the autonomic nervous system of patients with JHS might be overreactive to some environmental stimuli like the weather.

However, under the "modern" name dysautonomia not only anxiety features can be found [49] but also many symptoms described for more than two centuries in the present group of anxiety disorders [50]. Anxiety manifestations are among the most difficult to identify in the clinical practice even in patients suffering from generalized anxiety disorder, in which only 13% present anxiety as main complaint. Although dysautonomia and anxiety disorders are not in the same spectrum, they probably overlap.

In this sense, Eccles et al. have studied associations between regional cerebral grey matter and hypermobility in healthy volunteers. They found that bilateral amygdala volume distinguished those with hypermobility from those without it. Their data implicate the amygdala as a likely neural substrate mediating previously reported clinical associations between hypermobility, anxiety and psychosomatic conditions. Anxiety is linked theoretically to the abnormal generation and mapping of bodily arousal through the engagement of amygdala and insula. Enhanced interoceptive sensitivity also points to a more finely tuned sensory representation of internal bodily signals within the hypermobile group. Finally, they suggest that hypermobility is a multisystem phenotype that could mediate clinical vulnerability to neuropsychiatric symptoms [51]. Therefore, the link between JHS and dysautonomia provides an interesting physiological connection to interpret this unexpected association between a "somatic" and a "psychiatric" condition.

Our results address the biological basis of anxiety and a common source of this condition with other constitutional disturbances in relation to connective tissue and the autonomic nervous system. Patients with a diagnosis of JHS provide a highly valuable opportunity for an in-depth study of the genetic basis of anxiety. Anxiety is also a comorbidity and a risk factor in itself for a poor prognosis in several psychiatric diseases, as is the case with schizophrenia and bipolar disorders. These diseases also provide opportunities to further explore the connection between joint hypermobility and the development of anxiety in these conditions.

It is also important to point out a possible application of this evidence; as patients with JHS are at greater risk of suffering from anxiety conditions, it would be desirable to prevent the development of anxiety disorders by means of community programs at the very early stages of development. We strongly recommend screening for joint hypermobility in routine health assessment protocols in teenagers and early adulthood subjects. Even though the clinical evaluation of JHS is not extremely difficult, it does inevitably require formal training and an external validation of the procedure. In this context, some anamnestic questions might be useful for detecting positive cases at risk of suffering from anxiety disorders.

7. Conclusions

Finally, several conclusions can be made after more than 30 years of active research and clinical work in that field.

First, the association between anxiety (clinical and non clinical) and JHS is strong and replicated in several setting and samples.

Second, both conditions carry high genetic and heritable load. This is clinically very well established, but at the genetic level, there is no clear conclusion yet. Our finding of an interstitial duplication of human chromosome 15 (named DUP 25) as responsible for this association (with a non-Mendelian mechanism of disease-causing mutation) is now actively revisited.

Third, according to the type and number of somatic conditions found in the otherwise named "endogenous" anxiety disorders (panic, agoraphobia and social phobia), it seems that these patients tend to suffer from a particular cluster of disorders, particularly, osteo-muscular, irritable bowel, hypo/hyperthiroid, migraine, asthma, etc. It might well be that all these conditions share some common abnormalities in the autonomic nervous system as well as in the collagen structure as found in JHS. This may be a diathesis not yet identified, but worthy to investigate.

And fourth, the autonomic disregulation, although very difficult to assess at that level, may be one of the clues to understand the association, and also to develop appropriate treatments.

In summary, this intriguing relationship gives rise to several physio-pathological questions and prevention-related issues. JHS is a risk factor for anxiety disorders, worthy of evidence-based identification in the context of preventive psychiatry not only among adults but also among at-risk pediatric populations.

Acknowledgements

This work was supported by grant from Fondo de Investigación Sanitaria ISCIII (PI052381)

Author details

Guillem Pailhez and Antonio Bulbena

*Address all correspondence to: 97590@hospitaldelmar.cat

Anxiety Disorders Unit – INAD. Hospital del Mar., IMIM (Hospital del Mar Medical Research Institute), Barcelona, Spain

References

[1] Bulbena A, Pailhez G. Somatic conditions intrinsic to anxiety disorders. In: Szirmai A. (ed.) Anxiety and related disorders. Rijeka: InTech; 2011. p103-116.

[2] Muller JE, Koen L, Stein DJ. Anxiety and medical disorders. Curr Psychiatry Rep 2005;7:245-51.

[3] Wells KB, Golding JM, Burnam MA. Chronic medical conditions in a sample of the general population with anxiety, affective, and substance use disorders. Am J Psychiatry 1989;146:1440-6.

[4] Zaubler TS, Katon W. Panic disorder in the general medical setting. Journal of Psychosomatic Research 1998;44:25-42.

[5] Katon W, Roy-Byrne P. Panic disorder in the medically ill. J Clin Psychiatry 1989; 50:299-302.

[6] Stein MB. Panic disorder and medical illness. Psychosomatics 1986; 27:833-40.

[7] Wise MG, Taylor SE. Anxiety and mood disorders in medically ill patients. J Clin Psychiatry 1990;51:27-32.

[8] Härter MC, Conway KP, Merikangas KR. Associations between anxiety disorders and physical illness. Eur Arch Psychiatry ClinNeurosci 2003;253:313-20.

[9] Roy-Byrne PP, Davidson KW, Kessler RC, Asmundson GJ, Goodwin RD, Kubzansky L, Lydiard RB, Massie MJ, Katon W, Laden SK, Stein MB. Anxiety disorders and co-morbid medical illness. Gen Hosp Psychiatry 2008;30:208-25.

[10] Sareen J, Cox BJ, Clara I, Asmundson GJ. The relationship between anxiety disorders and physical disorders in the U.S. National Comorbidity Survey. Depress Anxiety 2005;21:193-202.

[11] Kessler RC, Ormel J, Demler O, Stang PE. Comorbid mental disorders account for the role impairment of commonly occurring chronic physical disorders: results from the National Comorbidity Survey. J Occup Environ Med 2003; 45:1257-66.

[12] Katon W. Panic disorder: Relationship to high medical utilization, unexplained physical symptoms, and medical costs. J Clin Psychiatry 1996;57:11-18.

[13] Simon NM, Fischmann D. The implications of medical and psychiatric comorbidity with panic disorder. J Clin Psychiatry 2005;66:8-15.

[14] Rogers MP, White K, Warshaw MG, Yonkers KA, Rodriguez-Villa F, Chang G, Keller MB. Prevalence of medical illness in patients with anxiety disorders. Int J Psychiatry in Medicine 1994;24:83-96.

[15] Pascual JC, Castaño J., Espluga N, Diaz B, Garcia-Ribera C, Bulbena A. Medical conditions in patients suffering from anxiety disorders. Med Clin (Barc) 2008;130:281-5.

[16] Linn BS, Linn MW, Gurel L. Cumulative Illness Rating Scale. J Am GeriatrSoc 1968;16:622-26.

[17] Collier DA. FISH, flexible joints and panic: are anxiety disorders really expressions of instability in the human genome? Br J Psychiatry 2002;181:457-9.

[18] Gratacos M, Nadal M, Martín-Santos R, Pujana M, Gago J, Peral B, Armengol L, Ponsa I, Miró R, Bulbena A, Estivill X. A polymorphic genomic duplication on human chromosome 15 is a susceptibility factor for panic and phobic disorders. Cell 2001; 1106:367-79.

[19] Pailhez G, Bulbena A, Fullana MA, Castaño J. Anxiety disorders and joint hypermobility syndrome: the role of collagen tissue. Gen Hosp Psychiatry 2009;31:299.

[20] Talati A, Ponniah K, Strug LJ, Hodge SE, Fyer AJ, Weissman MM. Panic disorder social anxiety disorder and a possible medical syndrome previously linked to chromosome 13. Biol Psychiatry 2001;63:594-601.

[21] Bulbena A, Duró JC, Porta M, Martín-Santos R, Mateo A, Molina L, Vallescar R, Vallejo J (1993) Anxiety disorder in the joint hypermobility syndrome Psychiatric Res Vol43 pp59-68

[22] Bulbena A, Gago J, Martín-Santos R, Porta M, Dasquens J, Berrios GE. Anxiety disorder & joint laxity a definitive link. Neurology Psychiatry and Brain Research 2004;111:137-40.

[23] Bulbena A, Gago J, Pailhez G, Sperry L, Fullana MA, Vilarroya O. Joint Hypermobility Syndrome is a Risk Factor Trait for Anxiety Disorders: a 15-year follow-up cohort study. General Hospital Psychiatry 2011;133:363-70.

[24] Rotés J, Argany A. La laxitud articular como factor de alteraciones del aparatolocomotor. Rev EspReumatol 1957;1:59-62.

[25] Beighton P, Solomon L, Soskolne C. Articular mobility in an African population. Ann Rheum Dis 1973;32:413-8.

[26] Bulbena A, Duró JC, Porta M, Faus S, Vallescar R, Martín-Santos R. Clinical assessment of Hypermobility of joints: Assembling criteria. J Rheumatol 1992;19:115-22.

[27] Beighton P, Grahame R, Bird H. Hypermobility of joints. London: Springer; 1999.

[28] Bravo JF. Síndrome de Ehlers-Danlos con especial énfasis en el síndrome de hiperlaxitud articular. Rev Med Chile 2009;137:1488-97.

[29] Keer R, Grahame R. Hypermobility Syndrome: Recognition and Management for Physiotherapists. London: Butterworth – Heinemann; 2003.

[30] Mishra MB, Ryan P, Atkinson P, Taylor H, Bell J, Calver D, Fogelman I, Child A, Jackson G, Chambers JB, Grahame R. Extra-articular features of benign joint hypermobility syndrome. Br J Rheumatol 1996;35:861-6.

[31] Flanders H. Diagnóstico y tratamientopsicosomáticos. Buenos Aires: José Janés; 1950.

[32] Carlsson C, Rundgren A. Hypermobility of the joints in women alcoholics. J Stud Alcohol 1980;41:78-81.

[33] Martín-Santos R, Bulbena A, Porta M, Gago J, Molina L, Duró JC. Association between the joint hypermobility syndrome and panic disorder. Am J Psychiatry 1998;155:1578-83.

[34] Bulbena A, Gago J, Sperry L, Berge D. The relationship between frequency and intensity of fears and a collagen condition. Depress Anxiety 2006;23:412-7.

[35] Pailhez G, Rosado S, BulbenaCabre A, Bulbena A. Joint Hypermobility Fears and Chocolate Consumption. Journal of nervous and mental disease 2011;199:903-6.

[36] Bulbena A, Agullo A, Pailhez G, Martin-Santos R, Porta M, Guitart J, Gago J. Is joint hypermobility related to anxiety in a nonclinical population also? Psychosomatics 2004; 45:432-7.

[37] Bulbena A, Anguiano JB, Gago J, Basterreche E, Ballesteros J, Eguiluz I, González Torres ME, Reddy DP, Coplan JD, Berrios GE. Panic/phobic anxiety in schizophrenia: a positive association with joint hypermobility syndrome. Neurology Psychiatry and Brain Research 2005;12:1-6.

[38] Bulbena A, Sperry L, Anguinano B, Pailhez G, Gago J. Joint hypermobility in schizophrenia: a potential marker for co-morbid anxiety. The open psychiatry journal 2007;1:31-3.

[39] Picado M, Carmona S, Pailhez G, Cortizo R, Planet R, Bergé D, Hoekzema E, Moreno A, Rovira M, Tobeña A, Bulbena A, Vilarroya O. Specific structural Abnormalities in schizophrenia anxiety and the comorbidity among them, June 6-10, 2010, Barcelona, Spain. 16th Annual Meeting of the Organization for Human Brain Mapping.

[40] García-Campayo J, Asso E, Alda M, Andres EM, Sobradiel N. Association between joint hypermobility syndrome and panic disorder: a case-control study. Psychosomatics 2010;51:55-61.

[41] Gulpek D, Bayraktar E, Akbay SP, Capaci K, Kayikcioglu M, Aliyev E, Soydas C. Joint hypermobility syndrome and mitral valve prolapse in panic disorder. Prog-NeuropsychopharmacolBiol Psychiatry 2004;28:969-73.

[42] Gulsun M, Yilmaz MB, Pinar M, Tonbul M, Celik C, Ozdemir B, Dumlu K, Erbas M. Thorax deformity joint hypermobility and anxiety disorders. Saudi Med J 2007;28:1840-4.

[43] Baeza-Velasco C, Bulbena A. Ansiedad social y alteracióndelcolágeno en personas de gran estatura. CuadernosPsicosomática y Psiquiatria de Enlace 2009;89/90:40-46.

[44] Wang H, Sekine M, Chen X, Kagamimori S. A study of weekly and seasonal variation of stroke onset. Int J Biometeorol 2002;47:13-20.

[45] Larcan A, Gilgenkrantz JM, Stoltz JF, Lambert H, Laprevote-Heully MC, Evrard D, Kempf JB, Lambert J. Climatologic parameters and myocardial infarction. Ann CardiolAngeiol (Paris) 1983;32:83-9.

[46] Redelmeier DA, Tversky A. On the belief that arthritis pain is related to the weather. ProcNatlAcadSci 1996;93:2895-6.

[47] Bulbena A, Pailhez G, Aceña R, Cunillera J, Rius A, Garcia-Ribera C, Gutiérrez J, Rojo C. Panic anxiety under the weather? Int J Biometeorol 2005;49:238-243.

[48] Gazit Y, Nahir AM, Grahame R, Jacob G. Dysautonomia in the joint hypermobility syndrome. Am J Med 2003;115:33-40.

[49] Bulbena A, Pailhez G, Gago J. "Connective tissue" between panic disorder and dysautonomia. Am J Med 2004;116:783.

[50] Berrios GE. Anxiety disorders: a conceptual history. J Affect Disord 1999;56:83-94.

[51] Eccles JA, Beacher FDC, Gray MA, Jones CL, Minati L, Harrison NA, Critchley HD. Brain structure and joint hypermobility: relevance to the expression of psychiatric symptoms. Br J Psych 2012; 200: 508–509.

[52] Benjamin J, Ben-Zion IZ, Dannon P, Schreiber S, Meiri G, Ofek A, Palatnik A. Lack of association between joint hyperlaxity and I: panic disorder and II: reactivity to carbon dioxide in healthy volunteers. Hum Psychopharmacol 2001;16:189-192.

Chapter 5

Anxiety Disorders in Pregnancy and the Postpartum Period

Roberta Anniverno, Alessandra Bramante,
Claudio Mencacci and Federico Durbano

Additional information is available at the end of the chapter

1. Introduction

All new mothers are somewhat anxious. Being a mother is a new role, a new job, with a new person in your life and new responsibilities. Anxiety in response to this situation is very common and somewhat adaptive. However, for several reasons, some mothers have excessive worries and experience a severe (and invalidating) level of anxiety in perinatal period. Important gonadal steroid levels modifications have been reported, with as much as a 100-fold variation in serum estrogen levels and a 1000-fold change in serum proges- terone levels during pregnancy. These changes can exacerbate such emotional difficulties. Psychological factors may also have an important role to play in the development of anxiety disorders at this time. Often the expectant mother has concerns over the health of the child, the change in lifestyle likely to occur in her own life after the birth of the child (especially if the first child), her own ability to be a good mother, and finances. There are also instances where the pregnancy is unexpected or unwanted, which may further increase stress and anxiety [1].

The postpartum period too is recognized as a time of vulnerability to affective disorders, particularly postpartum depression. In contrast, the prevalence and clinical presentation of anxiety disorders during pregnancy and the postpartum period have received little re- search attention [2]. In contrast with common belief that pregnancy is a state of well-be- ing with low rates of mental health issues, pregnancy does not protect at all against anxiety and depression [3].

2. Epidemiology and outcomes

There is now a growing realization that many women suffer from either new onset or exacerbation of existing anxiety disorders during perinatal period [4]. Studies of anxiety in pregnancy women show that a significant portion of them are affected [5]. Heron et al., in a large community sample of pregnant women, found that 21% had clinically significant anxiety symptoms and, of these, 64% continued to have anxiety in postpartum [6]. Other studies have also shown higher prevalence rates of anxiety disorders in the postnatal period compared with the general population: 20.4% had an anxiety disorder (approximately two thirds with comorbid depression) and 37.7% of women with a major depressive episode (MDE) had a comorbid anxiety disorder, with a prevalence rate of CIDI diagnosis of 29.2% [7]; 11.1% screened for PAD and 6.1% for PDD, with comorbidity found in 2.1% [8].

Anxiety and depression often occur together, are often present in pregnancy and persist if not treated [9; 10 among others]. These disorders can have a wide range of effects not only for the mother but on the fetus, the infant, partner and other family members (11-13).

Several prospective studies have shown that a prenatal anxiety disorder is one of the strongest risk factors for developing postnatal depression [4;14].

Common themes of severe anxiety during pregnancy include fear of fetal loss or fetal abnormalities. The terrors of parturition have been greatly reduced by analgesia and obstetric care, but pain and injury are still among the fears expressed by over 50% of women. Fear of delivery is often expressed, and other intense fears include those of hemorrhaging to death, or being torn or mutilated. Some women mentioned complication of parturition including maternal death and many are afraid of being alone during delivery [15].

A variety of poor outcomes are associated with anxiety during pregnancy: pre-eclampsia, increased nausea and vomiting, longer sick leave during pregnancy, increased number of visits to obstetrician, spontaneous preterm labor, preterm delivery, low birth weight, low APGAR scores, breastfeeding difficulties, a more difficult labor and delivery with increase of PTSD symptoms related to birth, admission of infant to neonatal care, elective cesarean section (1; 16-18; 19 and 20 for previous reviews).

3. Clinical aspects

The symptoms of anxiety during pregnancy or postpartum might include:

- constant worry;
- nervousness;
- anxiety;
- fatigue;
- restless legs;

- hypervigilant concerns or attention for the baby;

- extreme lability;

- thoughts of worry regarding the future, or catastrophic events occurring;

- insomnia;

- distractibility and inability to concentrate;

- appetite and sleep disturbance;

- a sense of memory loss;

- physical symptoms like dizziness, hot flashes, vomiting and nausea. [14; 21; 22]

Research shows that there are some risk factors that may predispose some women to anxiety disorders in perinatal period that include:

- family history of anxiety disorders;

- personal history of depression or anxiety

- thyroid imbalance;

- low socioeconomic status;

- unplanned or unwanted pregnancy;

- child care stress;

- personal characteristics like guilt-prone, perfectionistic, feeling unable to achieve, low self-esteem. [23].

Intense postnatal anxiety impairs maternal functioning, causes significant distress and may seriously disturb mother-infant interaction, with consequences raging from maternal neglect and failure to thrive to infanticide [4].

Anxiety disorders can take different forms in perinatal period:

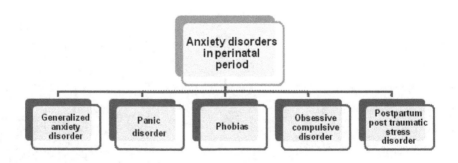

4. Generalized Anxiety Disorder (GAD)

There are few data on the epidemiology of GAD during pregnancy and postnatally. Wenzel et al. found that 4.4% of women in their study met diagnostic criteria for GAD and that over 30% reported subsyndromal symptoms [1, 32].

Sixty-five percent of patients with current GAD report comorbid disorders (most commonly depression, panic disorder, and agoraphobia). GAD, persistent and excessive worry of more than 6 months duration, may be more common in postnatal women than in the general population [23].

Pregnant women with GAD experience excessive worries about a number of life domains along with various physical symptoms such as tension headaches, muscle aches, irritability and poor concentration. Pregnancy itself is associated with role changes, health concerns for the fetus and bodily changes and may form the content of these worries. Diagnosing GAD poses special challenges in pregnancy, since it is normal to have a degree of worry and anxiety in this period of women's life [4].

There are no data on the course of pre-existing GAD in pregnancy. A large-scale community prospective study of around 8,300 women (based on the Avon Longitudinal Study of Parent and Child), which measured anxiety symptoms during pregnancy and postpartum period (from 18 weeks gestation to 8 months postnatally), found while 14.6% scored above threshold at 18 weeks gestation and 8% scored above threshold at 8 weeks postnatally, with 2.4% *de novo* presentation [24].

GAD main symptoms are:

- anxiety;
- apprehensive expectation;
- nervousness;
- fatigue;
- excessive, intrusive and persistent worries;
- a pervasive feeling of apprehension or dread;
- inability to tolerate uncertainty;
- difficulty concentrating or focusing on things;
- muscle tension;
- sleep disturbance;
- feeling edgy, restless, or jumpy;
- stomach problems, nausea, diarrhea.

5. Panic disorder

Panic disorder is an anxiety disorder characterized by recurring severe panic attacks, for at least one month. A panic attack may be a one-time occurrence, but many people experience repeated episodes.

Due to the physiological changes of pregnancy a woman may be at increased risk of onset or recurrence of panic disorder.

Physiological symptoms such as fear and autonomic arousal symptoms like shortness of breath, pounding heart and dizziness may be misinterpreted in catastrophic ways in relation to the pregnancy [3]

However, recent data suggest that pregnancy may confer some kind of protection against this disturb. In contrast the early postpartum period is reported to be a time of increased vulnerability to panic disorder, with figures ranging from 0.5% to 1.5% at 6 week postpartum [5]. In 1988, Metz and Sichel described panic disorder presenting for the first time in the early postpartum period. They showed that panic disorder affects approximately 10% of postpartum women [cited in 21]. Other important authors described cases of panic disorder presenting for the first time in the postnatal period [4 among others].

Wisner, Peindl and Hanusa, in 1996, found that 11% to 29% percent of women with panic disorder reported an onset during the postpartum period and women with a history of mild panic symptoms have experienced worsening of these symptoms in postpartum period (within the first 2 or 3 weeks and eventually being accompanied by depressive symptoms) [25].

Premenstrual hormonal changes may play a role in panic disorder, which would implicate the role of ovarian hormones in vulnerability to anxiety and panic in the postpartum period [4, 26].

In 1998 Beck conducted a phenomenological study to describe the experiences of the women with panic, in the postpartum period. Through interviews with mothers diagnosed with postpartum panic disorder, the author found six emerging themes describing the essence of the mother's experience:

- theme 1: the terrifying physical and emotional components of panic paralyzed women, leaving them feeling totally out of control;
- theme 2: during panic attacks, women's cognitive functioning abruptly diminished, whereas between these attacks women experienced a more insidious decrease in their cognitive functioning;
- theme 3: during the panic attack, women feverishly struggled to maintain their composure, leading to exhaustion;
- theme 4: because of the terrifying nature of panic, preventing further panic attacks was paramount in the lives of the women;

- theme 5: as a result of recurring panic attacks, negative changes in women's lifestyles ensued lowering their self-esteem and leaving them to bear the burden of disappointing not only themselves but also their families;

- theme 6: mothers were haunted by the prospect that their panic could have residual effect on themselves and their families.

Anticipatory anxiety about future attacks and consequences of these on the fetus can be significantly disabling. The symptoms of panic disorder in perinatal period my worse and some women becoming agoraphobic and socially isolated [23].

Panic disorder main symptoms are:

- shortness of breath or hyperventilation;

- palpitations, pounding heart, or accelerated heart rate;

- trembling or shaking;

- chest pain or discomfort;

- sweating;

- feeling unreal or detached from your surroundings;

- choking feeling

- nausea or abdominal distress;

- feeling dizzy, light-headed, or faint;

- numbness or tingling sensations;

- hot or cold flashes;

- fear of dying, losing control, or going crazy;

- paresthesias (numbness or tingling sensations). [3;4;27].

6. Phobias

"Fear" is the normal response to a genuine danger. Phobia is an irrational fear of an object or a situation leading to avoidance. It is an abnormally fearful response to a danger that is imagined or is irrationally exaggerated. People can develop phobic reactions to animals (e.g., spiders), activities (e.g., flying), or social situations (e.g., eating in public or simply being in a public environment).There is no literature on the exact prevalence and impact of specific phobias such as social phobia or agoraphobia during pregnancy. But there are two specific types of phobia that has been discussed in relation to pregnancy and child birth: tokophobia (intense fear of childbirth) and the phobia for the infant.

Tokophobia can lead to woman avoiding pregnancy, terminating pregnancy of a very much wanted baby or demanding caesarean section in subsequent pregnancies. It has been classified as: primary in a nulliparous woman, secondary if the woman has had previous traumatic deliveries or secondary to depressive illness or post-traumatic stress disorder (PTSD) during pregnancy. The prevalence of serious fear of childbirth was 5.5% in women. Is very important to consider factors influencing this fear:

- history of sexual or physical abuse;

- a traumatic gynecological examination;

- previous experience of childbirth and related anxiety;

- myths about labor and childbirth. [3;21]

Fear of childbirth may also be a symptom of PTSD associated with childbirth.

Phobia for the infant: a mother with infant-focused anxiety may develop a phobia for the infant. Brockington [28] describes the fear of cot death and says that a cause of severe chronic anxiety in the puerperium is fear of sudden infant death syndrome. They are mothers who will not let their infants sleep, for fear they stop breathing and other who waken them to see if they are alive. These mothers experience severe insomnia, because of the need to lie awake listening to the baby's breathing; they may check the infant 20-30 times every night.

Symptoms of a phobia include the following:

- feelings of panic, dread, horror, or terror;

- a persistent and overwhelming fear of the object or situation;

- recognition that the fear goes beyond normal boundaries and the actual threat of danger;

- reactions that are automatic and uncontrollable, practically taking over the person's thoughts;

- rapid heartbeat

- shortness of breath;

- trembling;

- an overwhelming desire to flee the situation, all the physical reactions associated with extreme fear;

- extreme measures taken to avoid the feared object or situation [27].

7. Obsessive–Compulsive Disorder (OCD)

Obsessive-compulsive disorder is a relatively common psychiatric disorder with lifetime prevalence rate of 0.8% to 3.2% in the community. It is an important health problem, because it leads to an impairment in the quality of life and functional status and to disabilities in occupational and social areas. Epidemiological studies show that OCD is more frequent in females compared to males. The mean age of onset of this disorder includes the childbearing years in women. Women with postpartum onset OCD often experience obsessions about harming their baby, they may avoid their infants due to their fear of acting on such thoughts. For this reason, their symptoms often impair their ability to care their infants. This situation may give rise to depressive symptoms [29-30].

The prevalence of OCD during pregnancy has been reported in the range of 0.2% to 5.2% in the literature, the relatively consistent rates among the studies are between 1% to 3%. Obsessive-compulsive symptoms are more frequently seen in pregnant women [29; 31].

The prevalence of OCD in postpartum period has been reported within wide range of 0.7% to 9.0%, and obsessive-compulsive symptoms were described in 14% to 63.5% of postpartum women [15; 32; 33; 34].

There are several case reports showing that pregnancy and postpartum period are associated with the onset of OCD more frequently than other life events [29].

The etiology of postpartum onset OCD is unknown. The acute onset may be due to the dramatic, rapid fall in the female hormones estrogen and progesterone, resulting in a dysregulation of serotonin, which than interacts with any predisposition to mental disorder. Another hypothesis regarding etiology, may be the rapid increase in oxytocin to a high level near the end of pregnancy and during postpartum, which may trigger an exacerbation or the onset of OCD [4].

In literature there are few studies analyzing risk factors for pregnancy induced OCD.

The main risk factors associated with pregnancy onset OCD are:

- primiparity;
- second or third trimester of gestation;
- number of gestations and live birth;
- miscarriage;
- gestational complication;
- positive family history of OCD. [29].

Compared to pregnancy onset OCD, the studies described above illustrate with more details the factors associated with postpartum onset OCD.

The main risk factors associated with pregnancy onset OCD are:

- primiparity (6.57% vs 1.81% multiparous ones);
- the first 4 weeks of postnatal period;
- higher levels of anxiety;
- obsessive-compulsive personality disorder;
- avoidant personality disorder;

- personal history of major depression;
- the existence of OCD related dysfunctional belief. [29-30].

Symptoms of perinatal OCD can include:

- obsessions, also called intrusive thoughts, which are persistent, repetitive thoughts or mental images related to the baby;
- compulsions, where the woman may do certain things over and over again to reduce her fears and obsessions;
- fear of being left alone with the infant;
- hypervigilance in protecting the infant;
- loss of appetite;
- tremendous guilt and shame;
- horrified by these things. [21; see also www.ppmdsupport.com]

Obsessions are defined as:

1. recurrent and persistent thoughts, impulses, or images that are experienced at some time during the disturbance, as intrusive and inappropriate and that cause marked anxiety or distress;

2. the thoughts, impulses, or images are not simply excessive worries about real-life problems;

3. the person attempts to ignore or suppress such thoughts, impulses, or images, or to neutralize them with some other thought or action;

4. the person recognizes that the obsessional thoughts, impulses, or images are a product of his or her own mind (not imposed from without as in thought insertion) [27].

Compulsions are defined as:

1. repetitive behaviors (e.g., hand washing, ordering, checking) or mental acts (e.g., praying, counting, repeating words silently) that the person feels driven to perform in response to an obsession, or according to rules that must be applied rigidly;

2. the behaviors or mental acts are aimed at preventing or reducing distress or preventing some dreaded event or situation; however, these behaviors or mental acts either are not connected in a realistic way with what they are designed to neutralize or prevent or are clearly excessive [27].

Compared with non-postpartum onset OCD, aggressive obsessions exhibit a tendency to be seen more frequently seen in postpartum onset OCD, and the most common obsessions were contamination and aggressive obsessions. Many authors noted that the aggressive obsessions had 9 times more chances of occurring in a postpartum woman with OCD than in a healthy postpartum woman. The aggressive obsessions mostly include fear of harming the baby [29,

33]. In some instances, sufferers report obsessions having to do with accidental harm, while in others the obsessions involve unwanted thoughts or ideas of intentionally harming the newborn. Some examples of the kinds of postpartum obsessions are as follows:

- the idea that the baby could die while sleeping (S.I.D.S);
- the thought of dropping the baby from a high place;
- the thought of putting the baby in the microwave;
- an image of the baby dead;
- thoughts of the baby choking and not being able to save him;
- unwanted impulses to shake the baby to see what would happen;
- thoughts of yelling at the baby;
- thoughts of poking the baby in the soft spot in her head (fontanel);
- thought of stabbing the baby;
- thoughts of drowning the baby during a bath. [29; 33 see also www.ocfoundation.org/ EO_Postpartum.aspx;].

Other women have contamination obsessions that are often focused on the baby:

- microorganisms;
- chemicals or dirt contaminations via her hand or the baby's bottles or foods. [30].

Compared with obsessions, the studies has less frequently focused on compulsive symptoms after the childbirth.

The most common compulsions are:

- cleaning/washing;
- checking.

Some compulsions were related to the baby:

- avoiding kitchen knives;
- not bathing the infant;
- staying physically isolated from the baby;
- checking the breathing or baby's body;
- excessive or ritualized washing or cleaning. [29; 33].

The important thing is that women with postpartum onset OCD, compared to psychotic women, have relatively good insight, do not exhibit psychotic features, don't want to harm the baby, recognize that thoughts/images are unhealthy and take step to protect the baby [32-34].

Less attention has been focused on the clinical characteristics of OCD in pregnancy [35]. Few reports suggest that contamination obsessions and cleaning/washing compulsions may be seen more frequently compared to other symptoms. Moreover, symmetry obsessions and checking compulsions are frequently observed in pregnant women. Aggressive and contamination obsessions in some pregnant women may be related to the fetus and some pregnant women experience thoughts of harming their unborn child. Often OCD is comorbid with other psychiatric disorders, in particular with major depression. Comorbid depression developed simultaneously or within 2 to 3 weeks after the onset of OCD. There are no studies that reported literature examining comorbid disorders in pregnant women with OCD [29; 34].

When undiagnosed and untreated, postpartum OCD can cause extreme distress in the mother and can also influence the type of care an infant receives, family relationships and interactions [30; 4].

These women run the risk of maternal-infant attachment difficulties [21].

8. Postpartum Post–Traumatic Stress Disorder (PTSD)

The term post-traumatic stress disorder (PTSD) refers to a disorder that can occur following the experience or witnessing of life-threatening events. We usually recognize events like terrorist incidents, serious accidents, or violent personal assaults as being capable of causing such trauma, so, it has proved difficult for people to understand that a "natural" process like childbirth can also be traumatizing. The fact is that a traumatic event can actually be any experience which involves the threat of death or serious injury to an individual or another person close to them (e.g. their baby). A person must then respond with intense fear, helplessness or horror for a diagnosis of PTSD to be made. The reported prevalence of diagnosed PTSD caused by childbirth ranges from 2-3% to 25% in the postpartum women [23].

Research into this field is limited and, to date, it has largely focused on the importance of the type of delivery a woman has undergone. However, recent studies have begun to look at the significance of women's perceptions of their birth experience. Then, it is now generally accepted that PTSD can be a consequence of a traumatic birth experience and important studies demonstrate that women did in fact suffer this type of traumatic stress after birth (see for more infos at www.birthtraumaassociation.org.uk). This type of PTSD are called postpartum post-traumatic stress disorder (PP PTSD) or post natal PTSD (PN PTSD) or "birth trauma".

Most often, this illness is caused by a real or perceived trauma during delivery or postpartum. These traumas could include:

• prolapsed cord;

• unplanned Caesarian section;

• cardiac arrest;

- postpartum hemorrhage;
- induction;
- use of vacuum extractor or forceps to deliver the baby;
- rapid delivery;
- severe toxemia;
- manual removal of placenta;
- premature birth;
- separation from infant in NICU;
- feelings of powerlessness, poor communication and/or lack of support and reassurance during the delivery. [26; 36; see also www.ppmdsupport.com].

Most significant risk factors for postpartum PTSD are therefore the following:

- domestic violence;
- history of sex trauma (e.g. sexual abuse, rape);
- previous adverse reproductive events (e.g. ectopic pregnancy, miscarriage, stillbirth);
- history of mental health problem;
- migration;
- mode of delivery;
- fear for their own safety or that of their child;
- lack of control;
- the attitudes of staff;
- inadequate pain relief;
- poor social support;
- previous traumatic events. [3,5,21, 27; 36; 37 see also www.birthtraumaassociation.org.uk].

A person who has been diagnosed with PTSD will find their normal life interrupted in many ways by a strong and powerful set of emotions and feelings over which they have no control.

Symptoms may start soon after childbirth or they could be delayed for months, and may persist for a long time and resulting in other problems such as depression [see for more infos at www.ppmsupport.com].

General symptoms of postpartum PTSD might include:

- anxiety and panic attack;
- intrusive re-experiencing of a past traumatic event;

- recurrent intrusive memories;

- flashbacks or nightmares;

- avoidance of stimuli associated with the event, including thoughts, feelings, people, places and details of the event;

- persistent increased arousal (irritability, outbursts of anger, difficulty sleeping an concentrating, hypervigilance, exaggerated startle response);

- reduced consciences status;

- feeling a sense of unreality and detachment;

- depressive symptoms;

- fear of sexual intimacy;

- restricted range of affect;

- sense of a foreshortened future. [21,23; 35 see also www.ppmsupport.com and www.birth-traumaassociation.org.uk].

It is important to understand that, following a traumatic event, sufferers of PTSD are left with a world view which has been altered profoundly and which often leaves them deeply afraid and anxious. The world is no longer considered to be a safe place and it can be difficult to trust the very individuals (health care professionals) who are supposed to be there to help. For those who develop PTSD, the future may look bleak as they struggle to liberate themselves from the images of the trauma they have endured. This can be particularly hard for women with 'birth trauma' because they often suffer these problems at a time when everyone expects them to be happy and positive. As a result, they often end up feeling guilty and this lowers self-esteem [36; 37; see for more info at www.ppmsupport.com].

If untreated, PTSD is associated with increased physical morbidity, subsequent psychiatric illness, accidental and non-accidental death. It may also have the following consequence:

- depression;

- suicide risk;

- an increased incidence of alcohol and other substance abuse;

- profound problems for a woman's relationship with her baby, problems with breast feeding and bonding;

- sexual avoidance;

- tokophobia (fear of childbirth);

- requests for otherwise unnecessary elective caesarean sections in subsequent pregnancies;

- over-vigilance and anxiety about a child's health;

- the impact on a woman's family

- avoidance of future medical care. [4; 36 see also www.ppmsupport.com].

9. Pharmacological and non-pharmacological treatments

Hereafter a short summary of the most commonly proposed treatment of anxiety in pregnancy and postpartum period, bearing in mind that pharmacological approaches, especially in pregnancy but also in breastfeeding period, are to be used with caution, collaborating with gynecologists, and weighting risks and benefits with greater attention than in "normal" patients; and bearing in mind, too, that until now there is a lack of evidence for the effectiveness of psychological therapies for anxiety disorder during the perinatal period (even if it is reasonable to consider that anxiety in pregnancy and postpartum differs little from the same disorders among non-pregnant women in both their presentation and course, and reasonably in the efficacy of its treatment).

Bear also in mind that there are some concerns about diagnostic criteria of anxiety disorders (and of depression, too) in pregnancy, as outlined in Matthey and Ross-Hamid [34] and McGuiness and al. [35], and these might be limitations in the correct use of medications in this period.

Psychological treatments

A detailed description of all the psychotherapies available for treating anxiety is beyond the scope of this chapter [see 24 and 36 for further details], anyway the most recent evidences are very well described elsewhere in this book . It is however useful to remind that cognitive-behavioral therapies are, at now, the golden standard based on efficacy and efficiency results compared to other form of psychological interventions. These therapies can be tailored on the client with more adequacy than other more structured (and ideologically based) form of psychotherapies, and can be of adequately short duration and time-sparing (in front of the time-consuming "job" of being mother, a short and time-sparing approach is desirable). Relaxation techniques are a specific application of CBT, are specifically symptom oriented, and can be proposed as the sole intervention for mild form of anxiety. CBT and relaxation can be exerted in groups, favouring indirect group support.

Interpersonal psychotherapy has gained a growing success, but its efficacy in anxiety problems is still questionable, lacking clinical evidence of efficacy, whereas its efficacy in depression is confirmed.

Psychodynamic psychotherapies, too, have questionable efficacy on anxious problems and require more commitment and time (and money too).

Pharmacological treatments

This section will describe the most frequently used pharmacological treatments to counteract anxiety and the most widely accepted evidences with regard to safety in pregnancy and post partum period.

Benzodiazepines

Earlier studies suggesting an increase in orofacial cleft defects following in utero exposure to benzodiazepines are counteracted by a recent large prospective study founding no significant association with such (or other) birth defects, although benzodiazepines are associated with negative obstetric outcomes like poor Apgar score at birth, tendency to preterm birth and low birth weight [38].

Nevertheless, benzodiazepines use in pregnancy has still contrasting evidences about safety for the newborn, due to methodological limits in the studies (not consideration of the consequences of maternal illness on fetus, familiar history of malformations, and so on) [39-40], even if the more recent data, considering a more wide spectrum of variables and a better quality in the design of the studies, seem to uphold the global safety of these molecules [41-42] except for anal atresia associated with lorazepam use in the I trimester [40] and for low weight at birth and preterm birth [43].

Regarding to the use of benzodiazepines in the III trimester of pregnancy and peripartum period, a floppy infant syndrome has been described, and also a transient slowing of growth (a complete normalization is however reached in the first year of life) [39,44].

There are some evidences pointing out the at now not yet clear balance risks / benefits of the use of benzodiazepines in pregnancy, especially with alprazolam [45].

According to available studies [45 amongst all], some indications on the use of benzodiazepines during pregnancy are the following:

- 'short-acting' benzodiazepines should be preferred and then can be used safely during pregnancy and breastfeeding if they are only used for a short period (less than 4 weeks)

- use the lowest dose, shorter treatment period, more fractioned dose (to avoid plasma peaks) as possible

- avoid multiprescriptions

- the use of 'long-acting' benzodiazepines should be avoided, in order to avoid accumulation reaction.

- use only benzodiazepines with safety records of long period

Antidepressants

There is a growing number of large prospective studies on **SSRI** in pregnancy and postnatal period, most of the evidence going against an association between any particular selective serotonin reuptake inhibitor (SSRI) and birth defects [48-53]. However some data evidenced an association between SSRI use and negative obstetric outcome like mild degrees of preterm birth and low birth weight [47; 54-56], and there are adverse neonatal outcomes reports including mild degrees of poor neonatal adaptation (neonatal withdrawal syndrome) following SSRI exposure [47,54,56-57], all of them transient. Fluoxetine is associated with a slight increase of negative obstetric outcomes but not of malformations after I trimester exposition [57], the study being supported by Lilly.

An increase of spontaneous abortions has been reported in some studies, even if not statistically significant [59-61].

In particular, these problems are evident using paroxetine. As for benzodiazepine studies, however, these studies suffer of methodological limitations [62-65] and sampling problems [63-64, 66-68,69-70].

Citalopram and escitalopram are associated with a slight increase of spontaneous abortions, comparable with any other antidepressant, and not significant low weight at birth but no increase of malformations [60, 70].

A link between neonatal persistent pulmonary hypertension and late exposure to SSRIs has initially been suggested [71-74] but not confirmed in following studies [75-78], even if some doubts already emerged [79]. An association between paroxetine exposure (especially in the I trimester) and infant cardiovascular malformations has recently been reported [50; 68, 80-83], even if a recent meta-analysis [84] and a large cohort study [85] found no significant association. Despite these results, and having other more "sure" SSRI, it is better and precautionary not to prescribe paroxetine as first line treatment.

There is limited evidence on the use of **SNRIs**, with most available evidence concerning venlafaxine, showing a lack of significative association with an increased risk of major birth defects [46, 50, 59], but a mild association with 'neonatal withdrawal syndrome' [85], neonatal seizures [86] and low weight at birth [87], and transient (resolving in less than 1 week) behavioral signs, but there was also an increase of use of tobacco and alcohol in treated women [88].

Mirtazapine has associated with an increase of spontaneous abortions but not with any increase of malformations [89]. The same results are for **bupropione** [90], **nefazodone** and **trazodone** [91]

Side effects of in utero exposure to **TCAs** are similar to those of SSRIs (i.e. premature delivery, low birth weight, neonatal distress, respiratory problems, hypoglycemia, cyanosis, jitteriness, convulsions, decreased Apgar score and the need for special-care nurseries) but have been reported to be more severe [80-81, 92].

Duration of treatments with antidepressants is not associated with teratogenic risk [93], as well as with gestation period of exposition [94].

Antipsychotics

In relation to antipsychotics, to be avoided as first line treatment of anxiety but useful in certain resistant subtypes of GAD, there are sparse evidence of non significant association with any birth defect, both for first generation antipsychotics [95-96] and for new generation antipsychotics [97-98]. First- and second-generation antipsychotics however have been associated with obesity in pregnancy [97] and high or low birth weight [98-99].

Postpartum and breastfeeding

In relation to breastfeeding, current evidences suggest that SSRIs [51, 100-102] and benzodiazepines with short half-lives [102] are transferred in only low concentrations to breast milk. During lactation, benzodiazepine use is not associated with adverse events in new-borns [102]. Regarding the use of benzodiazepines during breastfeeding, the little infor-mations available derive from a low number of studies, but the data are converging to a relative safety in their use, even if their use needs some cautions since neonatal metabo-lism and global clearance is very slow, and benzodiazepines in the long term tend to ac-cumulate [103-104].

A recent review on antidepressants use during breastfeeding period showed an acceptable safety using SSRI and nortryptiline, a cautious use of fluoxetine, and suggesting doxepine and nefazodone to be avoided [105], even if a recent review on antidepressants and breast-feeding suggests as first choice, due to their low degree of excretion into human milk, sertra-line, paroxetine and fluvoxamine, not recommending (for their long half life) citalopram escitalopram and fluoxetine [103]. For a complete review about limits and methodological problems in available studies on breastfeeding and use of psychiatric drugs see in particular Llewellin and Stowe [106], Fortinguerra et al. [103] and Moretti [104].

Final considerations about psychopharmacological treatments

As previously described, therefore, there are some (even if acceptable) risks associated with the use of psychotropic medications in this delicate period, but the clinician – GP, psychia-trist, gynecologist (and the mother, and her relatives) have to bear in mind that it should not be assumed that it is always better to avoid medication. Untreated mental health disorders in this period, as seen before, can significantly (and sometimes dramatically) affect the phys-ical and/or mental wellbeing of the woman, the fetus/infant, and significant other(s) and family [24,107-109] (see Table 2 for a summary). So, a careful evaluation of risks (compre-hending the naturalistic prevalence and incidence of birth defects - the background risk of birth defects in the general population is between 2% and 4% - compared to the, often low, increase linked to treatments) and benefits has to be carried on, in order to reach a real in-formed consent of the woman and her significant others to an adequate pharmacological treatment of the most invalidating form of anxiety disorders.

When prescribing a medication for a woman with a mental health disorder who is planning a pregnancy, pregnant or breastfeeding, the following recommendations, even if not new (2007) have to be followed [24]:

• choose medications with lower risk profiles for the mother and the fetus or infant;

• start low and increase slow to the lowest effective dose for the shortest time needed for treatment;

• monotherapy better than combination treatment;

• consider additional precautions for preterm, low birth weight or sick infants

• adequate monitoring of relapse, and discontinuation/withdrawal symptoms

TREATMENT	IN PREGNANCY AND IN POSTPARTUM PERIOD
NON-PHARMACOLOGICAL TREATMENTS	a. Psychoeducational interventions b. Psychotherapy • Cognitive-behavioral therapy (CBT) • Interpersonal therapy (IPT) • Psychodynamic therapy • Mother-infant psychotherapy c. Psychological support d. Progressive muscle relaxation
PHARMACOLOGICAL TREATMENTS	a. Anxyolitics b. Antidepressant c. Antipsychotics
COMBINED TREATMENT	An integrated approach where pharmacological treatment and psychotherapy work together is the best therapeutic intervention to achieve the most successful recovery from symptoms

(from: Beyondblue, 2011) [36].

Table 1.

Fetal/obstetrical outcomes	• Preterm delivery, prolongation of gestation • Lower birth weight, fetal distress • Spontaneous abortion higher risk • Pre-eclampia higher risk • Labour complications
Neonatal outcomes	• Neonatal maladaptation • Higher risk of admission in neonatal ICU • Lower Apgar • Growth retardation, slowed mental development • Behavioral disturbances
Child development	• Maternal-fetal / maternal-infant bonding disturbances • Affect disregulations (tantrums) • Alterations in the development of cognitive, relational, behavioral domains • Higher risk of separation anxiety and disorganized attachment styles • Higher impulsivity and lower QI at 14-15 yrs
Risk to mother	• Poor nutrition and impaired self care • Non compliance to medical advices • Worsening of comorbid medical illnesses • Increased use of substances (tobacco, alcool, drugs) • Postpartum psychiatric complications • Impact of family members

Table 2. Untreated anxiety and aoutcomes (adapted from 107-109)

Author details

Roberta Anniverno[1], Alessandra Bramante[1], Claudio Mencacci[2] and Federico Durbano[2]

1 Center for the prevention of depression in women – Neuroscience Department, A.O. Fate-benefratelli e Oftalmico, Milan, Italy

2 Neuroscience Department, A.O. Fatebenefratelli e Oftalmico, Milan, Italy

References

[1] Rubinchik S.M., Kablinger A.S., Gardner J.S., Medications for Panic Disorder and Generalized Anxiety Disorder During Pregnancy, Prim Care Companion J Clin Psychiatry. 2005; 7(3): 100–105.

[2] Austin M.P., Priest S.R., Clinical issue in perinatal mental health: new developments in the detection and treatment of perinatal mood and anxiety disorders, Acta Psychiatry Scand, 2005, 112(2): 97-104.

[3] Tyano S., Keren M., Herrman H., Cox J., Parenthood and Mental Health. A bridge between infant and adult psychiatry, Wiley-Blackwell, Oxford, 2010.

[4] Beck C.T., Driscoll J.W., Postpartum Mood and Anxiety Disorders. A Clinician's Guide, Jones and Bartlett Publishers, Sudbury, 2006.

[5] Vythilingum B., Anxiety disorders in pregnancy. Curr Psychiatry Rep, 2008, 10:331-335.

[6] Heron J., O'Connor T.G., Golding J., Glover V., The ALSPAC Study Team. The course of anxiety and depression through pregnancy and the postpartum in a community sample, J. Affect Disorders 2004; 80(1): 65-73.

[7] Austin MP; Hadzi-Pavlovic D; Priest SR; Reilly N; Wilhelm K; Saint K; Parker G. Depressive and anxiety disorders in the postpartum period: how prevalent are they and can we improve their detection? Arch Womens Ment Health. 2010; 13(5):395-401

[8] Reck C; Struben K; Backenstrass M; Stefenelli U; Reinig K; Fuchs T; Sohn C; Mundt C. Prevalence, onset and comorbidity of postpartum anxiety and depressive disorders. Acta Psychiatr Scand. 2008; 118(6):459-68

[9] Skouteris H; Wertheim EH; Rallis S; Milgrom J; Paxton SJ. Depression and anxiety through pregnancy and the early postpartum: an examination of prospective relationships. J Affect Disord. 2009; 113(3):303-8

[10] Mauri M; Oppo A; Montagnani MS; Borri C; Banti S; Camilleri V; Cortopassi S; Ramacciotti D; Rambelli C; Cassano GB. Beyond "postpartum depressions": specific anxiety diagnoses during pregnancy predict different outcomes: results from PND-ReScU. J Affect Disord. 2010; 127(1-3):177-84

[11] Ross L.E., McLean L.M., Anxiety Disorders during pregnancy and postpartum period: a systematic review. Journal Clinical Psychiatry, 2006; 67(8): 1285-1298.

[12] Misri S; Kendrick K; Oberlander TF; Norris S; Tomfohr L; Zhang H; Grunau RE. Antenatal depression and anxiety affect postpartum parenting stress: a longitudinal, prospective study. Can J Psychiatry. 2010; 55(4):222-8

[13] Britton JR. Infant temperament and maternal anxiety and depressed mood in the early postpartum period. Women Health. 2011; 51(1):55-71

[14] Milgrom J., Gemmil A.W., Bilszta J.L., et al., Antenatal risk factors for postnatal depression. A large prospective study. J Affect Disorders, 2007; 108: 147-157.

[15] Brockington I.F., Motherhood and Mental Health, Oxford medical Publication, Oxford, 1996.

[16] Field T; Diego M; Hernandez-Reif M; Figueiredo B; Deeds O; Ascencio A; Schanberg S; Kuhn C Comorbid depression and anxiety effects on pregnancy and neonatal outcome. Infant Behav Dev. 2010; 33(1):23-9

[17] Martini J; Knappe S; Beesdo-Baum K; Lieb R; Wittchen HU Anxiety disorders before birth and self-perceived distress during pregnancy: associations with maternal depression and obstetric, neonatal and early childhood outcomes. Early Hum Dev. 2010; 86(5):305-10

[18] Qiao Y; Wang J; Li J; Wang J Effects of depressive and anxiety symptoms during pregnancy on pregnant, obstetric and neonatal outcomes: a follow-up study. J Obstet Gynaecol. 2012; 32(3):237-40

[19] Alder J; Fink N; Bitzer J; Hösli I; Holzgreve W Depression and anxiety during pregnancy: a risk factor for obstetric, fetal and neonatal outcome? A critical review of the literature. J Matern Fetal Neonatal Med. 2007; 20(3):189-209

[20] Littleton HL; Breitkopf CR; Berenson AB Correlates of anxiety symptoms during pregnancy and association with perinatal outcomes: a meta-analysis. Am J Obstet Gynecol. 2007; 196(5):424-32

[21] Stone S.D., Menken A.E., Perinatal and postpartum mood disorders. Prospective and treatment guide for the health care practitioner, Springer Publishing Company, New York, 2008.

[22] Marcus S.M., Herringhausen J.E., Depression in childbearing women: when depression complicates pregnancy, Prim Care Clin Office Pract, 2009, 36:151-165.

[23] South Australian Perinatal Practice Guidelines, 2010, in http:// www.health.sa.gov.au/ppg/Default.aspx?tabid=35

[24] NICE Antenatal and Postnatal Mental Health: The NICE Guideline on Clinical Management and Service Guidance. Leicester: The British Psychological Society & The Royal College of Psychiatrists, 2007.

[25] Wisner K.L., Peindl K.S., Hanusa B.H., Effects of childbearing on the natural history of panic disorder with comorbid mood disorder. Journal of Affective Disorders,1996; 41: 173-180.

[26] Beck CT A checklist to identify women at risk for developing postpartum depression. Journal of Obstetric, Gynecologic, and Neonatal Nursing 1998; 27: 39-46

[27] DSM-IV-TR, Diagnostic and Statistical Manual of Mental Disorders, Text Revised, American Psychiatric Association Press, 2000.

[28] Brockington I.F., Macdonald E, Wainscott G, Maternal rejection of the young child: present status of the clinical syndrome. Psychopathology, 2011, 44:329-336

[29] Uguz F., Ayhan M.G., Epidemiology and clinical features of obsessive-compulsive disorder during pregnancy and postpartum period: a review. Journal of Mood Disorders, 2011; 1(4): 178-186.

[30] Timpano KR, Abramowitz JS, Mahaffey BL, Mitchell MA, Schmidt NB. Efficacy of a prevention program for postpartum obsessive-compulsive symptoms. J Psychiatr Res. 2011 Nov;45(11):1511-7.

[31] Faisal-Cury A, Menezes P, Araya R, Zugaib M. Common mental disorders during pregnancy: prevalence and associated factors among low-income women in São Paulo, Brazil: depression and anxiety during pregnancy. Arch Womens Ment Health. 2009;12(5):335-43

[32] Anniverno R., Bramante A., "Interventi clinici per il trattamento della psicopatologia in postpartum: pensieri sul proprio bambino" In Abstracts Book, Corso di aggiorna-mento "Disturbi affettivi in un mondo in rapido cambiamento", Bormio (Italy), 1-4 aprile 2012.

[33] Wenzel A, Haugen EN, Jackson LC, Brendle JR. Anxiety symptoms and disorders at eight weeks postpartum. J Anxiety Disord. 2005;19(3):295-311.

[34] Zambaldi CF, Cantilino A, Montenegro AC, Paes JA, de Albuquerque TL, Sougey EB. Postpartum obsessive-compulsive disorder: prevalence and clinical characteristics. Compr Psychiatry. 2009 Nov-Dec;50(6):503-9

[35] Matthey S, Ross-Hamid C. The validity of DSM symptoms for depression and anxiety disorders during pregnancy.J Affect Disord. 2011;133(3):546-52.

[36] McGuinness M, Blissett J, Jones C. OCD in the perinatal period: is postpartum OCD (ppOCD) a distinct subtype? A review of the literature. Behav Cogn Psychother. 2011;39(3):285-310

[37] Beyondblue: Clinical practice guidelines for depression and related disorders – anxiety, bipolar disorder and puerperal psychosis – in the perinatal period. A guideline for primary care health professionals (Austin M-P, Highet N and the Guidelines Expert Advisory Committee Eds.). Melbourne: beyondblue: the national depression initiative, 2011.

[38] Beck, C. Post-Traumatic Stress Disorder Due to Childbirth, The Aftermath. Nursing Research 2004; 53(4):216-224

[39] Wikner BN, Stiller CO, Bergman U et al Use of benzodiazepines and benzodiazepine receptor agonists during pregnancy: neonatal outcome and congenital malformations. Pharmacoepidemiol Drug Saf 2007; 16(11): 1203–10.

[40] McElhatton PR. The effects of benzodiazepine use during pregnancy and lactation. Reprod Toxicol. 1994;8(6):461-75

[41] Bonnot O, Vollset SE, Godet PF, d'Amato T, Dalery J, Robert E. [In utero exposure to benzodiazepine. Is there a risk for anal atresia with lorazepam?]. Encephale. 2003;29(6): 553-9

[42] Dolovich LR, Addis A, Vaillancourt JM, Power JD, Koren G, Einarson TR. Benzodiazepine use in pregnancy and major malformations or oral cleft: meta-analysis of cohort and case-control studies. BMJ. 1998;317(7162):839-43.

[43] Ornoy A, Arnon J, Shechtman S, Moerman L, Lukashova I. Is benzodiazepine use during pregnancy really teratogenic? Reprod Toxicol. 1998;12(5):511-5

[44] Wikner BN, Stiller CO, Bergman U, Asker C, Källén B. Use of benzodiazepines and benzodiazepine receptor agonists during pregnancy: neonatal outcome and congenital malformations. Pharmacoepidemiol Drug Saf. 2007;16(11):1203-10

[45] Kanto JH. Use of benzodiazepines during pregnancy, labour and lactation, with particular reference to pharmacokinetic considerations. Drugs. 1982;23(5):354-80.

[46] Iqbal MM, Sobhan T, Ryals T. Effects of commonly used benzodiazepines on the fetus, the neonate, and the nursing infant. Psychiatr Serv. 2002;53(1):39-49

[47] Einarson TR & Einarson A Newer antidepressants in pregnancy and rates of major malformations: a meta-analysis of prospective comparative studies. Pharmacoepidemiol Drug Saf 2005; 14(12): 823–27.

[48] de las Cuevas C & Sanz EJ Safety of selective serotonin reuptake inhibitors in pregnancy. Curr Drug Saf 2006; 1(1): 17–24.

[49] Rahimi R, Nikfar S, Abdollahi M Pregnancy outcomes following exposure to serotonin reuptake inhibitors: a meta-analysis of clinical trials. Reprod Toxicol 2006; 22(4): 571–75.

[50] Bellantuono C, Migliarese G, Gentile S Serotonin reuptake inhibitors in pregnancy and the risk of major malformations: a systematic review. Hum Psychopharmacol 2007; 22(3): 121–28.

[51] Cipriani A, Geddes JR, Furukawa TA et al Metareview on shortterm effectiveness and safety of antidepressants for depression: an evidence-based approach to inform clinical practice. Can J Psychiatry 2007; 52(9): 553–62.

[52] Louik C, Lin AE, Werler MM, Hernandez-Diaz S, Mitchell AA. Fist-trimester use of selective serotonin-reuptake inhibitors and the risk of birth defects. N Engl J Med 2007; 356:2675-83

[53] Alwan S, Reefhuis J, Rasmussen SA, Olney RS, Friedman JM. Use of selective serotonin-reuptake inhibitors in pregnancy and the risk of birth defects. N Engl J Med 2007; 356:2684-92

[54] Lattimore KA, Donn SM, Kaciroti N et al Selective serotonin reuptake inhibitor (SSRI) use during pregnancy and effects on the fetus and newborn: a meta-analysis. J Perinatol 2005; 25(9): 595–604.

[55] Wisner KL, Sit DKY, Hanusa BH, Moses-kolko EL, Bogen DL, Hunker DF, Perel JM, Jones-Ivy S, Bodnar LM, Singer LT. Major depression and antidepressant treatment: impact on pregnancy and neonatal outcomes. Am J Psychiatry 2009; 166:557-566

[56] Gentile S Serotonin reuptake inhibitor-induced perinatal complications. Pediatr Drugs 2007; 9(2): 97–106.

[57] Galbally M, Lewis AJ, Lum J et al Serotonin discontinuation syndrome following in utero exposure to antidepressant medication: prospective controlled study. Aust N Z J Psychiatry 2009; 43(9): 846–54.

[58] Goldstein DJ, Corbin LA, Sundell KL. Effects of first-trimester fluoxetine exposure on the newborn. Obstet Gynecol. 1997;89(5 Pt 1):713-8.

[59] Einarson A, Fatoye B, Sarkar M, Lavigne SV, Brochu J, Chambers C, Mastroiacovo P, Addis A, Matsui D, Schuler L, Einarson TR, Koren G. Pregnancy outcome following gestational exposure to venlafaxine: a multicenter prospective controlled study. Am J Psychiatry. 2001;158(10):1728-30.

[60] Klieger-Grossmann C, Weitzner B, Panchaud A, Pistelli A, Einarson T, Koren G, Einarson A. Pregnancy outcomes following use of escitalopram: a prospective comparative cohort study. J Clin Pharmacol. 2012;52(5):766-70

[61] Roca A, Garcia-Esteve L, Imaz ML, Torres A, Hernandez S, Botet F, Gelabert E, Subira S, Plaza A, Valdés M, Martin-Santos R. Obstetrical and neonatal outcomes after prenatal exposure to selective serotonin reuptake inhibitors: the relevance of dose. J Affect Disord. 2011;135(1-3):208-15

[62] Bar-Oz B, Einarson T, Einarson A, Boskovic R, O'Brien L, Malm H, Bérard A, Koren G. Paroxetine and congenital malformations: meta-Analysis and consideration of potential confounding factors. Clin Ther. 2007;29(5):918-26

[63] Tuccori M, Montagnani S, Testi A, Ruggiero E, Mantarro S, Scollo C, Pergola A, Fornai M, Antonioli L, Colucci R, Corona T, Blandizzi C. Use of selective serotonin reuptake inhibitors during pregnancy and risk of major and cardiovascular malformations: an update. Postgrad Med. 2010;122(4):49-65.

[64] Tuccori M, Testi A, Antonioli L, Fornai M, Montagnani S, Ghisu N, Colucci R, Corona T, Blandizzi C, Del Tacca M. Safety concerns associated with the use of serotonin

reuptake inhibitors and other serotonergic/noradrenergic antidepressants during pregnancy: a review. Clin Ther. 2009;31 Pt 1:1426-53.

[65] Gentile S, Bellantuono C.Selective serotonin reuptake inhibitor exposure during early pregnancy and the risk of fetal major malformations: focus on paroxetine. J Clin Psychiatry. 2009;70(3):414-22

[66] Gentile S. Pregnancy exposure to serotonin reuptake inhibitors and the risk of spontaneous abortions. CNS Spectr. 2008;13(11):960-6.

[67] Udechuku A, Nguyen T, Hill R, Szego K. Antidepressants in pregnancy: a systematic review. Aust N Z J Psychiatry. 2010;44(11):978-96.

[68] Maschi S, Clavenna A, Campi R, Schiavetti B, Bernat M, Bonati M. Neonatal outcome following pregnancy exposure to antidepressants: a prospective controlled cohort study. BJOG. 2008;115(2):283-9

[69] Gentile S. Selective serotonin reuptake inhibitor exposure during early pregnancy and the risk of birth defects. Acta Psychiatr Scand. 2011;123(4):266-75

[70] Einarson A, Choi J, Einarson TR, Koren G. Incidence of major malformations in infants following antidepressant exposure in pregnancy: results of a large prospective cohort study. Can J Psychiatry. 2009 Apr;54(4):242-6

[71] Sivojelezova A, Shuhaiber S, Sarkissian L, Einarson A, Koren G. Citalopram use in pregnancy: prospective comparative evaluation of pregnancy and fetal outcome.Am J Obstet Gynecol. 2005;193(6):2004-9.

[72] Chambers CD, Hernandez-Diaz S, Van Marter LJ et al. Selective serotonin-reuptake inhibitors and risk of persistent pulmonary hypertension of the newborn. New Engl J Med 2006, 354: 579–87.

[73] Källén B & Olausson PO Maternal use of selective serotonin reuptake inhibitors and persistent pulmonary hypertension of the newborn. Pharmacoepidemiology & Drug Safety 2008; 17: 801–06.

[74] Kieler H, Artama M, Engeland A, Ericsson O, Furu K, Gissler M, Nielsen RB, Nørgaard M, Stephansson O, Valdimarsdottir U, Zoega H, Haglund B. Selective serotonin reuptake inhibitors during pregnancy and risk of persistent pulmonary hypertension in the newborn: population based cohort study from the five Nordic countries. BMJ. 2011;344:d8012

[75] Andrade SE, McPhillips H, Loren D et al (2009) Antidepressant medication use and risk of persistent pulmonary hypertension of the newborn. Pharmacoepidemiol Drug Saf 18(3): 246–52.

[76] Wichman CL, Moore KM, Lang TR et al Congenital heart disease associated with selective serotonin reuptake inhibitor use during pregnancy. Mayo Clinic Proc 2009; 84: 23–27.

[77] Nordeng H, van Gelder MM, Spigset O, Koren G, Einarson A, Eberhard-Gran M. Pregnancy outcome after exposure to antidepressants and the role of maternal depression: results from the Norwegian Mother and Child Cohort Study. J Clin Psychopharmacol. 2012;32(2):186-94.

[78] Wogelius P, Nørgaard M, Gislum M, Pedersen L, Munk E, Mortensen PB, Lipworth L, Sørensen HT. Maternal use of selective serotonin reuptake inhibitors and risk of congenital malformations. Epidemiology. 2006;17(6):701-4.

[79] Occhiogrosso M, Omran SS, Altemus M. Persistent pulmonary hypertension of the newborn and selective serotonin reuptake inhibitors: lessons from clinical and translational studies. Am J Psychiatry. 2012;169(2):134-40.

[80] Looper KJ Potential medical and surgical complications of serotonergic antidepressant medications. Psychosomatics 2007; 48(1): 1–9.

[81] Reis M & Källén B Delivery outcome after maternal use of antidepressant drugs in pregnancy: an update using Swedish data. Psychol Med 2010; 5: 1–11.

[82] Oberlander TF, Misri S, Fitzgerald CE, Kostaras X, Rurak D, Riggs W. Pharmacologic factors associated with transient neonatal symptoms following prenatal psychotropic medication exposure. J Clin Psychiatry. 2004;65(2):230-7

[83] Oberlander TF, Warburton W, Misri S, Aghajanian J, Hertzman C. Neonatal outcomes after prenatal exposure to selective serotonin reuptake inhibitor antidepressants and maternal depression using population-based linked health data. Arch Gen Psychiatry. 2006;63(8):898-906.

[84] O'Brien L, Einarson TR, Sarkar M et al Does paroxetine cause cardiac malformations? J Obstet Gynaecol Can 2008; 30(8): 696–701.

[85] Einarson A, Pistelli A, DeSantis M et al Evaluation of the risk of congenital cardiovascular defects associated with use of paroxetine during pregnancy. Am J Psychiatry 2008; 165(6): 749–52.

[86] Moses-Kolko EL, Bogen D, Perel J et al Neonatal signs after late in utero exposure to serotonin reuptake inhibitors: Literature review and implications for clinical applications. J Am Med Assoc 2005; 293(19): 2372–83.

[87] Pakalapati RK, Bolesetty S, Austin M-P et al Neonatal seizures from in utero venlafaxine exposure. J Paediatr Child Health 2006; 42(11): 737–38.

[88] Ramos É, St-André M, Bérard A. Association between antidepressant use during pregnancy and infants born small for gestational age. Can J Psychiatry. 2010;55(10): 643-52.

[89] Ferreira E, Carceller AM, Agogué C, Martin BZ, St-André M, Francoeur D, Bérard A. Effects of selective serotonin reupatake inhibitors and venlafaxine during pregnancy in term and preterm neonates. Pediatrics 2007; 119:1 52-59

[90] Djulus J, Koren G, Einarson TR, Wilton L, Shakir S, Diav-Citrin O, Kennedy D, Voyer Lavigne S, De Santis M, Einarson A. Exposure to mirtazapine during pregnancy: a prospective, comparative study of birth outcomes. J Clin Psychiatry. 2006;67(8):1280-4.

[91] Chun-Fai-Chan B, Koren G, Fayez I, Kalra S, Voyer-Lavigne S, Boshier A, Shakir S, Einarson A. Pregnancy outcome of women exposed to bupropion during pregnancy: a prospective comparative study. Am J Obstet Gynecol. 2005;192(3):932-6.

[92] Einarson A, Bonari L, Voyer-Lavigne S, Addis A, Matsui D, Johnson Y, Koren G. A multicentre prospective controlled study to determine the safety of trazodone and nefazodone use during pregnancy. Can J Psychiatry. 2003;48(2):106-10.

[93] Källén B Neonate characteristics after maternal use of antidepressants in late pregnancy. Arch Pediatrics Adolesc Med 2004; 158: 312–16.

[94] Ramos E, St-André M, Rey E, Oraichi D, Bérard A. Duration of antidepressant use during pregnancy and risk of major congenital malformations. Br J Psychiatry. 2008;192(5):344-50.

[95] Oberlander TF, Warburton W, Misri S, Aghajanian J, Hertzman C. Effects of timing and duration of gestational exposure to serotonin reuptake inhibitor antidepressants: population-based study. Br J Psychiatry. 2008;192(5):338-43.

[96] Diav-Citrin O, Shechtman S, Ornoy S et al Safety of haloperidol and penfluridol in pregnancy: a multicenter, prospective, controlled study. J Clin Psychiatry 2005; 66(3): 317–22.

[97] Reis M & Källén B (2008) Maternal use of antipsychotics in early pregnancy and delivery outcome. J Clin Psychopharm 28(3): 279–88.

[98] Einarson A & Boskovic R Use and safety of antipsychotic drugs during pregnancy. J Psychiatr Pract 2009; 15: 183–92.

[99] Newham JJ, Thomas SH, MacRitchie K et al Birth weight of infants after maternal exposure to typical and atypical antipsychotics: prospective comparison study. Brit J Psychiatry 2008; 192: 333–37.

[100] Newport DJ, Calamaras MR, DeVane CL et al Atypical antipsychotic administration during late pregnancy: placental passage and obstetrical outcomes. Am J Psychiatry 2007; 164: 1214–20.

[101] Weissman AM, Levy BT, Hartz AJ et al Pooled analysis of antidepressant levels in lactating mothers, breast milk, and nursing infants. Am J Psychiatry 2004; 161(6): 1066–78.

[102] Eberhard-Gran M, Eskild A, Opjordsmoen S Use of psychotropic medications in treating mood disorders during lactation: practical recommendations. CNS Drugs 2006; 20(3): 187–98.

[103] Kelly LE, Poon S, Madadi P, Koren G. Neonatal Benzodiazepines Exposure during Breastfeeding. J Pediatr. 2012;161(3):448-51

[104] Fortinguerra F, Clavenna A, Bonati M. Psychotropic drug use during breastfeeding: a review of the evidence. Pediatrics 2009; 124:e547-e556

[105] Moretti ME. Psychotropic drugs in lactation. Can J Clin Pharmacol, 2009; 16(1):e49-e57

[106] Davanzo R, Copertino M, De Cunto A, Minen F, Amaddeo A. Antidepressant drugs and breastfeeding: a review of the literature. Breastfeed Med. 2011;6(2):89-98

[107] Llewellyn A, Stowe ZN. Psychotropic medications in lactation. J Clin Psychiatry. 1998;59 Suppl 2:41-52.

[108] Qiao Y, Wang J, Li J, Wang J. Effects of depressive and anxiety symptoms during pregnancy on pregnant, obstetric and neonatal outcomes: a follow-up study. J Obstet Gynaecol. 2012;32(3):237-40

[109] Field T, Diego M, Hernandez-Reif M, Figueiredo B, Deeds O, Ascencio A, Schanberg S, Kuhn C. Comorbid depression and anxiety effects on pregnancy and neonatal outcome. Infant Behav Dev. 2010;33(1):23-9

[110] Fishell A. Depression and anxiety in pregnancy. J Popul Ther Clin Pharmacol 2010, 17(3):e363-e369

Therapies: New Approaches and Insights

Chapter 6

Current State of the Art in Treatment of Posttraumatic Stress Disorder

Ebru Şalcıoğlu and Metin Başoğlu

Additional information is available at the end of the chapter

1. Introduction

Posttraumatic stress disorder (PTSD) is the most common mental health problem among people exposed to traumatic events. Since its introduction into the psychiatric classification system in the 1980s various treatments have been tested for PTSD. Meta-analyses based on randomized controlled trials (RCTs) concluded that trauma-focused psychotherapies are most effective treatments for PTSD [1-3]. The most widely used trauma-focused psychotherapies are exposure treatment, cognitive therapy, cognitive behavioural treatment (CBT) involving a combination of exposure and cognitive interventions, and Eye Movement Desensitization and Reprocessing (EMDR). In this chapter we briefly review these treatments in terms of their theoretical background, application, efficacy, tolerability, and length of delivery.

2. Trauma-focused psychotherapies

2.1. Exposure treatment

Exposure based interventions have the largest evidence base and received the strongest empirical support for efficacy in treatment of PTSD as well as other anxiety disorders [4, 5]. Exposure treatment has its theoretical foundation in learning theory of fear acquisition and extinction. Basically, learning theory holds that fear is learned through classical conditioning and system-atic exposure to feared stimulus without any adverse consequence results in progressive reduction in the fear response (i.e. extinction or habituation of fear response). The mechanism of exposure treatment is now explained with the concept of habituation and corrective learn-ing in the widely known *emotional processing theory* developed by Foa and colleagues [6, 7]. According to this theory, fear is represented in memory as a structure consisting of information about (a) the feared stimulus, (b) verbal, physiological, and motor responses, and (c) their interpreted meaning [8, 9]. Exposure therapy exerts its effect through activation of the 'fear structure' and integration of corrective information that is incompatible with it (e.g. disconfirmation of overestimated probability of harm) [6]. Successful exposure therapy does not abolish pathological associations in the fear structure, but rather establishes new, non-pathological ones [7]. In other words, fear reduction implies new learning, not unlearning. Three indicators of emotional processing determine successful learning and thus outcome of exposure therapy: (a) initial fear activation (i.e. physiological arousal in response to feared stimulus), (b) within-session habituation of anxiety (i.e. fear reduction during exposure to feared stimulus), and (c) between-session habituation (i.e. reduction in initial fear response across sessions) [6]. Within-session habituation helps dissociating the stimulus from fear response and between-session habituation forms the basis for long-term learning by providing opportunities of change in the meaning of the association between stimulus and fear response (i.e. lowered expectation of harm and lessened valence, negativity, of the stimulus). Within-session habituation is a necessary prerequisite for between-session habituation.

Although the contemporary learning theory provides the most validated, comprehensive, and plausible theory of anxiety disorders [10, 11], the emotional-processing theory has received partial support. In an extensive review of clinical studies that examined the contribution of three indicators of learning to treatment outcome, Craske and colleagues found only weak support for the premises of emotional processing theory [12]. The authors found no consistent evidence to support or refute the role of initial fear activation. While within session-habituation often occurs, the amount by which fear declines or the level of fear on which a given exposure trial ends does not predict overall improvement. Hence, within session-habituation appears to be mediated by mechanisms that are different than the mechanisms responsible for long-term outcomes. Although some studies show that the amount by which fear is reduced across occasions of exposure (between-session habituation) predicts treatment outcome, other studies indicate that improvement occurs despite lack of significant reductions in parameters of fear (e.g. heart rate or skin conductance) between exposure sessions. Finally, the authors found no evidence for the premise that within session-habituation is a necessary precursor to between-session habituation. On the basis of these findings and the literature documenting the context-specific nature of fear extinction [13], it has been suggested that that there is a need to shift away from an emphasis on fear reduction during exposure therapy to a new exposure paradigm which emphasizes attenuating avoidance behaviour and strengthening anxiety and fear tolerance [12, 14]. This is consistent with experimental work with animals which show that unpredictable and uncontrollable stressors play an important role in the development of anxiety and fear responses [15, 16] and the evidence from research with trauma survivors suggesting that lack of sense of control over traumatic stressors is the critical mediating factor in PTSD [11, 17-20]. Thus, helping the person regain control over traumatic stressors might therefore reduce traumatic stress [15, 21].

The goal of classic exposure therapy in PTSD as practised today is to promote anxiety reduction through habituation and emotional processing of trauma memory [22]. This is achieved by imaginal exposure to trauma memory and live exposure to trauma reminders. In imaginal exposure the survivor recounts anxiety evoking memories about the traumatic event in a systematic, prolonged and repetitive manner, while in live exposure s/he confronts anxiety evoking reminders of the traumatic event. Most treatment protocols combine imaginal and live exposure, while a few incorporate only imaginal exposure [23-25]. The way imaginal and live exposure is implemented shows great variability across programmes. For instance, in the widely used *Prolonged Exposure* programme developed by Foa and colleagues [26], live exposure is introduced simultaneously with imaginal exposure and imaginal exposure is followed by a discussion of emotional responses to trauma memory. In the *Exposure Therapy* protocol of Marks and colleagues [27], on the other hand, live exposure is introduced midway in the treatment following 5 sessions of imaginal exposure and emotional responses to trauma memory are not discussed at any stage. Many treatment programmes that are largely based on these two protocols also employed additional interventions such as anxiety management techniques (e.g. relaxation training, coping skills training, breathing training, thought stopping, and guided self-dialogue) [28, 29], cognitive restructuring [30-33], supportive counselling [23] and imagery rescripting (i.e. developing a positive alternative visual representation of oneself coping more effectively with the trauma during and / or after its occurrence) [34, 35]. Relatively little research has been conducted to examine the contribution of these techniques to improvement. While some evidence suggests that adding cognitive restructuring to exposure enhances treatment effects [23], other studies show that cognitive interventions [27, 36, 37] or various anxiety management techniques [38] do not confer additional benefits when used in combination with exposure.

Considering the problems associated with the habituation model and the findings on the importance of sense of control in trauma survivors (reviewed above), Basoglu and colleagues [21, 39-41] modified exposure treatment by: (a) focusing on only behavioural avoidance in treatment (i.e. live exposure to trauma cues), thereby eliminating treatment ingredients that rely on heavy therapist input and pose challenges of practicability in different post-disaster and cross-cultural settings; and (b) shifting treatment focus from habituation to feared stimuli to enhancement of 'sense of control' over them. The underlying principle of the new *Control-Focused Behavioural Treatment* is to enhance a person's resilience against traumatic stressors by helping them to develop sense of control over them. This can be achieved by exposure to either (a) unconditioned stimuli in a safe and controlled environment (i.e. the original traumatic stressor in simulated form or in virtual reality settings) or (b) conditioned stimuli (e.g. trauma reminders) that possess the distress-evoking characteristic of the unconditioned stimuli until the person is able tolerate and control associated distress [42]. To this end treatment targets behavioural avoidance of trauma reminders and mainly involves therapist-delivered instructions for self-exposure to feared and avoided situations until the survivor is able to tolerate and feel in control of anxiety or fear (rather than until 'fear is reduced'). The findings from clinical trials (reviewed below) showed that *Control Focused Behavioural Treatment* has promise in treatment of mass trauma survivors.

2.2. Cognitive therapy

Cognitive therapy of anxiety disorders is based on the understanding that anxiety occurs due to selective processing of information in the environment perceived as signalling threat or danger to the individual and such cognitive biases can be corrected through conscious reasoning [43, 44]. The cognitive model of PTSD views anxiety as an outcome of maladaptive appraisals about trauma and its consequences and attributions centring on danger and threat [45]. In addition, traumatic events are believed to shatter people's basic beliefs and assumptions about themselves, the world, and others [46]. Therapy is thus designed to restructure or correct dysfunctional ways of thinking that cause distress, anxiety, or fear. The survivor is taught to challenge dysfunctional thoughts or beliefs through Socratic reasoning, test their accuracy through behavioural experiments in situations perceived threatening or dangerous, and replace them with alternative ones that better reflect reality.

Empirical support for cognitive theory of PTSD is rather weak. No prospective study with pre- to post-trauma assessments tested whether traumatic events shatter basic beliefs and assumptions. Although survivors with PTSD tend to report more negative beliefs [47-49] or information processing biases [50-52], there is not sufficient evidence to refute the argument that these may be epiphenomena of traumatic stress problems, rather than being a cause of them. Research on this issue that employed statistical controls to examine the role of all possible contributing factors to the disorder (e.g. demographic, personal history, trauma exposure characteristics etc.) did not indeed find a strong association between beliefs and PTSD [18, 20]. Furthermore, exposure, though referred to as *behavioural experiment*, is considered a necessary component of cognitive therapy for successful treatment because it allows better processing of threat [43, 44]. As exposure's efficacy is already established in anxiety disorders, it is difficult to attribute successful treatment outcome in cognitive therapy to cognitive change. Furthermore, even when treatment protocols do not directly involve an exposure component, they may indirectly trigger it. Similarly, exposure therapy alone may provide an opportunity to test dysfunctional appraisals about trauma and thereby lead to cognitive change. Comparative studies found cognitive therapy as effective as exposure [27, 53, 54]. However, the fact that no study examined whether cognitive therapy instigated self-exposure in between sessions among treated cases preclude a definitive conclusions about the importance of cognitive change in treatment. On the other hand, there is evidence showing that exposure treatment without cognitive restructuring produce as much cognitive change as exposure with cognitive restructuring [37, 55, 56]. Reductions in negative cognitions were significantly related to reductions in PTSD symptoms in these studies, suggesting that cognitive change occurs as a response to improvement in PTSD and not vice versa. These findings support the view that cognitive responses to trauma are epiphenomena of traumatic stress.

As exposure protocols, cognitive therapy programmes for PTSD differ in their specifics. The *Cognitive Therapy* programme developed by Ehlers and colleagues [57, 58] and *Cognitive Processing Therapy* developed by Resick and colleagues [53] involve imaginal exposure to the traumatic memory, but this is limited to only a few sessions and the focus of imaginal reliving is to teach the survivor modify their beliefs about the meaning of the traumatic event. The Ehlers et al programme also involves some unsystematic live exposure (e.g. visiting the site where the trauma happened). Other cognitive therapy protocols do not involve any exposure elements [24, 27].

2.3. Eye Movement Desensitization and Reprocessing (EMDR)

The field of PTSD treatment witnessed a rapid growth of new treatment protocols, the most studied of which is undoubtedly EMDR. EMDR is an information processing therapy during which the patient recounts trauma story with its cognitive, affective, and physiological features while simultaneously focusing visually on bilateral movements of an external stimulus until the distress evoked by traumatic memory subsides [59]. The EMDR theorists maintain that the eye movements reduce the distress associated with trauma memories and help cognitive and emotional reprocessing of the traumatic event. EMDR combines multiple theoretical perspectives and techniques, most pronouncedly imaginal exposure and cognitive restructuring. Proponents of EMDR hold that the very brief and interrupted nature of imaginal exposure in EMDR sessions is at stark contrast with the behaviour therapists' requirement of prolonged and uninterrupted exposure to achieve habituation and disconfirmation of fear-expectancies [5, 6]. However, research on the processes of change in exposure treatment has not been conclusive regarding these requirements [12, 60]. EMDR proponents also contend that the use of directed eye movements distinguishes this form of therapy from other cognitive behavioural approaches. However, the role of eye movements in treatment has not been theoretically clarified and the findings of dismantling studies (reviewed in a meta-analysis) suggest that the eye movements are neither necessary nor sufficient to treatment outcome [61].

2.4. Other trauma focused interventions

Some treatment programmes for PTSD combined different components of existing treatment protocols under a different name (e.g. *Cognitive-Behaviour Trauma Treatment Protocol* [62], *Trauma Focused Group Psychotherapy* [32], *Direct Therapeutic Exposure* [33]. Some other new protocols, on the other hand, mainly embodied some form of exposure and cognitive restructuring, but these were presented with a different rationale for efficacy and they varied in the procedures of implementation (e.g. *Narrative Exposure Therapy* [63], *Imagery Rehearsal Therapy* [64], *Image Habituation Training* [65, 66], etc.). Although they look like new treatment approaches, these are mainly modified forms of existing treatments for PTSD. Also, few are grounded in theories of actiology of PTSD and related empirical support.

2.5. Evidence base of trauma-focused psychotherapies

As noted earlier, several meta-analyses of randomised controlled trials showed comparable efficacies for various trauma-focused psychotherapies [1-3]. These meta-analyses, however, did not examine the efficacy of various treatment packages with respect to their main components. Such examination is important in clarifying the ingredients that are most useful for achieving maximum efficacy. Such knowledge also has important implications for refining theories of PTSD. To identify the contribution of each component to treatment efficacy we conducted a comprehensive literature review of randomized controlled trauma-focused treatment studies of PTSD. These studies were selected through a literature search of randomized controlled trials of CBT in PsycInfo (1806 – 2009), PILOTS (1960 – 2009), and PubMed (1966 – 2009) databases. To be included in the meta-analysis the study must have (a) tested the efficacy of a treatment for PTSD against a control group, waitlist or placebo treatment or alternative intervention, or combination of any of these, using a randomized controlled trial design, (b) included adults who met diagnostic criteria for acute (1 to 3 months post-trauma) or chronic (more than 6 months post trauma) PTSD as defined by DSM-III, DSM-IIIR, DSM-IV, or DSM-IVTR, (c) used valid structured interview forms and / or self-rated instruments for the assessment of PTSD, (d) its sample size was large enough to allow sufficient power in analyses (i.e. at least 8 patients in each group), (e) provided sufficient data in the article for calculation of effect sizes or through contact with authors, and (f) has been published in English. This search revealed 41 studies that met the inclusion criteria. We analysed them meta-analytically by combining their findings using the standardised effect size statistic. Effect size is a measure of the strength or magnitude of a treatment effect and one way to calculate it is by computing the difference between pre- and post-treatment means on outcome measures and dividing this by the pooled standard deviation of those means [67]. This method can also be used to calculate the effect size between two treatment conditions. Effect size values of 0.20 indicate small, 0.50 moderate, and 0.80 large treatment effects. Larger effect sizes indicate more symptom reduction and less residual symptoms at the end of treatment. As various clinician-rated and / or self-rated instruments were used to assess PTSD we computed an aggregate effect size over all PTSD measures employed in a study. Data were analysed using SPSS 14.

Table 1 shows the number of participants, attrition rates, treatment duration (number of sessions and total hours spent), and effect sizes for PTSD and depression from baseline to post-treatment for main treatment components of 41 randomized controlled trials. Studies involving *Control-Focused Behavioural Treatment* [21] are excluded from this meta-analysis due to its theoretical difference from other treatment protocols and brevity (i.e. single-session application). These studies are reviewed separately in Section 2.6. Treatments in Table 1 were tested with survivors from a wide range of trauma events, including war veterans, rape victims and survivors of childhood abuse, survivors of civilian trauma (e.g. physical assault, crime, traffic accident, etc.), and refugees. Exposure-based interventions were tested with all these trauma survivors, whereas cognitive treatments and EMDR were mainly tested with survivors of rape and civilian trauma. Control conditions involved waiting list and non-specific treatments such as relaxation, supportive counselling, and present-centred therapy (i.e. coping and problem solving skills training).

	N conditions	Sample Size	Attrition rate	N sessions	Treatment duration		Effect size[a] Mean (SD)
Main treatment components			%	Mean (range)	Hours Mean (SD)	Weeks Mean (Range)	PTSD
Imaginal exposure[1]	6	105	20	8.5 (4-14)	11.8 (6.6)	9 (3-23)	0.86 (0.39)
Imaginal + live exposure[2]	11	317	25	10 (5-20)	16.5 (9.2)	9 (4.5-16)	1.98 (0.69)

	N conditions	Sample Size	Attrition rate	N sessions	Treatment duration		Effect size[a] Mean (SD)
Main treatment components			%	Mean (range)	Hours Mean (SD)	Weeks Mean (Range)	PTSD
Imaginal exposure + cognitive restructuring[3]	4	165	20	17 (8-30)	29.6 (21.7)	17 (9-30)	1.29 (1.11)
Live exposure + cognitive restructuring[4]	2	64	16	11 (--)	16.5 (0.0)	5.5 (--)	3.80 (0.83)
Imaginal + live exposure + cognitive restructuring[5]	10	193	32	11 (4-20)	18.5 (9.9)	12 (4-18)	1.74 (0.48)
Cognitive therapy without exposure[6]	2	51	8	11 (10-12)	13.5 (2.1)	21 (16-26)	1.41 (0.35)
Cognitive therapy with limited imaginal / live exposure[7]	4	107	19	16 (12-27)	18.1 (11.6)	12 (6-17)	2.42 (0.67)
Imaginal & live exposure + anxiety management[8]	2	34	17	8 (7-9)	12.0 (2.1)	6 (5-7)	1.78 (0.30)
Imaginal exposure + skills training[9]	2	33	32	25 (16-34)	37.5 (19.1)	15 (12-17)	1.16 (0.87)
Imaginal exposure + imaginal rescripting[10]	2	76	31	6.5 (3-10)	11.0 (5.7)	7.5 (5-10)	1.09 (0.31)
EMDR[11]	12	199	16	6 (2-12)	8.5 (4.6)	6 (2-10)	1.66 (0.94)
Control Conditions							

	N conditions	Sample Size	Attrition rate	N sessions	Treatment duration		Effect size[a] Mean (SD)
Main treatment components			%	Mean (range)	Hours Mean (SD)	Weeks Mean (Range)	PTSD
Relaxation[12]	4	59	11	10 (8-12)	11.7 (3.5)	10 (6-16)	0.75 (0.61)
Supportive counseling[13]	4	66	18	8 (5-10)	11.4 (3.0)	6 (4-10)	0.60 (0.32)
Present centered therapy[14]	3	268	18	18 (9-30)	27.8 (15.8)	20 (10-30)	0.70 (0.48)
Treatment as usual[15]	2	47	7	--	--	--	0.69 (0.58)
Waitlist / minimal attention control[16]	25	516	11	--	--	--	0.27 (0.38)

[a] Calculated from the raw data reported in the articles. Where data were provided only in graphic form, raw data were obtained from the authors. For articles reporting effect sizes without reporting any data, effect sizes as reported in the published article were used.

1= [23, 25, 34, 54, 63, 65], 2 = [26, 27, 36-38, 53, 89, 107-110], 3 = [23, 32, 33, 111], 4 = [112, 113], 5 = [27, 30, 31, 36, 37, 62, 114-117], 6 = [27, 54], 7 = [53, 57, 118, 119], 8 = [29, 38], 9 = [28, 33], 10 = [34, 64], 11 = [29, 62, 65, 108, 110, 116, 120-125], 12 = [27, 65, 110, 120], 13 = [23, 26, 63, 114], 14 = [32, 115, 126], 15 = [31, 123], 16 = [25, 26, 28, 30, 33, 36, 38, 53, 57, 63, 64, 89, 108, 111-116, 118-122, 124]

Table 1. Evidence base for trauma-focused interventions

All active treatments yielded larger effects on PTSD than did control conditions. Although all treatments achieved clinically large effect sizes (over 0.80) in PTSD, they differed in their efficacy. Imaginal exposure and cognitive therapy had limited efficacy compared with other treatments when they were used alone. Although the addition of cognitive restructuring, skills training, and imagery rescripting enhanced the efficacy of imaginal exposure, treatment effects still remained limited. On the other hand, the efficacy of both imaginal exposure and cognitive therapy reached their maximum when they were combined with live exposure (1.98 and 3.80, respectively). These findings imply that live exposure is the critical ingredient in CBT packages. Cognitive therapy programmes involving an exposure component also performed significantly better than cognitive therapy alone, suggesting that cognitive interventions by themselves are not sufficient for successful treatment outcome. The addition of other interventions to full exposure programmes did not lead to better outcomes (they even compromised treatment gains). EMDR was also effective in PTSD, however it was associated with more residual symptoms than the potent forms of exposure based treatments with or without cognitive restructuring. It is also noteworthy that the evidence base for exposure treatments involves more methodologically rigorous studies than that of EMDR.

It is worth noting that the effect sizes reported in Table 1 are based on cases that completed a given programme during a RCT. As 8% to 32% of the patients dropped out of the studies, the composition of the experimental groups can no longer be considered random, which creates a selection bias reflecting the outcome of those who remain in the study or who respond to the specific treatment [68]. Findings based on more conservative intent-to-treat (or last observation carried forward) analyses, which include non-treated or non-treatment-responder cases, are more attenuated. For example, the effect sizes for imaginal and live exposure and cognitive therapy with limited exposure programmes in studies that reported intent-to-treat analyses were 1.23 (n = 4) and 1.80 (n = 3), respectively. We selected to report findings based on completers analyses because we were interested in seeing treatment outcome among those who received the full treatment. Also, intent-to-treat analyses were not consistently reported in all articles.

Tolerability of a treatment as indicated by attrition rates is an important parameter in evaluating treatment protocols. Attrition rates varied across treatment protocols but the differences were not statistically significant. When we grouped interventions, the average rate of dropout was 25% from treatment packages involving an exposure component (including cognitive therapy with limited exposure), 8% from cognitive therapy and, 16% from EMDR. Although it seemed that interventions involving exposure were less tolerable, this finding needs to be cautiously interpreted because they were examined in a total of 43 trial conditions compared with only 2 cognitive therapy and 12 EMDR conditions. In addition, the number of participants in exposure was 5.5 to 21 times higher than those in EMDR and cognitive therapy (1094 vs 199 and 51, respectively).

Treatments showed great variability with respect to number of sessions and time to recovery they required. Interventions involving exposure and cognitive therapy were delivered in a mean 12 sessions, while EMDR was administered in an average of 6 sessions. Treatment lasted an average of 16 hours (SD = 11) in exposure, 20 (SD = 12) hours in exposure with cognitive interventions, 13.5 (SD = 2.1) in cognitive therapy, and 8.5 (SD = 4.6) in EMDR. Treatment delivery in these interventions took a mean of 9 (SD = 5), 12 (SD = 6), 21 (SD = 7), and 6 (SD = 3) weeks, respectively. Although delivered in about the same number of sessions, cognitive interventions required more time in treatment than did exposure alone. Cognitive therapy alone achieved relatively limited effects in a longer period of time than did all other treatments. EMDR appeared to be the briefest treatment.

Treatment programmes reported in Table 1 vary in their complexity for training. Although practice varies, more complex treatment programmes require more time for training and supervision and they are therefore more difficult to disseminate. There is not much information on the duration of various training programmes. The most common exposure protocol used with trauma survivors, prolonged exposure [26] and cognitive therapy [58] require 5 days of training each [36]. Combined treatments take longer time for training. EMDR Institute's website states that EMDR basic training is completed in 40 hours and 2-day workshops are held for advanced training. The complex procedures involved in conducting imaginal exposure and cognitive restructuring pose challenges in training of lay therapists. All these treatments also require continuous supervision. Furthermore, they rely on heavy therapist input and as such they are not suitable for dissemination on a self-help basis.

The cross-cultural applicability of these interventions is largely unknown as they were mostly tested in western countries. As exposure therapy targets universals of human behaviour (fear and avoidance) it would be expected to have promise in different cultural settings. On the other hand, it is difficult to make predictions about cognitive interventions, because cross-cultural validity of the so called maladaptive / faulty thinking patterns about trauma and its sequelae is not known. Furthermore, requirements of keeping homework sheets [26, 53] and heavy writing tasks involved in some treatment protocols [53] may complicate their practicability among survivors with low level of education that characterize populations of developing countries. They also pose challenges of use under difficult post-disaster or post-war settings, where survivors deal with day-to-day survival problems. Finally, the efficacy of these treatments has rarely been examined in survivors of natural disasters and war.

2.6. Control-focused behavioural treatment

Control-Focused Behavioural Treatment was tested in two open and two randomized clinical trials involving 331 earthquake survivors with chronic PTSD. In an open trial [39], among survivors with a PTSD diagnosis, the probability of clinically significant improvement was 76% after one session and 88% after two sessions, reaching 100% after four sessions. This improvement corresponded to a mean 57% reduction in PTSD symptoms, 69% in fear and avoidance behaviours, and 50% in depression. The mean number of sessions required for improvement was 1.7. In a subsequent randomized controlled trial *Control-Focused Behavioural Treatment* achieved improvement in 80% of survivors when delivered in a *single session* [40]. In the latter study, behavioural avoidance was the first symptom to improve early in treatment (6 weeks), followed by improvement in re-experiencing and hyperarousal symptoms [69]. Thus, reduction in avoidance appeared to be the critical factor that initiated the process of improvement in other symptoms. Further studies showed that treatment effect could be enhanced by 20% by an additional session involving therapist aided exposure to simulated earthquake tremors in an earthquake simulator [41, 70]. Improvement was maintained in the long-term in all studies, despite further exposure to numerous aftershocks and expectations of another major earthquake. An average of 6 sessions of *Control-Focused Behavioural Treatment* achieved similar improvement rates in asylum-seekers and refugees in Turkey, despite adverse psychosocial and economic circumstances [21, 71]. These findings suggested that *Control-Focused Behavioural Treatment* has promise in treatment of mass trauma survivors in non-western settings. The single-session application of *Control-Focused Behavioural Treatment*, which emphasizes self-conducted exposure in survivors' daily routine, has promise of easy distribution to large number of survivors in mass disaster settings. Further studies are needed to confirm these findings in different trauma populations living in different cross-cultural settings.

3. Pharmacotherapy of PTSD

According to pathophysiological theories, PTSD symptoms occur as an outcome of excessive activation of the amygdala by stimuli that are perceived to be threatening. The key psychobiological systems that are believed to be altered in PTSD are adrenergic, hypothalamic-pituitary-adrenocortical (HPA), glutametergic, serotenergic, and dopaminergic systems. Various pharmacological agents therefore aim to intervene disruptions in these systems. Before 2000 a handful of randomized controlled trials reported some beneficial effects of tricyclic antidepressants. With the introduction of *Selective Serotonin Reuptake Inhibitors* (SSRI) in the treatment of anxiety disorders, researchers lost interest in studying these medications because SSRIs had more tolerable side effects and pharmaceutical companies are more eager to provide funding for research on these medications [72]. SSRIs are now indicated as the pharmacotherapy of choice in several clinical practice guidelines for PTSD [72-74]. Recently, the efficacy of newer antidepressants, including serotonin-norepinephrine reuptake inhibitors (SNRIs, venlafaxine) and noradregenic and specific serotonergic agents (NaSSA, mirtazaine) has also been examined. In addition, some atypic antipsychotic medications (risperidone and olanzapine) have been tested as adjunctive agents for refractory patients who have failed to respond to antidepressants. In this section we review the evidence from double-blind placebo controlled randomized clinical trials of SSRIs, SNRIs, NaSSa, and atypical antipsychotics. These agents are selected for the review because other drugs (e.g. anticonvulsant / antikindling agents, monoamine oxidase inhibitors, etc.) have been mostly tested in case studies or open label trials. Benzodiazepines are not included in the review because they were not found to be effective in PTSD [72]. The same methodology described above for trauma-focused therapy protocols was followed.

Table 2 lists 21 studies that tested the efficacy of antidepressants and antipsychotics combined with antidepressants in double-blind placebo controlled randomized controlled design. Treatment duration varied between 4 to 16 weeks. The attrition rates for drug and placebo were 31% (SD = 7%, range 13-47%) and 29% (SD = 14%, range 0-59%), respectively. These figures were slightly higher than those reported in psychotherapy trials. Mean reduction in PTSD symptoms was 38% (SD = 16.5) in cases treated with active drugs, while it was 28% (SD = 14.1) in cases given pill placebo. Thus, drug-placebo difference was only 10%. This pattern of improvement was also noted in effect sizes (these were calculated using change scores as described by Kazis et al. [75], because drug trials did not always report post-treatment scores). Although the majority of the drugs achieved large pre- to post-treatment effects, so did the pill placebo. Indeed, the between-treatment effect sizes rarely exceeded the threshold (i.e. 0.50) necessary to detect a clinically significant difference between an active drug and placebo. This is in contrast with exposure-based treatments which yielded much larger effect sizes. It is worth noting, however, drug trials based their findings on all cases that completed at least one assessment after baseline, thus including the cases that dropped-out from treatment by carrying their last observation forward in the data set. Even though this conservative analysis strategy may counteracted drug efficacy compared to trauma-focused psychological treatments, evidence shows that treatment effects are more stable in the latter. There are no studies that examined relapse rates in drug-free follow-ups. Few double-blind placebo controlled

| | Drug | | | Placebo | | | Drug vs Placebo |
| | | | | | | | |
	N studies	n	% Change[b]	Effect Size Mean (SD)	n	% Change[b]	Effect Size Mean (SD)	Effect Size Mean (SD)
Sertraline[1]	5	471	36	1.54 (0.69)	474	29	1.30 (0.63)	0.31 (0.20)
Fluoxetine[2]	5	464	44	2.35 (0.38)[c]	245	32	1.83 (0.39)[c]	0.62 (0.37)[d]
Paroxetine[3]	3	541	44	1.77 (0.69)	363	30	1.22 (0.41)	0.57 (0.31)
Venlafaxine[4]	2	340	57	3.16 (0.54)	347	48	2.61 (0.40)	0.48 (0.04)
Mirtazapine[5]	1	17	35	1.06 (--)	9	17	0.86 (--)	0.60 (--)
Risperidone augmentation[6]	4	67	26	0.99 (0.60)	63	21	0.87 (0.44)	0.26 (0.53)
Olanzapine augmentation[7]	1	10	17	0.67 (--)	9	3	0.16 (--)	0.75 (--)

[a] Effect sizes calculated from the raw data reported in the articles. Within group effect sizes calculated as mean change score divided by the standard deviation of the baseline score. Between-groups effect sizes were calculated as mean change score between drug and pill placebo groups divided by standard deviation of the baseline score for placebo group.

[b] Percent reductions in PTSD symptoms pre- to post-treatment

[c] Within treatment effect sizes for one study (van der Kolk et al, 1994) were not available and thus excluded.

[d] Drug vs placebo effect size for one study (van der Kolk et al, 1994) taken from [127]

1 = [128-132], 2 = [125, 133-136], 3 = [137-139], 4 = [132, 140], 5 = [141], 6 = [142-145], 7 = [146]

Table 2. Effect sizes in double-blind randomized controlled trials of pharmacotherapy for PTSD[a]

maintenance studies involving survivors treated with SSRIs found that discontinuation of drug treatment is associated with return of PTSD symptoms [76-78].

The augmentation of antidepressant treatments with atypical antipsychotics in treatment refractory patients did not also result in better outcomes, except for one study which involved only a small number of survivors. Antidepressant treatment (paroxetine) did not also augment treatment effects in patients who remained symptomatic after 12 weeks of exposure treatment [79](not listed in Table 2). On the other hand, adding exposure treatment to SSRI treatment conferred additional benefits in patients who did not respond to previous pharmacotherapy [80, 81].

A problem concerning pharmacotherapy clinical trials in PTSD is that the findings have limited generalizability because most studies involved middle-aged females sexually abused as children or Vietnam Veterans [72]. There is also less evidence on the efficacy of medications in different age groups, because concerns about increased suicides among children and adolescents treated with SSRIs for depression and concerns about safety, age-related pharmacokinetic capacity, drug-drug interactions, and comorbid medical conditions in elderly people, pose obstacles to pharmacotherapy research in these populations [72]. Finally, when used in combination with exposure-based treatments, drugs may undermine the efficacy of the latter by facilitating attributions of improvement to the tablets rather than to personal efforts. In view of these findings, use of antidepressants as a first-line intervention in treatment of trauma survivors could hardly be justified.

4. Other psychological treatments

There are various other interventions used with trauma survivors, which vary greatly in their emphasis in treatment. Some of these treatments aim to increase general well-being of survivors (e.g. psychosocial support, psychoeducation, normalisation, art therapy or other expressive recreational activities, etc.) or alleviate general psychological distress (e.g. coping skills training, affect management, counselling, family therapy, etc.), while others target specific psychopathology such as PTSD and depression (e.g., interpersonal psychotherapy, school based intervention for children, brief eclectic psychotherapy, etc.). Most of these treatments involve a mixture of diverse interventions without a well-defined theoretical framework. This is an important problem because a treatment could only achieve partial effects unless its mechanisms of action match the causal processes that underlie a mental health problem [82]. Furthermore, as they do not specifically target trauma induced anxiety and fear reactions, many treatments achieve low improvement rates. One example of such treatments is school-based intervention programme developed for children. This treatment mainly involves psychoeducation, normalisation of trauma reactions through creative-expressive activities (e.g. play, art therapy), and skills training. Two RCTs that tested the efficacy of this intervention in child survivors of war in Bosnia [83] and political violence in Indonesia [84] found only small to moderate treatment effects in PTSD symptoms compared to waitlist controls (effect sizes = 0.22 and 0.51, respectively). Similar moderate treatment effects were obtained in other RCTs of a psychosocial intervention program for female survivors of war in Bosnia [85] and an affect management treatment in child sexual abuse survivors [86].

A misplaced focus in treatment also occurs when specific psychiatric disorders other than PTSD are targeted. The findings of two RCTs are cases in point. In one of the studies [87], depressive symptoms were targeted with group interpersonal psychotherapy and creative play in Ugandan adolescent war survivors. Creative play showed no effect on depression severity, while interpersonal group psychotherapy reduced depression in girls but not in boys. Neither treatment resulted in significant improvement in anxiety, conduct problems, and psychosocial functioning. Targeting depression with a self-management treatment also failed to reduce depression, PTSD, and psychosocial functioning in adult male veterans [88]. These limited treatment effects could be explained by a misplaced focus in treatment.

There is some evidence suggesting that trauma focused psychodynamic therapy and brief eclectic psychotherapy combining psychodynamic therapy with cognitive restructuring and imaginal exposure are effective in PTSD. In three RCTs, compared to waitlist controls, these treatments achieved medium to large treatment effects in PTSD symptoms (range 0.66-0.94)

[89-91]. Methodological problems preclude definitive conclusions about the effects of these treatments. It is also worth noting that treatment was delivered in 16 to 20 sessions. Considering that exposure based treatments achieve higher treatment effects when delivered in a mean of 12 sessions, the usefulness of psychodynamic or eclectic approaches become questionable.

A widely used treatment approach for refugees and survivors of torture in rehabilitation centres around the world is multi-disciplinary treatment, including social, legal, medical, and psychological aid for survivors. An open outcome evaluation study based on 55 persons admitted to the Research Centre for Torture Victims in Denmark in 2001 and 2002 showed no improvement in PTSD, depression, anxiety or health-related quality of life after 9 months of treatment, leading the authors to conclude that future studies are needed to explore effective interventions for traumatised refugees [92]. In a more recent non-random quasi experimental study of torture survivors in Nepal, multi-disciplinary treatment reduced non-specific somatic problems related to torture, but not more severe specific mental health problems, including PTSD and depression, and associated disability [93]. The authors concluded that evidence-based treatments that are able to address specific mental health problems and associated disability need to be investigated for torture survivors.

5. Interventions to prevent the development of PTSD

5.1. Critical incident stress debriefing

Critical Incident Stress Debriefing has been a widely used psychological intervention after mass trauma events. In this approach survivors exposed to similar traumatic experiences participate in a structured session where they talk about the traumatic event in detail. This session, which takes place soon after the trauma, is said to allow venting of survivors' emotions about the traumatic incident within the context of psychosocial support from others and attenuate the intensity of acute stress reactions, thereby reducing the risk of developing PTSD [94]. Two RCTs with individual trauma survivors [95, 96] and one RCT with deployed soldiers [97] did not find beneficial effects of debriefing in preventing or improving PTSD symptoms. These findings led major clinical guidelines for Acute Stress Disorder (ASD) and PTSD not to recommend the use of debriefing following traumatic events [73, 98].

5.2. Brief CBT

Condensed forms of treatment based on cognitive-behavioural principles have been tested in survivors with ASD (i.e. within 1-month post-trauma) or acute PTSD (i.e. within 3 months post-trauma). Treatment packages, usually delivered in 4 to 5 sessions, involved psychoeducation; breathing, relaxation, anxiety management training; cognitive restructuring; imaginal and live exposure. A meta-analysis of the efficacy of these interventions in ASD with respect to control groups is reported in Table 3. The latter included repeated assessment (1 study), supportive counselling (5 studies), and waiting list (1 study). As the outcome was similar across all controls they were pooled for the meta-analysis. Brief CBT and prolonged exposure (imaginal + live exposure) achieved large treatment effects in PTSD severity and moderate effects in depression both at post-treatment and 6-months post-trauma. More survivors in the control groups met diagnostic criteria for PTSD at post-treatment and follow up. It is worth noting that the effect sizes in Table 3 are based on those who completed treatment and more conservative intent-to-treat analyses do not always yield favourable outcome for treatment [99]. Also, between-groups differences disappeared at follow-up in some studies [100]. The generalizability of these findings is limited because they are mainly based on survivors of assault and traffic accident. Furthermore, although treatment is relatively brief, the applicability of a 5-session treatment following mass trauma events is questionable. Nevertheless, these findings suggest that brief exposure-based interventions delivered early after the trauma accelerate recovery process in survivors and prove effective in preventing chronic PTSD.

				Post-Treatment		Follow-up	
	N conditions	n Treatment	n Control	Effect Size	PTSD diagnosis (Tx vs control)	Effect Size	PTSD diagnosis (Tx vs control)
Acute Stress Disorder							
Brief CBT[1]	4	58	56	1.21	8 13% vs 46-83%	0.83	10-22% vs 22-67%
Imaginal + live exposure[2]	3	54	53	1.13	12-14% vs 56-71%	1.15	15% vs 67%
Cognitive restructuring[3]	1	23	21	0.59	52% vs 71%	--	
Acute PTSD							
Brief CBT[a, 4]	--	76	76	0.30	30% vs 30%	0.61	10% vs 15%
Brief CBT[5]	--	61	52	0.63	38% vs 61%	0.34	26% vs 44%
Cognitive restructuring + coping skills training[6]	--	10	10	0.82	20% vs 50%	1.03	0 vs 20%

Effect Size = between-groups Cohen's d effect size index

[a] Effect sizes reflect outcome in intent-to-treat analyses.

1 = [99-102], 2 = [23, 103, 147], 3 = [147], 4 = [104], 5 = [148], 6 = [149]

Table 3. Efficacy of brief cognitive-behavioural treatment programmes in ASD and Acute PTSD in randomised controlled trials

Treatment outcome in early intervention studies of acute PTSD was not as good as that obtained in studies of ASD. Table 3 also shows findings from 3 RCTs. These studies are examined separately because their findings were not consistent, probably due to the fact that one study reported only intent-to-treat data. Compared to waiting list groups two studies of brief CBT found only small to moderate treatment effects in PTSD and small effect in depression at both post-treatment and follow-up (conducted about 6 to 13 months post-trauma). More favourable treatment effects were obtained with cognitive restructuring combined with coping skills training relative to relaxation control, however this study was based on a very small sample.

Interestingly, early interventions produced greater reductions in avoidance behaviour and, whereas significant improvement occurred in reexperiencing and arousal symptoms, negligible reductions occurred on avoidance symptoms in control groups [99, 101-104]. These findings points to the important role played by avoidance symptoms in the maintenance of PTSD. More studies need to be conducted on diverse survivor populations and different cultural settings.

5.3. Propranolol

It has been proposed that the beta-adrenergic antagonist propranolol may have promise in preventing the later development of PTSD by reducing enhancement of traumatic memories. Two RCTs that tested this hypothesis yielded inconsistent results. In one of these studies [105] 41 emergency department patients who had experienced a trauma likely to precipitate PTSD were treated orally with 40 mg of propranolol within six hours of the occurrence of the traumatic event. The drug dose was repeated four times daily for 10 days, with a nine-day taper period. After one month, 18% (2 / 11) of propranolol completers met diagnostic criteria for PTSD, in contrast to 30% (6 / 20) of placebo completers. The drop-out rate from propranolol and placebo was 39% and 13%, respectively. In the other study [106] 48 acute physical injury patients admitted to a surgical trauma centre were randomised to receive propranolol, the anxiolytic anticonvulsant gabapentin, or placebo within 48 hours of trauma. Although well tolerated, neither drug showed a significant benefit over placebo on posttraumatic stress symptoms or depressive symptoms. It is worth noting that 92% of the acutely injured patients refused to participate in the study, in part reflecting their reluctance to receive medication. These inconsistent findings on treatment efficacy considered together with high drop-out rate and refusal to take the medication suggest that medication is not a viable preventative option for PTSD.

6. Conclusion

In this chapter we reviewed critically current treatment approaches for PTSD. The evidence in the literature clearly shows that trauma-focused psychotherapies are the first line of choice in the treatment of PTSD. The question remains as to which trauma-focused treatment protocol is the best option. Exposure therapy involving live exposure and cognitive therapies incorporating an exposure component are the more efficacious treatments for PTSD. Exposure therapy has several advantages over cognitive therapy. Its theoretical background is more robust and experimentally validated than cognitive therapy. It also has larger evidence base, was tested with a wider range of trauma survivors, and has more promise in cross-cultural applicability. Furthermore, cognitive therapy involves elaborate procedures that require substantial training in its administration. Finally, exposure therapy requires relatively less time for observable improvement.

Despite these advantages exposure therapy is not without problems. About 40% to 50% of patients fail to achieve clinically significant improvement after exposure therapy. These modest improvement rates could be explained by a strong focus on anxiety reduction, rather than anxiety tolerance, which may be counterproductive in treatment. Indeed, the evidence indicates that the degree by which fear reduces or the level of fear following exposure is not related to treatment outcome. Furthermore, exposure therapy is not sufficiently brief for use in mass disaster settings. Although the procedures involved in exposure do not require lengthy and costly training compared to other treatments, they are not suitable for delivery on a self-help basis. There is thus need for a simple and brief intervention that emphasises anxiety / fear tolerance and that can be easily delivered to masses. *Control-Focused Behavioural Treatment* has promise in meeting this need. This short and effective treatment, which emphasizes self-conducted exposure in survivors' daily routine with an aim to increase anxiety tolerance and promote resilience, is suitable for easy distribution to large number of survivors in mass disaster settings.

Author details

Ebru Şalcıoğlu[1,2,3] and Metin Başoğlu[1,2]

*Address all correspondence to: Ebru.Salcioglu@kcl.ac.uk, ebrusalcioglu@halic.edu.tr, esalcioglu@dabatem.org

1 Institute of Psychiatry, King's College London, University of London, UK

2 Istanbul Centre for Behaviour Research and Therapy, Istanbul, Turkey

3 Department of Psychology, Haliç University, Istanbul, Turkey

References

[1] Bradley, R., et al., *A multidimensional meta-analysis of psychotherapy for PTSD.* American Journal of Psychiatry, 2005. 162(2): p. 214-227.

[2] Bisson, J.I., et al., *Psychological treatments for chronic post-traumatic stress disorder - Systematic review and meta-analysis.* British Journal of Psychiatry, 2007. 190: p. 97-104.

[3] Van Etten, M.L. and S. Taylor, *Comparative efficacy of treatments for post-traumatic stress disorder: A meta-analysis.* Clinical Psychology & Psychotherapy, 1998. 5(3): p. 126-144.

[4] Barlow, D.H., *Anxiety and its Disorders: The Nature and Treatment of Anxiety and Panic.* 2nd ed. 2002, New York: Guilford Press.

[5] Marks, I.M., *Fears, Phobias, and Rituals.* 1987, Oxford: Oxford University Press.

[6]   Foa, E.B. and M.J. Kozak, *Emotional processing of fear: exposure to corrective information.* Psychological Bulletin, 1986. 99(1): p. 20-35.

[7]   Foa, E.B. and R.J. McNally, *Mechanisms of change in exposure therapy,* in *Current Controversies in the Anxiety Disorders,* R.M. Rapee, Editor. 1996, Guilford Press: New York. p. 329-343.

[8]   Lang, P.J., *Imagery in therapy: an information processing analysis of fear.* Behavior Therapy, 1977. 8: p. 862-888.

[9]   Lang, P.J., *A bio-informational theory of emotional imagery.* Psychophysiology, 1979. 16: p. 495-512.

[10] Mineka, S. and J. Sutton, *Contemporary Learning Theory Perspectives on the Etiology of Fears and Phobias,* in *Fear and Learning: From Basic Principles to Clinical Implications,* M.G. Craske, D. Hermans, and D. Vansteenwegen, Editors. 2006, American Psychological Association: Washington, DC. p. 75-97.

[11] Mineka, S. and R. Zinbarg, *A contemporary learning theory perspective on the etiology of anxiety disorders - It's not what you thought it was.* American Psychologist, 2006. 61(1): p. 10-26.

[12] Craske, M.G., et al., *Optimizing inhibitory learning during exposure therapy.* Behaviour Research and Therapy, 2008. 46(1): p. 5-27.

[13] Bouton, M.E., *Learning and Behavior: A Contemporary Synthesis.* 2007, Sunderland: Sinauer Assiciates, Ic.

[14] Craske, M.G. and J.L. Mystkowski, *Exposure therapy and extinction: Clinical studies,* in *Fear and Learning: From Basic Principles to Clinical Implications,* M.G. Craske, D. Hermans, and D. Vansteenwegen, Editors. 2006, American Psychological Association: Washington, DC. p. 217-233.

[15] Başoğlu, M. and S. Mineka, *The role of uncontrollable and unpredictable stress in posttraumatic stress responses in torture survivors,* in *Torture and its Consequences: Current Treatment Approaches,* M. Başoğlu, Editor. 1992, Cambridge University Press: Cambridge. p. 182-225.

[16] Foa, E.B., R. Zinbarg, and B.O. Rothbaum, *Uncontrollability and unpredictability in posttraumatic stress disorder: an animal-model.* Psychological Bulletin, 1992. 112(2): p. 218-238.

[17] Başoğlu, M., M. Livanou, and C. Crnobarić, *Torture vs other cruel, inhuman, and degrading treatment - Is the distinction real or apparent?* Archives of General Psychiatry, 2007. 64(3): p. 277-285.

[18] Başoğlu, M., et al., *Psychiatric and cognitive effects of war in former Yugoslavia - Association of lack of redress for trauma and posttraumatic stress reactions.* Journal of the American Medical Association, 2005. 294(5): p. 580-590.

[19] Başoğlu, M., et al., *Psychological preparedness for trauma as a protective factor in survivors of torture*. Psychological Medicine, 1997. 27(6): p. 1421-1433.

[20] Şalcıoğlu, E., *The effect of beliefs, attribution of responsibility, redress and compensation on posttraumatic stress disorder in earthquake survivors in Turkey*, in *Institute of Psychiatry*. 2004, King's College London: London.

[21] Basoglu, M. and E. Salcioglu, *A Mental Healthcare Model for Mass Trauma Survivors: Control-Focused Behavioral Treatment of Earthquake, War, and Torture Trauma*. 2011, Cambridge: Cambridge University Press.

[22] Foa, E.B., G. Steketee, and B.O. Rothbaum, *Behavioral and cognitive conceptualizations of post-traumatic stress disorder*. Behavior Therapy, 1989. 20(2): p. 155-176.

[23] Bryant, R.A., et al., *Imaginal exposure alone and imaginal exposure with cognitive restructuring in treatment of posttraumatic stress disorder*. Journal of Consulting and Clinical Psychology, 2003. 71: p. 706-712.

[24] Tarrier, N., et al., *Cognitive therapy or imaginal exposure in the treatment of post-traumatic stress disorder - Twelve-month follow-up*. British Journal of Psychiatry, 1999. 175: p. 571-575.

[25] Keane, T.M., et al., *Implosive (flooding) therapy reduces symptoms of PTSD in Vietnam combat veterans*. Behavior Therapy, 1989. 20(2): p. 245-260.

[26] Foa, E.B., et al., *Treatment of posttraumatic stress disorder in rape victims: A comparison between cognitive-behavioral procedures and counseling*. Journal of Consulting and Clinical Psychology, 1991. 59(5): p. 715-723.

[27] Marks, I.M., et al., *Treatment of posttraumatic stress disorder by exposure and/or cognitive restructuring - A controlled study*. Archives of General Psychiatry, 1998. 55(4): p. 317-325.

[28] Cloitre, M., et al., *Skills training in affective and interpersonal regulation followed by exposure: A phase-based treatment for PTSD related to childhood abuse*. Journal of Consulting and Clinical Psychology, 2002. 70(5): p. 1067-1074.

[29] Lee, C., et al., *Treatment of PTSD: Stress inoculation training with prolonged exposure compared to EMDR*. Journal of Clinical Psychology, 2002. 58(9): p. 1071-1089.

[30] Fecteau, G. and R. Nicki, *Cognitive behavioural treatment of posttraumatic stress disorder after a motor vehicle accident*. Behavioural and Cognitive Psychotherapy, 1999. 27: p. 201-214.

[31] Difede, J., et al., *A randomized controlled clinical treatment trial for World Trade Center attack-related PTSD in disaster workers*. Journal of Nervous and Mental Disease, 2007. 195: p. 861-865.

[32] Schnurr, P.P., et al., *Randomized Trial of Trauma-Focused Group Therapy for Posttraumatic Stress Disorder: Results From a Department of Veterans Affairs Cooperative Study.* Archives of General Psychiatry, 2003. 60(5): p. 481-489.

[33] Glynn, S.M., et al., *A test of behavioral family therapy to augment exposure for combat-related posttraumatic stress disorder.* Journal of Consulting and Clinical Psychology, 1999. 67(2): p. 243-251.

[34] Arntz, A., M. Tiesema, and M. Kindt, *Treatment of PTSD: A comparison of imaginal exposure with and without imagery rescripting.* Journal of Behavior Therapy and Experimental Psychiatry, 2007. 38(4): p. 345-370.

[35] Grunert, B.K., et al., *Imagery rescripting and reprocessing therapy after failed prolonged exposure for post-traumatic stress disorder following industrial injury.* Journal of Behavior Therapy and Experimental Psychiatry, 2007. 38(4): p. 317-328.

[36] Foa, E.B., et al., *Randomized trial of prolonged exposure for posttraumatic stress disorder with and without cognitive restructuring: outcome at academic and community clinics.* Journal of Consulting and Clinical Psychology, 2005. 73(5): p. 953-964.

[37] Paunovic, N. and L.-G. Öst, *Cognitive-behavior therapy vs exposure therapy in the treatment of PTSD in refugees.* Behaviour Research and Therapy, 2001. 39(10): p. 1183-1197.

[38] Foa, E.B., et al., *A comparison of exposure therapy, stress inoculation training, and their combination for reducing posttraumatic stress disorder in female assault victims.* Journal of Consulting and Clinical Psychology, 1999. 67(2): p. 194-200.

[39] Başoğlu, M., et al., *A brief behavioural treatment of chronic post-traumatic stress disorder in earthquake survivors: results from an open clinical trial.* Psychological Medicine, 2003. 33(4): p. 647-654.

[40] Başoğlu, M., et al., *Single-session behavioral treatment of earthquake-related posttraumatic stress disorder: A randomized waiting list controlled trial.* Journal of Traumatic Stress, 2005. 18(1): p. 1-11.

[41] Başoğlu, M., E. Şalcıoğlu, and M. Livanou, *A randomized controlled study of single-session behavioural treatment of earthquake-related post-traumatic stress disorder using an earthquake simulator.* Psychological Medicine, 2007. 37(2): p. 203-213.

[42] Şalcıoğlu, E. and M. Başoğlu, *Control-focused behavioral treatment of earthquake survivors using live exposure to conditioned and simulated unconditioned stimuli.* Cyberpsychology, Behavior, and Social Networking, 2010. 13(1): p. 13-19.

[43] Beck, A.T., G. Emery, and R. Greenberg, *Anxiety Disorders and Phobias: A Cognitive Perspective.* 1985, New York: Basic Books.

[44] Beck, A.T. and D.A. Clark, *An information processing model of anxiety: Automatic and strategic processes.* Behaviour Research and Therapy, 1997. 35(1): p. 49-58.

[45] Ehlers, A. and D.M. Clark, *A cognitive model of posttraumatic stress disorder.* Behaviour Research and Therapy, 2000. 38(4): p. 319-345.

[46] Janoff-Bulman, R., *Shattered Assumptions: Towards a New Psychology of Trauma.* 1992, New York: Free Press.

[47] Dunmore, E., D.M. Clark, and A. Ehlers, *Cognitive factors involved in the onset and maintenance of posttraumatic stress disorder (PTSD) after physical or sexual assault.* Behaviour Research and Therapy, 1999. 37(9): p. 809-829.

[48] Foa, E.B., et al., *The Posttraumatic Cognitions Inventory (PTCI): Development and validation.* Psychological Assessment, 1999. 11(3): p. 303-314.

[49] Steil, R. and A. Ehlers, *Dysfunctional meaning of posttraumatic intrusions in chronic PTSD.* Behaviour Research and Therapy, 2000. 38(6): p. 537-558.

[50] Smith, K. and R.A. Bryant, *The generality of cognitive bias in acute stress disorder.* Behaviour Research and Therapy, 2000. 38(7): p. 709-715.

[51] Zoellner, L.A., et al., *Are trauma victims susceptible to false memories?* Journal of Abnormal Psychology, 2000. 109(3): p. 517-524.

[52] Foa, E.B., et al., *Processing of threat-related information in rape victims.* Journal of Abnormal Psychology, 1991. 100(2): p. 156-162.

[53] Resick, P.A., et al., *A comparison of cognitive-processing therapy with prolonged exposure and a waiting condition for the treatment of chronic posttraumatic stress disorder in female rape victims.* Journal of Consulting and Clinical Psychology, 2002. 70(4): p. 867-879.

[54] Tarrier, N., et al., *A randomized trial of cognitive therapy and imaginal exposure in the treatment of chronic posttraumatic stress disorder.* Journal of Consulting and Clinical Psychology, 1999. 67(1): p. 13-18.

[55] Foa, E.B. and S.A.M. Rauch, *Cognitive changes during prolonged exposure versus prolonged exposure plus cognitive restructuring in female assault survivors with posttraumatic stress disorder.* Journal of Consulting and Clinical Psychology, 2004. 72(5): p. 879-884.

[56] Livanou, M., et al., *Beliefs, sense of control and treatment outcome in post-traumatic stress disorder.* Psychological Medicine, 2002. 32(1): p. 157-165.

[57] Ehlers, A., et al., *Cognitive therapy for post-traumatic stress disorder: development and evaluation.* Behaviour Research and Therapy, 2005. 43(4): p. 413-431.

[58] Ehlers, A., et al., *A randomized controlled trial of cognitive therapy, a self-help booklet, and repeated assessments as early interventions for posttraumatic stress disorder.* Archives of General Psychiatry, 2003. 60(10): p. 1024-1032.

[59] Shapiro, F., *Eye Movement Desensitization and Reprocessing: Basic Principles, Protocols, and Procedures.* 2001, New York: The Guilford Press.

[60] Craske, M. and J.L. Mystkowski, *Exposure therapy and extinction: Clinical studies,* in *Fear and Learning: From Basic Principles to Clinical Implications,* M.G. Craske, D. Her-

mans, and D. Vansteenwegen, Editors. 2006, American Psychological Association: Washington, DC. p. 217-233.

[61] Davidson, P.R. and K.C. Parker, *Eye movement desensitization and reprocessing (EMDR): a meta-analysis 2001.* Journal of Consulting and Clinical Psychology, 2001. 69: p. 305-316.

[62] Devilly, G.J. and S.H. Spence, *The Relative Efficacy and Treatment Distress of EMDR and a Cognitive-Behavior Trauma Treatment Protocol in the Amelioration of Posttraumatic Stress Disorder.* Journal of Anxiety Disorders, 1999. 13(1-2): p. 131-157.

[63] Neuner, F., et al., *A Comparison of Narrative Exposure Therapy, Supportive Counseling, and Psychoeducation for Treating Posttraumatic Stress Disorder in an African Refugee Settlement.* Journal of Consulting and Clinical Psychology, 2004. 72(4): p. 579-587.

[64] Krakow, B., et al., *Imagery rehearsal therapy for chronic nightmares in sexual assault survivors with posttraumatic stress disorder: A randomized controlled trial.* Journal of the American Medical Association, 2001. 286(5): p. 537-545.

[65] Vaughan, K., et al., *A trial of eye movement desensitization compared to image habituation training and applied muscle relaxation in post-traumatic stress disorder.* Journal of Behavior Therapy and Experimental Psychiatry, 1994. 25(4): p. 283-291.

[66] Vaughan, K. and N. Tarrier, *The use of image habituation training with post-traumatic stress disorders.* The British Journal of Psychiatry, 1992. 161(5): p. 658-664.

[67] Cohen, J., *Statistical Power Analysis for the Behavioral Sciences.* Second Edition ed. 1988, New Jersey: Lawrence Erlbaum Associates.

[68] Kazdin, A.E., *Research Design in Clinical Psychology.* 2003, Boston: Allyn and Bacon.

[69] Şalcıoğlu, E., M. Başoğlu, and M. Livanou, *Effects of live exposure on symptoms of posttraumatic stress disorder: The role of reduced behavioral avoidance in improvement.* Behaviour Research and Therapy, 2007. 45(10): p. 2268-2279.

[70] Başoğlu, M., M. Livanou, and E. Şalcıoğlu, *A single session with an earthquake simulator for traumatic stress in earthquake survivors.* American Journal of Psychiatry, 2003. 160(4): p. 788-790.

[71] Salcioglu, E. and M. Basoglu, *Control-focused behavioural treatment of female war survivors with torture and gang rape experience: four case studies.* European Journal of Psychotraumatology, 2011. 2 Suppl 1: p. S192.

[72] Friedman, M.J. and J.R.T. Davidson, *Pharmacotherapy for PTSD*, in *Handbook of PTSD: Science and Practice*, M.J. Friedman, T.M. Keane, and P.A. Resick, Editors. 2007, The Guilford Press: New York. p. 376-405.

[73] American Psychiatric Association, *Practice guideline for the treatment of patients with acute stress disorder and posttraumatic stress disorder.* 2004, Arlington, VA: American Psychiatric Association Practice Guidelines.

[74] Friedman, M.J., et al., *Pharmacotherapy*, in *Effective Treatments for PTSD*, E.B. Foa, T.M. Keane, and M.J. Friedman, Editors. 2000, The Guilford Press: New York. p. 84-105.

[75] Kazis, L.E., J.J. Anderson, and R.F. Meenan, *Effect sizes for interpreting changes in health status*. Medical Care, 1989. 27(3): p. S178-S189.

[76] Davidson, J., et al., *Efficacy of Sertraline in Preventing Relapse of Posttraumatic Stress Disorder: Results of a 28-Week Double-Blind, Placebo-Controlled Study*. American Journal of Psychiatry, 2001. 158(12): p. 1974-1981.

[77] Martenyi, F., et al., *Fluoxetine v. placebo in prevention of relapse in post-traumatic stress disorder*. The British Journal of Psychiatry, 2002. 181(4): p. 315-320.

[78] Rapaport, M.H., J. Endicott, and C.M. Clary, *Posttraumatic stress disorder and quality of life: Results across 64 weeks of sertraline treatment*. Journal of Clinical Psychiatry, 2002. 63(1): p. 59-65.

[79] Simon, N.M., et al., *Paroxetine CR augmentation for posttraumatic stress disorder refractory to prolonged exposure therapy*. Journal of Clinical Psychiatry, 2008. 69: p. 400-405.

[80] Otto, M.W., et al., *Treatment of pharmacotherapy-refractory posttraumatic stress disorder among Cambodian refugees: a pilot study of combination treatment with cognitive-behavior therapy vs sertraline alone*. Behaviour Research and Therapy, 2003. 41(11): p. 1271-1276.

[81] Rothbaum, B.O., et al., *Augmentation of sertraline with prolonged exposure in the treatment of posttraumatic stress disorder*. Journal of Traumatic Stress, 2006. 19(5): p. 625-638.

[82] Başoğlu, M., *Treatment for depression symptoms in Ugandan adolescent survivors of war and displacement*. Journal of the American Medical Association, 2007. 298(18): p. 2138-.

[83] Layne, C.M., et al., *Effectiveness of a school based group psychotherapy program for war-exposed adolescents: a randomized controlled trial*. Journal of the American Academy of Child and Adolescent Psychiatry, 2008. 47(9): p. 1048-1062.

[84] Tol, W.A., et al., *School-Based Mental Health Intervention for Children Affected by Political Violence in Indonesia: A Cluster Randomized Trial*. Journal of the American Medical Association, 2008. 300(6): p. 655-662.

[85] Dybdahl, R., *Children and mothers in war: an outcome study of a psychosocial intervention program*. Child Development, 2001. 72(4): p. 1214-1230.

[86] Zlotnick, C., et al., *An affect-management group for women with posttraumatic stress disorder and histories of childhood sexual abuse*. Journal of Traumatic Stress, 1997. 10(3): p. 425-436.

[87] Bolton, P., et al., *Interventions for depression symptoms among adolescent survivors of war and displacement in Northern Uganda: a randomized controlled trial*. Journal of the American Medical Association, 2007. 298(5): p. 519-527.

[88] Dunn, N.J., et al., *A randomized trial of self-management and psychoeducational group therapies for comorbid chronic posttraumatic stress disorder and depressive disorder.* Journal of Traumatic Stress, 2007. 20(3): p. 221-237.

[89] Brom, D., R.J. Kleber, and P.B. Defares, *Brief psychotherapy for posttraumatic stress disorders.* Journal of Consulting and Clinical Psychology, 1989. 57(5): p. 607-612.

[90] Gersons, B.P.R., et al., *Randomized clinical trial of brief eclectic psychotherapy for police officers with posttraumatic stress disorder.* Journal of Traumatic Stress, 2000. 13(2): p. 333-347.

[91] Lindauer, R.J.L., et al., *Effects of brief eclectic psychotherapy in patients with posttraumatic stress disorder: randomized clinical trial.* Journal of Traumatic Stress, 2005. 18(3): p. 205-212.

[92] Carlsson, J.M., E.L. Mortensen, and M. Kastrup, *A follow-up study of mental health and health-related quality of life in tortured refugees in multidisciplinary treatment.* Journal of Nervous and Mental Disease, 2005. 193: p. 651-657.

[93] Tol, W.A., et al., *Brief multi-disciplinary treatment for torture survivors in Nepal: a naturalistic comparative study.* International Journal of Social Psychiatry, 2009. 55(1): p. 39-56.

[94] Mitchell, J.T., *When disaster strikes...The Critical Incident Stress Debriefing process.* Journal of Emergency Medical Services, 1983. 8: p. 36-39.

[95] Bisson, J.I., et al., *Randomized controlled trial of psychological debriefing for victims of acute burn trauma.* British Journal of Psychiatry, 1997. 171: p. 78-81.

[96] Hobbs, M., et al., *A randomized trial of psychological debriefing for victims of road traffic accidents.* British Medical Journal, 1996. 313: p. 1438-1439.

[97] Adler, A.B., et al., *A group randomized trial of critical incident stress debriefing provided to U.S. peacekeepers.* Journal of Traumatic Stress, 2008. 21(3): p. 253-263.

[98] National Institute of Clinical Excellence (NICE), *Posttraumatic Stress Disorder (PTSD): The management of PTSD in adults and children in primary and secondary care.* National Clinical Practice Guideline Number 26. 2005, London: Gaskel and the British Psychological Society.

[99] Bryant, R.A., et al., *The additive benefit of hynosis and cognitive-behavioral therapy in treating acute stress disorder.* Journal of Consulting and Clinical Psychology, 2005. 73(2): p. 334-340.

[100] Foa, E.B., D. Hearstikeda, and K.J. Perry, *Evaluation of a brief cognitive-behavioral program for the prevention of chronic PTSD in recent assault victims.* Journal of Consulting and Clinical Psychology, 1995. 63(6): p. 948-955.

[101] Bryant, R.A., et al., *Treating acute stress disorder following mild traumatic brain injury.* American Journal of Psychiatry, 2003. 160(3): p. 585-587.

[102] Bryant, R.A., et al., *Treatment of acute stress disorder: a comparison of cognitive-behavioral therapy and supportive counseling.* Journal of Consulting and Clinical Psychology, 1998. 66(5): p. 862-866.

[103] Bryant, R.A., et al., *Treating acute stress disorder: an evaluation of cognitive behavior therapy and supportive counseling techniques.* American Journal of Psychiatry, 1999. 156(11): p. 1780-1786.

[104] Bisson, J.I., et al., *Early cognitive-behavioural therapy for post-traumatic stress symptoms after physical injury.* British Journal of Psychiatry, 2004. 184: p. 63-69.

[105] Pitman, R.K., et al., *Pilot study of secondary prevention of posttraumatic stress disorder with propranolol.* Biological Psychiatry, 2002. 51(2): p. 189-192.

[106] Stein, M.B., et al., *Pharmacotherapy to prevent PTSD: Results from a randomized controlled proof-of-concept trial in physically injured patients.* Journal of Traumatic Stress, 2007. 20(6): p. 923-932.

[107] Ironson, G., et al., *Comparison of two treatments for traumatic stress: A community-based study of EMDR and prolonged exposure.* Journal of Clinical Psychology, 2002. 58(1): p. 113-128.

[108] Rothbaum, B.O., M.C. Astin, and F. Marsteller, *Prolonged exposure versus eye movement desensitization and reprocessing (EMDR) for PTSD rape victims.* Journal of Traumatic Stress, 2005. 18(6): p. 607-616.

[109] Schnurr, P.P., et al., *Cognitive behavioral therapy for posttraumatic stress disorder in women - A randomized controlled trial.* Journal of the American Medical Association, 2007. 297(8): p. 820-830.

[110] Taylor, S., et al., *Comparative efficacy, speed, and adverse effects of three PTSD treatments: Exposure therapy, EMDR, and relaxation training.* Journal of Consulting and Clinical Psychology, 2003. 71(2): p. 330-338.

[111] Hinton, D.E., et al., *A randomized controlled trial of cognitive-behavior therapy for Cambodian refugees with treatment resistant PTSD and panic attacks: A cross-over design.* Journal of Traumatic Stress, 2005. 18(6): p. 617-629.

[112] Kubany, E.S., E.E. Hill, and J.A. Owens, *Cognitive trauma therapy for battered women with PTSD: Preliminary findings.* Journal of Traumatic Stress, 2003. 16(1): p. 81-91.

[113] Kubany, E.S., et al., *Cognitive trauma therapy for battered women with PTSD (CTT-BW).* Journal of Consulting and Clinical Psychology, 2004. 72(1): p. 3-18.

[114] Blanchard, E.B., et al., *A controlled evaluation of cognitive behaviorial therapy for posttraumatic stress in motor vehicle accident survivors.* Behaviour Research and Therapy, 2003. 41(1): p. 79-96.

[115] McDonagh, A., et al., *Randomized trial of cognitive-behavioral therapy for chronic post-traumatic stress disorder in adult female survivors of childhood sexual abuse.* Journal of Consulting and Clinical Psychology, 2005. 73(3): p. 515-524.

[116] Power, K., et al., *A controlled comparison of eye movement desensitization and reprocessing versus exposure plus cognitive restructuring versus waiting list in the treatment of post-traumatic stress disorder.* Clinical Psychology & Psychotherapy, 2002. 9(5): p. 299-318.

[117] Cottraux, J., et al., *Randomized Controlled Comparison of Cognitive Behavior Therapy with Rogerian Supportive Therapy in Chronic Post-Traumatic Stress Disorder: A 2-Year Follow-Up.* Psychotherapy and Psychosomatics, 2008. 77(2): p. 101-110.

[118] Chard, K.M., *An evaluation of cognitive processing therapy for the treatment of posttraumatic stress disorder related to childhood sexual abuse.* Journal of Consulting and Clinical Psychology, 2005. 73(5): p. 965-971.

[119] Monson, C.M., et al., *Cognitive processing therapy for veterans with military-related post-traumatic stress disorder.* Journal of Consulting and Clinical Psychology, 2006. 74(5): p. 898-907.

[120] Carlson, J.G., et al., *Eye movement desensitization and reprocessing (EDMR) treatment for combat-related posttraumatic stress disorder.* Journal of Traumatic Stress, 1998. 11(1): p. 3-24.

[121] Devilly, G.J., S.H. Spence, and R.M. Rapee, *Statistical and reliable change with eye movement desensitization and reprocessing: Treating trauma within a veteran population.* Behavior Therapy, 1998. 29(3): p. 435-455.

[122] Jensen, J.A., *An investigation of eye movement desensitization and reprocessing (EMD/R) as a treatment for posttraumatic stress disorder (PTSD) symptoms of Vietnam combat veterans.* Behavior Therapy, 1994. 25(2): p. 311-325.

[123] Marcus, S.V., P. Marquis, and C. Sakai, *Controlled study of treatment of PTSD using EMDR in an HMO setting.* Psychotherapy: Theory, Research, Practice, Training, 1997. 34(3): p. 307-315.

[124] Rothbaum, B.O., *A controlled study of eye movement desensitization and reprocessing in the treatment of posttraumatic stress disordered sexual assault victims.* Bulletin of the Menninger Clinic, 1997. 61(3): p. 317-334.

[125] Van der Kolk, B.A., et al., *A randomized clinical trial of eye movement desensitization and reprocessing (EMDR), fluoxetine, and pill placebo in the treatment of posttraumatic stress disorder: Treatment effects and long term maintenance.* Journal of Clinical Psychiatry, 2007. 68(1): p. 37-46.

[126] Scholes, C., G. Turpin, and S. Mason, *A randomised controlled trial to assess the effectiveness of providing self-help information to people with symptoms of acute stress disorder following a traumatic injury.* Behaviour Research and Therapy, 2007. 45(11): p. 2527-2536.

[127] Friedman, M.J., *Drug Treatment for PTSD*. Annals of the New York Academy of Sciences, 1997. 821(The Psychobiology of Posttraumatic Stress Disorder): p. 359-371.

[128] Brady, K., et al., *Efficacy and Safety of Sertraline Treatment of Posttraumatic Stress Disorder: A Randomized Controlled Trial*. Journal of the American Medical Association, 2000. 283(14): p. 1837-1844.

[129] Davidson, J.R.T., et al., *Multicenter, Double-blind Comparison of Sertraline and Placebo in the Treatment of Posttraumatic Stress Disorder*. Archives of General Psychiatry, 2001. 58(5): p. 485-492.

[130] Friedman, M.J., et al., *Randomized, double-blind comparison of sertraline and placebo for posttraumatic stress disorder in a Departmant of Veterans Affairs setting*. Journal of Clinical Psychiatry, 2007. 68(5): p. 711-720.

[131] Zohar, J., et al., *Double-blind placebo-controlled pilot study of sertraline in military veterans with posttraumatic stress disorder*. Journal of Clinical Psychopharmacology, 2002. 22(2): p. 190-195.

[132] Davidson, J., et al., *Venlafaxine extended release in posttraumatic stress disorder: A sertraline- and placebo-controlled study*. Journal of Clinical Psychopharmacology, 2006. 26(3): p. 259-267.

[133] Connor, K.M., et al., *Fluoxetine in post-traumatic stress disorder. Randomised, double-blind study*. The British Journal of Psychiatry, 1999. 175(1): p. 17-22.

[134] Martenyi, F., et al., *Fluoxetine versus placebo in posttraumatic stress disorder*. Journal of Clinical Psychiatry, 2002. 63(3): p. 199-206.

[135] Martenyi, F., E.B. Brown, and C.D. Caldwell, *Failed efficacy of fluoxetine in the treatment of posttraumatic stress disorder*. Journal of Clinical Psychopharmacology, 2007. 27(2): p. 166-170.

[136] Van der Kolk, B.A., et al., *Fluoxetine in post-traumatic stress disorder*. Journal of Clinical Psychiatry, 1994. 55: p. 517-522.

[137] Tucker, P., et al., *Paroxetine in the treatment of chronic posttraumatic stress disorder: Results of a placebo-controlled, flexible dosage trial*. Journal of Clinical Psychiatry, 2001. 62(11): p. 860-868.

[138] Marshall, R.D., et al., *Efficacy and Safety of Paroxetine Treatment for Chronic PTSD: A Fixed-Dose, Placebo-Controlled Study*. American Journal of Psychiatry, 2001. 158(12): p. 1982-1988.

[139] Marshall, R.D., et al., *A controlled trial of paroxetine for chronic PTSD, dissociation, and interpersonal problems in mostly minority adults*. Depression and Anxiety, 2007. 24(2): p. 77-84.

[140] Davidson, J., et al., *Treatment of Posttraumatic Stress Disorder With Venlafaxine Extended Release: A 6-Month Randomized Controlled Trial.* Archives of General Psychiatry, 2006. 63(10): p. 1158-1165.

[141] Davidson, J.R.T., et al., *Mirtazapine vs. placebo in posttraumatic stress disorder: a pilot trial.* Biological Psychiatry, 2003. 53(2): p. 188-191.

[142] Hamner, M.B., et al., *Adjunctive risperidone treatment in post-traumatic stress disorder: A preliminary controlled trial of effects on comorbid psychotic symptoms.* International Clinical Psychopharmacology, 2003. 18: p. 1-8.

[143] Bartzokis, G., et al., *Adjunctive risperidone in the treatment of chronic combat-related posttraumatic stress disorder.* Biological Psychiatry, 2005. 57(5): p. 474-479.

[144] Reich, D.B., et al., *A preliminary study of risperidone in the treatment of posttraumatic stress disorder related to childhood abuse in women.* Journal of Clinical Psychiatry, 2004. 65(12): p. 1601-1606.

[145] Rothbaum, B.O., et al., *Placebo-controlled trial of risperidone augmentation for selective serotonin reuptake inhibitor-resistant civilian posttraumatic stress disorder.* Journal of Clinical Psychiatry, 2008. 69(4): p. 520-525.

[146] Stein, M.B., N.A. Kline, and J.L. Matloff, *Adjunctive olanzapine for SSRI-resistant combat-related PTSD: A double-blind, placebo-controlled study.* American Journal of Psychiatry, 2002. 159(10): p. 1777-1779.

[147] Bryant, R.A., et al., *Treatment of acute stress disorder: a randomized controlled trial.* Archives of General Psychiatry, 2008. 65(6): p. 659-667.

[148] Sijbrandij, M., et al., *Treatment of acute posttraumatic stress disorder with brief cognitive behavioral therapy: a randomized controlled trial.* American Journal of Psychiatry, 2007. 164(1): p. 82-90.

[149] Echeburúa, E., et al., *Treatment of acute posttraumatic stress disorder in rape victims: An experimental study.* Journal of Anxiety Disorders, 1996. 10(3): p. 185-199.

Chapter 7

Using Hypnosis in the Treatment of Anxiety Disorders: Pros and Cons

Catherine Fredette, Ghassan El-Baalbaki,
Sylvain Neron and Veronique Palardy

Additional information is available at the end of the chapter

1. Introduction

In psychotherapy outcome research, many empirical studies have shown that cognitive behavioural treatments are efficacious for many disorders [1]. In a recent systematic review of 27 studies, Hofmann and Smits [2] show that cognitive behavioural therapy (CBT) has proven to be an unquestionably efficacious treatment for adult anxiety disorder when compared to both pharmacological and psychological placebos. However, they conclude that there was considerable room for improvement. Moreover, the high complexity and co-morbidity that is often found with anxiety disorders sometimes requires the use of two or more treatment methods that are flexible and adjustable to one other [3]. According to Kirsch, Lynn, and Rue [4] and Schoenberger [5], hypnosis can be integrated easily into current cognitive and behavioural interventions in clinical practice. Indeed, CBT and hypnosis share a number of aspects that render their combination natural; for example, imagery and relaxation, which are found in both techniques [6]. Hypnosis has been used effectively in a variety of medical settings (surgery, dentistry, chronic pain management, labour etc.) and several studies report its efficacy in the treatment of anxiety disorders [7-13]. A recent systematic review of randomized controlled trials concludes that current evidence is not sufficient to support the use of hypnosis as a sole treatment for anxiety [14]. However, in a meta-analysis, Kirsch, Montgomery, and Sapirstein [15] found that the addition of hypnosis to CBT substantially enhanced the treatment outcome for several problems (anxiety, obesity, pain, etc.). The addition of hypnosis to CBT helps the patient in several aspects of therapy, such as the preparation for in-vivo exposure, imagery exposure, developing coping skills, and cognitive restructuring [6, 16-18]. Moreover, patients using hypnosis effectively develop a better sense of self-efficacy, which is known to enhance self-regulation and is linked to lower psychological distress and better quality of life. Hence, hypnosis is worth exploring as an additional tool to improve traditional CBT.

In this chapter, we offer a comprehensive review of the literature regarding the use of hypnosis in the treatment of anxiety disorders. We will present evidence that supports its use or not as an adjunct treatment to CBT, also known as cognitive-behavioral hypnotherapy (CBH). We will also present evidence that does not justify its use as an independent treatment for anxiety disorders. Due to the amount of research on Post-Traumatic Stress Disorder (PTSD) and hypnosis, the reader will notice that a lot of the information will be related to PTSD. We will conclude by giving a simple guideline for practitioners interested in developing and using hypnosis as an adjunctive therapeutic tool in their practice.

2. Description and definition

Although under different names and applications, hypnosis has been depicted, described and documented in ancient civilizations (e.g. Egyptians, Greeks, Chinese, Indians, Sumerians, Persians and others) and was mostly used by healers. In his book *Ash Shifa* (Healing), Ibn Sina (Avecenna) wrote about the mind–body relationship and accepted the reality of hypnosis, naming it "al Wahm al-Amil" [19]. He differentiated it from sleep and described the impact of imagination on sensation and perception [20]. More recently, the British physician James Braid [1795-1960], who is recognized for conducting many research studies and experiments on hypnotic phenomena, coined the words *neurypnology and neuro-hypnosis* [21, 22]. In fact, he observed his patients while in trance and concluded that they were in a "nervous sleep." The Greek word for sleep is hypnos [21]. These terms were quickly transformed into the word *hypnosis*. Hypnosis lost its appeal with the rise of psychoanalysis during the first half of the 20th century [23]. Indeed, after a short interest in the practice of hypnosis, Freud abandoned and rejected the idea [21]. As a valid form of psychotherapy, hypnotherapy only regained its popularity with the advent of the First and Second World Wars [23]. During this time, psychiatrists were faced with a new disease, called *shell shock or war fatigue*, and used hypnosis as a way to relieve the symptoms [21]. Today, this disorder is known as PTSD. Subsequently, the modern study of hypnosis began to flourish. Throughout the years, hypnosis has been represented in various ways, whether good or bad, and many popular misconceptions around this phenomenon remain [22]. Indeed, people under hypnosis are sometimes viewed as robots who do things that they would not normally do [22]. Even though individuals under hypnosis are more prone to suggestions, they still remain in control of what they say and do [24]. In fact, despite the perception that experiences under hypnosis often contain automatic or involuntary actions, hypnotised patients ultimately act in congruity with their goals and in accordance with their points of view [25]. Another mistaken belief is that hypnosis is not real. However, recent scientific studies (e.g. brain imaging studies) go beyond these mainstream conceptions and expose the true nature of hypnosis and its possible uses [25].

Burrows, Stanley, and Bloom [26] describe hypnosis as a technique that induces, through relaxed and focused attention, an elevated state of suggestibility. During this state, reduction in critical thinking, reality testing and tolerance of reality distortion allow the person to experience different phenomena (vivid imagery, drug free anaesthesia, drug free analgesia, and so on) that might otherwise be hard to attain [26]. Contrary to common perceptions, hypnosis is a natural phenomenon which people experience in a lighter way several times a day [27]. Daydreaming, being so absorbed by a book or movie that you do not hear someone calling your name or absent-mindedly driving past an expressway exit are all examples of shallow hypnotic states [27]. According to the division 30 of the American Psychological Association (APA), a procedure becomes a hypnotic one when the following two components are present: an introduction in which a person is told that suggestions for imaginative experiences will come, and the first suggestion, which functions as the induction [22]. Examples of suggestions during the introduction include: "I am going to ask you to imagine some changes in the way you think and feel. Is that ok? Let's see what happens" [22]. The formulation of hypnotic suggestions is different from other types of suggestions (e.g. placebo, social influence), given the fact that it requests the patient to participate [22].The first suggestion might come directly after the introduction and is usually a suggestion to close the eyes, move the arm or hand or alter perception [22]. Given that there are many types of hypnotic suggestions, standardized scales of suggestibility can be applied before someone undergoes formal hypnotherapy to see how suggestible the person is to all kinds of hypnotic suggestions [28]. During ideomotor suggestions, a certain action, such as arm levitation occurs automatically without awareness of volitional effort by the person [28]. Challenge suggestions occur when the hypnotised person is unable to execute an act that is ordinarily under voluntary control such as bending an arm [28]. Cognitive suggestions also can be used to create various cognitive or visual distortions such as pain reduction, selective amnesia, and hallucinations [28]. These different types of suggestions were characterized by Hilgard [29] as the domain of hypnosis.

Hypnotic experiences take place in the realm of imagination of the person under hypnosis [30]. However, it is interesting to note that hypnotic mental imageries and ordinary ones do not have the same experiential qualities [30]. Indeed, the construction of a mental imagery is both intentionally and consciously created, whereas imaginary experiences under hypnosis are generally involuntary [30]. People are suggested or informed about an image and it naturally comes to them. This difference seems to be supported by the fact that neurocognitive activations differ from normal and hypnotic imaginary experiences [31]. Another characteristic of hypnotic experiences, including the ideomotor ones, is that they are cognitive in nature [30]. Indeed, participants simply experience alterations in cognitive processes such as perception and memory. People differ in their abilities to experience hypnosis and it might be that some hypnotic responses require specific underlying abilities that are not shared by everyone, or that many individual components might be needed to experience a hypnotic phenomenon [32]. The ability to dissociate, cognitive flexibility, susceptibility to suggestions, fantasy proneness, and imaginative abilities were identified as possible traits that make an individual more amenable to experience hypnosis [33-36].

3. Theories of hypnosis

Hypnotic techniques became popular long before people knew what they were and how they worked. In the past, theorists viewed hypnosis as an altered state of consciousness or trance, but the quest to find evidence of this presumed state remained fruitless [28]. Indeed, it was discovered that people can respond in a similar yet slightly diminished way to non-hypnotic suggestions, suggesting that hypnosis is just another normal experience [28]. More-over, since people under hypnosis are able to execute a full range of behaviours, theories needed to be able to encompass all of these aspects [28]. Due to the failure to explain such phenomena, several theories of hypnosis were developed, such as the psychoanalytic theo-ry, the reality-testing theory, and more recently, the cold control theory and the discrepan-cy-attribution theory [21, 37, 38]. However, toward the end of the 20th century, two theories stood out as the most researched and influential ones: the dissociative theory and the socio-cognitive theory.

Dissociative theories were first developed based on speculations about links between hyp-nosis and the phenomenon of dissociation [28]. Although a clear definition of dissociation is lacking, the first proponent of the dissociation theory described it as a split in the subunits of mental life, resulting in one or more parts left out from conscious awareness and voluntary control [39]. The neodissociative theory, developed by Hilgard, posits that hypnotic behav-iours are produced by a "division of consciousness into two or more parts" [28] in which "part of the attentive effort and planning may continue without any awareness of it all" (p.2, 40]. Additionally, these subsystems are coordinated by a higher-order executive system, the 'executive ego' [39]. According to this theory, hypnosis alters the functioning of the execu-tive ego, which tricks the mind about what is really going on. For example, when someone is asked to raise their arm under hypnosis, the executive ego might be responsible for the movement; however, because the awareness component of this has been separated into an-other part, this appears as an involuntary act to the hypnotised person [28].

Akin to dissociative theories, sociocognitive theories reject the idea that hypnosis requires an altered state of consciousness [41]. In fact, the same individualized social and cognitive variables that shape complex social behaviours are thought to determine hypnotic responses and experiences [41]. These variables are (a) a positive experience (attitudes, expectations, beliefs) with hypnosis in general, (b) good motivation to respond to suggestions, (c) clear in-dications that signal how to respond to hypnotic suggestions, and (d) implicit or explicit in-structions in which to become absorbed or to imagine suggestions provided by the hypnotist. It is thought that when all of these variables are working together in a given indi-vidual, the person is under hypnosis [25]. Moreover, sociocognitive theories state that re-sponses under hypnosis are goal-directed and that hypnotised people continue to act according to their aims and values, just as they ordinarily behave according to a socialized role [42]. Finally, rather than being attributed to an altered state of mind, the enhanced re-sponses seen in people under hypnosis are merely a reflection of increased motivation and expectations [42].

Beyond differences and resulting controversy steaming from the dissociative and sociocognitive theory perspectives, new findings from psychophysiological and brain imaging studies have allowed the scientific community to support the hypothesis that experiences under hypnosis are "genuine" [24]. Indeed, studies demonstrated that there are distinctive patterns of activation (anterior cingulate cortex and frontal cortical areas) attributable to hypnosis and that these patterns comprise mechanisms used in other familiar cognitive tasks (focused attention, imagination, absorption) [24, 31]. Furthermore, there are specific psychophysiological correlates for suggested experiences [24, 31]. Some studies demonstrated that there is a qualitative distinction between neurocognitive activations that occur when people are asked to imagine certain images under hypnosis and in ordinary conditions [31]. Also, the hypnotic experiences appear to create brain states closer to the real experience, a phenomenon corroborated by the subjective reports of individuals [31]. Finally, brain imaging and psychophysiological studies might also enrich our understanding of the respective contribution of the social context, the subject's aptitudes, expectations, and intrasubjective experience of hypnotic phenomena.

4. The clinical use of hypnosis

4.1. Medical conditions

4.1.1. Hypnosis alone

Thus far, the value of hypnosis has already been recognized for many physical and medical conditions. Indeed, in 1996, the National Institute of Health Technology Assessment Panel Report considered hypnosis as a viable and effective solution to treat pain associated with cancer and many other chronic pain conditions [43]. It was even found that in certain conditions, the degree of analgesia resulting from hypnosis matched or even exceeded that provided by morphine [43]. These findings are supported by the results of Montgomery, DuHamel, and Redd's[44] meta-analytic review, which found that 75% of the people experienced pain reduction due to hypnosis, and these reductions were found in both a clinical and a healthy population. In their review of the literature, Neron and Stephenson [45] also present evidence on the effectiveness of hypnotherapy for emesis, analgesia, and anxiolysis in acute pain. Montgomery et al. [46] found that when compared to empathic listening, presurgery hypnosis was more effective in reducing pain intensity and pain unpleasantness for breast cancer patients. In addition to reducing the pain associated with cancer, hypnosis was also found to effectively reduce the affective morbidities (anxiety, discomfort, and emotional upset) associated with the medical procedures [46-48], as well as reduce fatigue [46, 49], sleep problems [49], nausea [46] and the quantity of medication needed [46]. Similar results (reduction in pain, anxiety and medication and better satisfaction) were found for plastic surgery patients [50], severe burn care patients [51], women giving birth [52], breast biopsy patients [53] and patients undergoing dental procedures [54]. Hypnosis also served as a sole anaesthetic ingredient for thousands of surgeries [43]. Other medical conditions that have been found to be responsive to hypnosis are preoperative preparations for surgery, a subgroup of patients with asthma, dermatological disorders, irritable bowel syndrome, hemophillia, post-chemotherapy nausea and emesis (Pinnell & Covino(2000) cited in 43). Of note is that in the medical environment, clinical hypnosis is provided as an adjunct to medical treatment. There is usually no time for multiple sessions based on skills acquisition and homework. Intervention is often provided at bedside, or in preparation and during medical procedures away from the usual office-based psychotherapy setting. The goal of care is often symptom relief and comfort during the medical procedure and not psychological therapeutic change, which is typically the end point of psychotherapy. Hypnosis is used because it is efficacious but most importantly it is practical (short: minimal practice, no homework or assignments; portable: self-hypnosis)[1].

4.1.2. CBH As an adjunct to CBT

Kirsch et al. [15] reported substantial effect sizes for problems such as weight loss, pain, anxiety, and insomnia. More specifically, it was found to be particularly effective for the treatment of obesity [15, 56]. Indeed, long-term weight loss was maintained at follow-ups, which is an issue for most people who gain their weight back soon after losing it [15]. In their review of the literature, Chambless and Ollendick [57] even identified hypnosis (in conjunction with CBT) as an empirically supported therapy for obesity, along with headaches and irritable bowel syndrome [57]. A study done with women suffering from chronic breast cancer pain revealed that cognitive hypnotherapy or CBH was effective not only in reducing pain, but also in decreasing pain over time as the cancer progressed [58]. As for cigarette smoking, many studies assessing the use of hypnosis as an adjunct to cognitive-behavioural interventions found good results [59], with the rate of abstinence varying from 31 to 91% at the end of treatment and 31 to 87% around the three-four month follow-ups [56]. However, these results should be interpreted with caution, as some research demonstrated considerable limitations such as the exclusive use of self-reports, small sample sizes, a lack of differentiation between hypnosis and relaxation techniques and no clear definition of cigarette smoking [56]. More recently, some studies using more reliable approaches showed promising results in the use of hypnosis for cigarette smoking. Indeed, results indicate that after treatment, at three month, six month and 12 month follow-ups, more participants in the hypnosis group were abstinent [60, 61]. Rather than using CBH, these studies either compared hypnosis to behavioural treatment or to a waiting-list control group. Hypnosis appears to be a promising avenue for many physiological and psychological problems but most importantly, hypnosis is a cost-effective alternative procedure [43]. However, as Schoenberger's review [62] indicates, more rigorous

---

1 Flory & Lang provide examples and data supporting this type of hypnotic intervention used as a flexible and practical tool to alleviate pain, anxiety, and treatment side effects while potentially reducing the need for sedation and stabilizing the vital signs [55].

methodologies as well as more studies comparing specifically the added benefit of hypnosis to CBT are needed to determine its real effects.

4.2. Anxiety disorders

4.2.1. Social anxiety disorder

The essential feature of social anxiety disorder (SAD) or social phobia is an important and persistent fear or worry about social and performance situations [63]. Social phobia can be divided into two types: generalized, in which individuals fear most social situations (e.g. having a conversation, facing authority, speaking in front of people and so on); and specific, when individuals only fear one particular situation (e.g. eating in front of people). According to different studies, the prevalence of SAD ranges from three to 13 % of the population. In their review of five meta-analyses that looked specifically at the treatment of SAD, Rodebaugh, Holaway, and Heimberg [64] found that CBT appears to provide benefits for adults diagnosed with SAD, with modest to large effect sizes when compared to waiting-list control, as well as moderate to large effect sizes from pre to post-treatment.

Hypnosis as a sole treatment. To our knowledge, there is only one randomized controlled trial testing the use of hypnosis as a sole treatment for social phobia. In early attempts to view the potential of hypnosis to treat social anxiety, Stanton [65] randomized 60 adults seeking help for handling their anxiety. Anxiety levels were assessed by the Willoughby Questionnaire. The author compared a hypnotic procedure consisting of positive suggestions and mental imagery to another group that listened to quiet music (movements from Mozart symphonies) and to a control group. Both experimental groups met in their respective groups for 30 minutes for three weeks. At the end of treatment, both experimental groups experienced a significant reduction in their anxiety, whereas the control group saw minor changes in their anxiety levels. Moreover, the reduction for the hypnosis group was larger. Finally, the therapeutic gains were maintained for the hypnosis group only at six month follow-ups. Although these results were encouraging, this study presented many limitations such as the fact that there was no statistical calculation of the difference between the hypnosis and music groups and that the validity of the instrument was not presented. One case report also indicated that hypnosis was useful in treating social phobia [66]. Although hypnosis was used as a sole treatment, the author pointed out that the patient had experience with typical phobia treatments such as systematic imaginal and in-vivo exposure and that this familiarity might have contributed to the successful outcome.

CBH. Schoenberger, Kirsch, Gearan, Montgomery, and Pastyrnak [67] conducted a randomized controlled study on public speaking anxiety in which they compared the efficacy of CBT to the same therapy combined with hypnosis and a waiting-list control group. The experimental treatments included cognitive restructuring and in-vivo exposure. The hypnosis component consisted of replacing relaxation training by hypnotic inductions and suggestions [67]. In terms of self-report measures of public speaking anxiety, both experimental treatments produced a reduction in anxiety compared to the control group. As for the subjective and behavioural measures of fear, only the hypnotic group differed significantly from the control group. These measures were taken by a blind observer during a impromptu speech that participants gave in front of two observers. Finally, the mean effect sizes calculated across the dependant measures revealed a significant difference between the two experimental groups in favor of the hypnotic treatment (mean effect for the nonhypnotic treatment is 0.80 standard deviation and 1.25 standard deviation for the hypnotic treatment, $t(5) = 3.75$, $p < .05$) [67].

4.2.2. Specific phobias

A phobia is characterized by a marked and persistent fear prompted by the presence or anticipation of an encounter with a specific object or situation [63]. This situation can create a sensation of panic, somatic manifestations of anxiety, fainting or even trigger a panic attack in the phobic person. According to the DSM-IV-TR [63], there are 5 subtypes of phobias: animal type, natural environment type, situational type, blood-injection-injury type, and other type, which includes all phobias that do not fit in the previous categories. The lifetime prevalence rate varies from 7.2 to 11.3%. CBT procedures (including in vivo-exposure and systematic desensitization) are considered the treatments of choice for specific phobias [68]. Even though these techniques apply to most phobias, certain ones require specific adaptation such as the applied tension technique for blood-injury-injection phobias [68].

Hypnosis as a sole treatment. We found two randomized controlled studies that utilized hypnosis as a stand-alone treatment for specific phobias. In the first one, Hammarstrand, Berggren, and Hakeberg [69] compared a group of women with dental phobias using two types of experimental treatments: a behavioural treatment based on psychophysiological principles, and hypnotherapy. The psychophysiological treatment consisted of progressive relaxation, videos of dental scenes and biofeedback training. As for the hypnotherapy, the participants were told to imagine different dental scenes, which corresponded to the videos of the psychophysiological group, and received suggestions. In addition, a control group who received general anaesthesia was added. Unlike the rest of the participants, this group was not randomized. The results showed that only the psychophysiological group experienced a significant reduction in anxiety. However, no significant difference between the two experimental and control groups was found. It should be noted that out of the 22 participants in this study, only 13 completed the treatments (eight in the psychophysiological treatment, five in hypnotherapy) and thus the sample was too small to draw real conclusions. Moreover, since the control group was not randomized, there is the possibility that these participants were different from the other two groups. In an exploratory study of four people suffering from specific phobias (i.e. fear of flying, snakes, driving, and heights), Llobet [21] assessed the effectiveness of group hypnotherapy. The hypnotherapy consisted of imaginary exposure with the use of the "magic bubble technique "[2], as well as the age regression technique[3] [21]. The author stated that behavioural techniques expose patients to the avoided stimuli in a "here and now" context [21]. Although these techniques have been proven efficacious, therapy should employ self-exploration in order for patients to understand their unique conscious and unconscious processes [21]. Age regression hypnotherapy can thus solve this problem [21]. Results of this study indicated that all participants saw their anxiety reduced in a significant way. Even though the participants' anxiety increased slightly at the two-week follow-up, participants still experienced on average a 56.46% decrease compared to their baseline score. The benefits of the group therapy might have been enhanced if it was combined with other well-recognized methods for treating phobias – a focus for future research.

CBH. As for the integration of hypnosis with CBT or behavioural protocols for specific phobias, we found several case reports and case studies and only one randomized controlled trial. Recently, Forbes [71] compared the relative effectiveness of systematic desensitization with hypnosis to the same treatment with relaxation in the management of animal phobias. His results showed that patients in the hypnosis group enjoyed greater anxiety reduction than the other group. Finally, case studies also corroborated the effectiveness of CBH for driving phobia [72], animal phobia [73], and airplane phobia [74]. This evidence tends to support the use of CBH as an effective therapy for different types of phobias.

4.2.3. Panic disorder with or without agoraphobia

The main feature of Panic Disorder with or without Agoraphobia (PD/A) is the presence of recurrent, unexpected panic attacks, accompanied by persistent concerns about having other panic attacks, worry about the possible implications or consequences of panic attacks, or a significant behavioural change related to the attacks [63]. As for panic attacks, they are discrete periods of intense fear or discomfort that are accompanied by both physical and cognitive symptoms such as heart palpitations, hyperventilation, dizziness, a fear of losing control or going crazy, depersonalization and so on. People who suffer from PD sometimes develop agoraphobia, which is an anxiety related to being in places or situations in which escape might be difficult or impossible and help difficult to receive. In community samples, rates vary between one and two percent, although higher rates [3.5%) were found in some studies (75]. When treating PDA, both the Canadian Psychological Association (CPA) and the APA recognize CBT as the first line of treatment [76]. Indeed, efficacious and robust treatment effects of this therapy have been verified across a variety of treatment settings for extended follow-up periods.

Hypnosis as a sole treatment or in conjunction with other non- cognitive and behavioural techniques. The use of hypnotic techniques to treat PD/A was successfully identified in some case reports [77-79]. Hypnotic techniques such as age regression, hypnoanalysis[4] [77], ego-strength-

---

2 In order to render exposures less distressing, patients under hypnosis are suggested to imagine themselves in a magic bubble when they revisit their feared object or situation, which acts as a protection.

3 During age regression, the person is guided back in time to a past experience in order to relive it, or the person can also be suggested to remember the experience in a here-and-now as vividly as possible [70].

ening suggestions [78], and the use of medication in conjunction in one case [79] led most patients to become panic free. However, no controlled trial studies could be found on hypnosis alone.

CBH. In the only controlled trial study on the efficacy of CBH in treating PDA, Dyck and Spinhoven [80] demonstrated that a combined therapy (self-hypnosis and exposure) was not superior to exposure alone in terms of time spent by agoraphobics walking on a prescribed route. In this case, the hypnotic technique employed was imaginary exposure plus suggestions from the therapist consisting of successful encounters with the feared situation (prescribed route). One problem with this study is that it used a cross-over design (exposure alone and then combined/ combined followed by exposure alone) and thus the eventuality that patients still continued to use hypnosis during the exposures alone cannot be ruled out. Thus, reservations must be kept in mind with regard to these latter results. Interestingly, the authors also found that preference for treatment shifted toward the combined treatment as the study went on [80]. Positive results for CBH were demonstrated in many case reports [18, 81, 82]. Indeed, hypnosis was found to enhance CBT protocols by facilitating exposures to both the symptoms of panic and situational anxiety. Moreover, it also was found to be successful in conjunction with Rational Emotive therapy (RE).

4.2.4. *Generalized anxiety disorder*

People who suffer from Generalized Anxiety Disorder (GAD) experience excessive and hardly controllable worry and anxiety most of the time. Contrary to some other anxiety disorders where the anxiety is focused on a specific event or thing (e.g. specific phobia), GAD individuals worry about different situations and activities. Many individuals also develop somatic symptoms such as muscle tension, nausea, and sweating. In community samples, approximately three percent of the population will develop GAD [63]. As for the treatment of GAD, traditional narrative reviews and meta-analyses have consistently found that CBT and applied relaxation are the most efficacious treatments [83].

Hypnosis as a sole treatment. Recently, a study investigated hypnosis as an alternative method for CBT in the treatment of GAD [27]. The hypnosis component was comprised of suggestions involving the lessening of anxiety. Based on the Beck Anxiety Inventory (BAI) scores of 60 patients, the author stated that there was evidence of hypnosis being as effective as CBT in the treatment of GAD [27]. These results were derived from the archived records of a local licensed mental health therapist's private practice. Although these results are positive, the patients were not randomized to the treatments but rather assigned to treatment based on their own desire to receive hypnotherapy or CBT. It is thus safer to say that hypnosis was as effective as CBT for patients who believed in and wished to be treated with hypnotherapy. Also, since this was a retrospective study, many aspects such as the number of sessions, and the integrity of therapy could not be controlled for.

---

4 Hypnoanalysis is a mix of hypnosis and psychoanalytic techniques

CBH. In a pilot randomized controlled study of 10 patients, Allen [84] assessed the compara-ble efficacy of a treatment incorporating CBT, hypnosis, and biofeedback to a waiting-list control group. All patients in the experimental group demonstrated a reduction in both trait and state anxiety. Most of them (four out of five) even obtained post-test state anxiety scores below the normative range. As for the control group, their anxiety remained at a clinically significant level [84]. CBH also came out as a successful aid in the treatment of GAD, as demonstrated by Baker's [85] case report.

4.2.5. Obsessive-compulsive disorder

Obsessive-Compulsive Disorder's (OCD) main features are recurrent obsessions and/or compulsions that are so severe that they are time-consuming and/or cause distress to the person. Obsessions may be persistent ideas, thoughts, impulses or images that can be relat-ed to many different topics such as contamination, religion, symmetry and repeated doubts. As for compulsions, they are repetitive behaviours or mental acts that people perform in or-der to diminish the anxiety associated with their obsessions. The estimated lifetime preva-lence of OCD is 2.5% [63]. In a recent review of the literature, Podea, Suciu, Suciu, and Ardelean [86] concluded that CBT is an effective treatment for OCD, that it is at least as ef-fective as medication and that it demonstrates good benefits at follow-ups.

CBH. So far, hypnosis has occupied a relatively restricted role in the treatment of OCD [87] and this is reflected in the few numbers of studies on this topic. Indeed, no well con-trolled studies on the efficacy of CBH have been completed so far to see the additive ef-fect of hypnosis to CBT [88]. Rather, the hypnosis literature only contains descriptions of clinical work done with a minimal number of patients and a series of case studies usual-ly unaccompanied by measurable data. Still, as a combination to CBT, hypnosis was found to be efficacious in many case reports and one case study [88-92]. For example, be-cause his patient did not respond to CBT and medication, Frederick [88] developed an in-tervention in which CBT and hypnoanalysis were incorporated. The hypnosis part was mainly aimed at the resolution of the dissociative symptoms. Other authors used hypno-sis during exposures (e.g. exposure-response prevention, flooding) in order to enhance its effect, relieve anxiety and ameliorate the patients' affect regulation [90-92]. Very recently, Meyerson and Konichezky [87] presented three single-case reports in which hypnotically-induced dissociation (HID) combined with CBT protocols was successfully used in order to treat patients with OCD. According to Yapko [93], HID is the ability to split a fully and unified experience into many different components, while amplifying awareness of one part and diminishing awareness of the others. For example, some patients report that they cannot recognize themselves without their disorder. HID can thus be used to help the person dissociate him or herself from the disorder and amplify their feeling of experienc-ing life without the disorder.

4.2.6. Post-traumatic stress disorder

In the DSM-IV-TR [63], PTSD is described as the development of characteristic symptoms after an individual is exposed to an extreme traumatic stressor (A1). The traumatic event must put at risk the physical integrity of the individual or others and the person's response must involve intense fear, helplessness, or horror (A2). The characteristic symptoms of PTSD include (B) stress and hyperarousal, (C) persistent avoidance of situations or reminders of the trauma and (D) vivid experiences of being back in the midst of the traumatic event, which are often referred to as a *flashback*. Finally, (E) these symptoms must last for at least one month. If the time is less than that, the diagnostic is labelled as Acute Stress Disorder (ASD). PTSD lifetime prevalence rates are approximately eight percent. In high risk populations such as veterans, these rates may rise to as high as 30% [94]. In terms of treatment, variations of CBT protocols such as cognitive processing therapy (CPT) and prolonged exposure are known to effectively treat PTSD symptoms [95].

Among all of the anxiety disorders, the addition of hypnosis to CBT in the treatment of PTSD is the most studied. This interest has been triggered by factors such as the evidence that PTSD patients seem to be more highly hypnotisable when compared to the general population and other patient populations [96-98]. Butler, Duran, Jasiukaitis, Koopman et al. [99] developed a diathesis-stress model of dissociation to explain this phenomenon which is that "highly hypnotisable/dissociative people would be more likely to develop posttraumatic/dissociative conditions rather than other psychiatric conditions". Evidence in support of this model are the fact that higher scores on hypnotisability scales are associated with avoidance symptoms, which is a core aspect of PTSD [96] as well as with better therapeutic success [100]. However, research is needed to exclude the possibility that it is the development and maintenance of PTSD that create a state of high hypnotisability. Moreover, clinical findings seem to suggest that there is a similarity in phenomenology between PTSD symptoms and the experience of hypnosis [101]. For example, during hypnosis, the person is entirely focused and absorbed into the suggestions and this absorption is also evidenced in PTSD sufferers, who sometimes focus so intensely on their traumatic memories that they are able to create physical and emotional responses. Another common factor is the phenomenon of dissociation, which can occur both during and after the trauma. Finally, both PTSD and hypnosis are experiences in which the person is hyper-responsive to both their environment (social, physical cues) and internal cues [101]. Because traditional interventions are mostly aimed at targeting the core symptoms of PTSD, the interest in hypnosis was also prompted by the fact that as a flexible form of treatment, it might be able to target important symptoms such as sleep and dream disturbance, pain, and emotional and anxiety withdrawal problems associated with traumas [100, 102].

Hypnosis as a sole treatment or in conjunction with relaxation training. A recent randomized controlled study tested the hypothesis that hypnosis could help relieve the cluster of hyperarousal symptoms in PTSD, in a group of women who had experienced sexual trauma [103]. This study compared the use of a hypnotic induction (Elkins Hypnotisability Scale) to a standard care intervention, which was a combination of supportive counselling, CBT, interpersonal therapy, and solution-focused technique [103]. Following the initial induction, a hypnotic induction recording for subjects in the treatment group was given to use at home over a period of one week. The author reported a statistically significant decrease in hyperarousal symptoms, general anxiety, and difficulty concentrating for the hypnotic group [103]. However, participants did not fall under the clinically significant line, and on many measures there was no significant difference between the control and treatment group. Some noticeable limitations of this study were that even though the groups were randomized, some of the baseline symptoms of the hypnosis group were more severe than that of the control group, which might explain the small differences between the two groups on some measures at the end of treatment. [103]. Even though it was the study's goal to create a short treatment, it came out that one week was probably too short of an interval to see the real effects of hypnosis and reach clinically significant results. It would have been interesting to see the added benefit of hypnosis to the standard treatment over a longer period of time. Moreover, in this study, there was minimal use of hypnosis. Indeed, the hypnotic induction did not include any suggestions to treat aspects of PTSD.

As part of their symptoms, PTSD sufferers often complain about sleep problems [17]. Some studies indicated that hypnosis can be helpful in reducing time to sleep onset in a group of individuals with chronic insomnia [104, 105]. A meta-analysis of 59 outcome studies also demonstrated that the short-term effects of hypnosis (one-two months) and relaxation training were comparable to the effects of short-term drug therapy and that the long-term outcomes even surpassed the drug therapy in certain instances [106]. Abramowitz, Barak, Ben-Avi, and Knobler [107] studied a group of chronic combat-related PTSD sufferers who experienced sleep problems even though they received supportive therapy and serotonin reuptake inhibitors (SSRIs). The participants had difficulty falling asleep as well as maintaining sleep and reported night terrors. The authors compared the efficacy of two weeks of one-and-a-half hour hypnotherapy sessions with the drug therapy Zolpidem to see the effects on PTSD symptoms and sleep problems. They found that in addition to see a reduction in the major PTSD symptoms, the hypnotic group reported better sleep quality, fewer awakenings, and less morning sleepiness.

CBH. There are many recent instances of case studies and reports that describe the success of hypnosis in conjunction with CBT for traumas associated with industrial accidents [108-110], motor-vehicle accident [111], sexual abuse and rape trauma [112-114], spouse abuse-related trauma [101, 114-116] and assault-related trauma [117]. For example, Degun-Mather [118] [119] reported the success of hypnosis in conjunction with CBT in two cases of patients suffering from different traumas (childhood and war). Hypnotherapy was used in order to activate and reconstruct the traumatic memories. On a larger scale, Brom, Kleber, and Defares [120] compared the effectiveness of four psychotherapeutic methods for the treatment of PTSD in 112 patients: hypnotherapy based on behavioural techniques, trauma desensitization, psychodynamic treatment, and a waiting-list control group, and determined that the treatment groups were significantly lower in trauma-related symptoms than the control group. However, the authors of the original study reported that there was still a lot of similarity between the three treatment conditions which could be due to similarities in the behaviours of the therapists, which they did not measure directly. No statistical measures were presented to compare the active treatment groups. In their systematic review, Coelho, Canter, and Ernst [14] reanalyzed the data and found that on some measures (STAI-S, STAI-T, IES), the hypnotic group obtained statistically better results compared to the other treatment groups both at post-test and follow-up. Bryant et al.'s [121] randomized study compared the effectiveness of CBT, hypnosis and CBT, and social counselling for trauma survivors who suffer from ASD. The rationale behind their study was that hypnotic techniques might be able to breach dissociative symptoms of ASD [121]. A hypnotic induction was thus given right before imaginal exposure, in an attempt to ease the emotional processing of the traumatic memories [121]. Their results indicated that at post-treatment and follow-ups (six months, three years), fewer patients in the CBT (2.11%) and hypnosis with CBT group (4.22%[5]) met criteria for PTSD [121]. Also, hypnosis with CBT resulted in fewer re-experiencing symptoms than CBT alone at post-treatment, but this difference was not found at follow-up [121]. Even though these results are positive, the authors used hypnosis in only one aspect of their therapy (imaginary exposure). Hypnosis has many functions and is exploitable in many parts of therapy (which will be described in details below) and thus a broader application of it might have generated more additive gains and yielded clearer results. Moreover, the literature on hypnosis and PTSD is filled with examples of how hypnosis can be used specifically in the treatment of PTSD, so that its benefits can be enhanced. For further reading, see Lynn et al. [17] and Degun-Mather [119].

Recently, a new hypnotic technique called hypnotherapeutic olfactory conditioning (HOC) showed promising potential in the treatment of PTSD. Based on CBT protocols, HOC is a technique that helps patients create new olfactory associations in order to surmount anxieties and dissociative states [102]. More precisely, it is the "development, under hypnosis, of a positive olfactory association which allows the patient to regain control of their symptoms, especially when they were created by olfactory stimuli" (p.317 102). This technique is based on the notion that the sense of smell has the ability to create vivid memories due to the particular position of the olfactory bulb in the brain [102]. In an exploratory study of three individuals suffering from needle phobia, panic disorder and PTSD respectively, Abramowitz and Lichtenberg [122] found a marked reduction in the symptoms, as attested by the rating scales and reduction in the use of medication. In a prospective study testing HOC with 36 patients suffering from chronic PTSD, results demonstrated significant reductions in symptoms, as assessed by the Impact of Events Scale (IES–R), Beck Depression Inventory, and Dissociative Experiences Scale [102]. The gains were maintained at six month and one year follow-ups. In this study, the authors did not compare the direct added benefits of HOC to standard protocols. However, the fact that most patients had already been in therapy for a mean time of more than two years and that baseline symptoms presented significant psychopathology indicates that HOC was able to provide additional benefits to the therapy. Still, replication studies are needed for HOC.

---

5 results for 3 year follow-up.

4.2.7. Other anxiety-related problems

Hypnosis as a sole treatment. A 1978 study looked at the difference between two non-pharmacological interventions in the treatment of what was then called "anxiety neurosis". The two treatments were either a meditational relaxation technique comprised of muscle relaxation and concentration on inner breathing and stillness, or a self-hypnosis treatment, also comprised of muscle relaxation and suggestions to send tingling feelings and light to the parts of the body where anxiety symptoms were manifested [123].The participants were tested on levels of hypnotisability and were then separated into two groups: medium-high hypnotisable subjects and low hypnotisable subjects. Then, the participants in each group were randomized to one of the two experimental treatments. Although more participants in the hypnotic group improved according to the Hamilton Anxiety Rating Scale, the results indicated that there was essentially no difference between the two techniques in terms of therapeutic efficacy [123]. However, participants in the medium-high group, independently of the type of treatment, significantly improved on the psychiatric assessment and demonstrated a decrease in their average systolic blood pressure [123]. One major limitation of this study is that at the beginning, the authors randomized 69 people to the four treatment conditions, however, 37 of them did not complete the protocol. Thus, in addition to providing no results on the drop-outs, the benefits of randomization cannot be assumed in this study. Moreover, the hypnosis treatment was very similar in content to the meditational group, which can explain the minute difference between the two. Stanton [124] randomly assigned a group of 40 students to either a self-hypnosis training group or a control group, which consisted of discussions on ways to reduce test anxiety. The participants were matched on sex and anxiety scores. After two sessions and at a six month follow-up, anxiety scores were significantly reduced for the hypnotic group only. More recently, O'Neill, Barnier, and McConkey [125] compared self-hypnosis training with progressive relaxation in a group of stressed, anxious, and worried patients. At a one month follow-up, both groups indicated significant improvement on the Beck Anxiety Inventory (BAI-State and Trait) but no significant difference was found between these two groups on the BAI. However, the hypnosis group surpassed the relaxation group on cognitive changes and perceptions of treatment efficacy [125]. Indeed, the hypnosis patients reported superior expectations of the success of therapy [125]. A closer look at the procedures revealed that the content of the instructions given to both groups were very similar. These results seem to indicate that the simple fact of defining certain aspects of therapy *hypnosis* provided confidence and better expectation in patients [16]. Finally, in an attempt to determine the effectiveness of hypnosis on test anxiety, Hyman [126] randomized 21 participants to a hypnotic-induction only group, a post-suggestion hypnotic group or a control group. The participants received only one session of hypnosis and the post-hypnotic suggestions consisted of suggestions for reduction of test anxiety [126]. The results showed that directly after the inductions, there was no significant difference between the three groups, as evidenced by the Test Anxiety Inventory (TAI). At one month follow-up though, a significant difference was observed between the post-hypnotic group and the control group in terms of anxiety. The post-hypnotic suggestion group was also the only group who experienced a significant decrease in test anxiety over time (between post and follow-up assessments). Although the sample size of this study was very small, this seems to indicate that post-hypnotic suggestions might be one of the active ingredients of hypnosis CBH.

A study comparing the effects of two hypnotic procedures (imagery and cognitive restructuring under hypnosis versus hypnotic induction only) with two control groups (attention placebo and no treatment) on the treatment of test anxiety supports the idea that the combination of hypnosis and CBT offers more therapeutic gains [127]. Indeed, results indicate that while the induction-only group had more improvements than the two control groups, only the group receiving imagery and cognitive restructuring under hypnosis obtained significant results on anxiety and academic performance [127].

4.2.8. Summary and conclusions on the clinical use of hypnosis

To date, except for PTSD, there is a very small number of randomized controlled studies assessing the impact of CBH for the treatment of anxiety disorders, which limits the conclusions that can be drawn about its external validity. However, the results presented above still indicate that CBH is a promising treatment modality. Indeed, in addition to demonstrating its efficacy as a complete intervention to reduce anxiety symptoms, all studies that compared the additive effect of hypnosis found positive results, except for one. As stated before, this study used a cross-over design which might explain the lack of superiority for the combined group (exposure and hypnosis). Also, Mellinger [128] and Scrignar [91] reported the success of hypnosis as a valuable adjunct to render exposure practices more viable. Finally, using non-leading methods, Degun-Mather [118] reported the successful use of hypnosis to transform the fragmented memories of a war veteran who suffered from chronic PTSD and dissociative fugues into a complete narrative, leading to re-appraisal and re-structuring of the trauma. As for the evidence supporting hypnosis as a stand-alone treatment, results are mixed. Indeed, some of the case reports and studies presented above found positive results [21, 27]. On the other hand, in 2003, the STEER [129] looked at four randomized controlled trials of hypnotherapy as a sole therapy for anxiety, coming to the conclusion that there was insufficient evidence regarding the efficacy of hypnotherapy and that it did not appear to be more effective than other treatments. In their conclusion, the authors of the STEER report also mentioned that the general quality of all studies was unsatisfactory. All of them presented major methodological flaws, such as a lack of established questionnaires, no use of imagery or suggestions during hypnosis, small sample sizes and no clear indications of qualification of competence of the therapists. This again renders it difficult to draw firm conclusions. More recently, a systematic review of controlled trial studies revealed that hypnosis as a sole treatment for anxiety was not superior than control conditions (waiting list controls, contact controls, or other non-standard treatments) [14], and though it is a powerful supportive tool, using it as a therapy by itself is an error [130]. Research on clinical hypnosis should reflect the clinical practice in psychotherapy, [56] and thus hypnosis should be viewed and studied as an adjunct to commonly used and recognized techniques. In fact, hypnotic technique can directly reinforce CBT strategies by helping patients to control and regulate the anxiety as well as the cognitive and attentional processes characteristic of many

Disorders	Hypnosis alone	CBH
Social anxiety disorder	Good outcomes [65-66]	Good outcomes [67]
	Significant reduction in anxiety at post-test and superiority of hypnosis at six-month follow-ups [66]	CBH more efficacious than CBT alone
Specific phobias	Mixed results [21][69]	CBH and HOC as an effective treatment [71-74]
	Significance was reached in the Llobet study [21] but not in the Stanton study [69]	CBH provided better results than CBT alone [71] HOC allowed patient to face the phobic situation with success [122]
Panic disorder with or without agoraphobia	Generally good results [77-79]	Mixed results [18][80-82][122]
	Only based on case studies and reports. Intensity of episodes is reduced while other patients are panic-free	No superiority of CBH compared to CBT in one study, but patients received both treatments in a cross-over design, which limits the conclusions [80] Effective relief of symptoms found in other studies [18][81-82][122]
Generalized anxiety disorder	Good outcomes [29]	Good outcomes [84-85]
	Hypnosis as effective as CBT (no randomization)	Most patients in hypnosis and CBT group obtained anxiety scores below the normative ranges at post-test [84]
Obsessive-compulsive disorder	Not applicable	Good results [88-92]
		Based on case reports
Post traumatic stress disorder	Good outcomes [103-107]	Good outcomes [102][108-122]
	Statistically significant reduction in hyperarousal symptoms but results did not reach clinical significance [103] Hypnosis effective for treating sleep problems [104-105] and equivalent or better than drugs [106-107]	CBH superior to CBT and other techniques on some measures [120-121] HOC found to be effective in reducing symptoms at post-test [102][122] and six-month follow-ups [102]
Other anxiety-related problems	Mixed results [123-126]	Good outcome [127]
	Improvement but no indication that hypnosis as a sole treatment is more efficacious than other methods or no treatment, except for one study [124]. Superiority only stood out at one-month follow-up in another study [126]	Superiority of CBH over hypnosis alone and control groups

Table 1.

anxiety disorders [87]. One point to note, however, is that the boundaries between hypnosis as a stand-alone treatment and as an adjunct are sometimes unclear, as some people view a hypnotic induction followed by suggestions as CBT in itself [14]. For a summary table of the data presented above, see table 1.

5. Guidelines and benefits of the application of hypnosis to CBT protocols

5.1. How to integrate hypnosis to CBT components

As a psychosocial treatment, CBT has roots in both the cognitive and behavioural traditions and is based on the idea that our thoughts influence our feelings and behaviours [131]. Important components of CBT include relaxation training, exposure (both imaginal and in-vivo), cognitive restructuring, the building of coping skills, ego-strengthening, and self-efficacy. In the following, based on what several authors described (William, Bryant, Lynn and colleagues, Alladin, Degun-Mather), we will report a summary of how hypnosis can enhance each of these components [6, 16, 17, 23, 119]

Developing a good therapeutic alliance and motivation toward the therapy. The benefits of adding hypnosis to standard treatments of anxiety are manifold. The basis of therapy is the development of a good therapeutic alliance. The goal-directed and generally positive environment surrounding hypnosis may promote a better rapport with the therapist, as well as enhance treatment adherence [17]. For example, successful experiences of facing fears under hypnosis can foster trust in the hypnotherapist [23]. Moreover, positive views toward hypnosis might increase confidence in the effectiveness of therapy for certain patients [17].

Developing a sense of self-efficacy and heightened ego strengthening. Hypnotic techniques such as Ego strengthening are used to foster self-efficacy, self-esteem and self-assurance in patients. Self-efficacy provides a better quality of life, self-regulation and control and is one of the essential components in the successful treatment of anxiety disorders [23].

Self-control. Similarly, a great advantage of hypnosis is that it creates a feeling in the patients that they are in control of their difficulties, instead of being at the mercy of their symptoms [132]. Indeed, people learn to surmount their fears in trance and obtain cognitive reinforcement of their ability to cope [18].

Relaxation training. Relaxation techniques are an integral part of CBT as they help patients control their feelings of anxiety and tension [133]. For example, with the high level of arousal that PTSD patients tend to display, it can become difficult for them to fully participate in their therapy [17]. Many hypnotic techniques can serve to soothe patients and help them build personal resources [17]. For example, the patients can be taught relaxation techniques and learn the use of a safe place imaginary technique, which they can further practice by themselves using self-hypnosis [17]. Other relaxation techniques may include deep breathing, muscular relaxation and suggestions for relaxation. Hypnosis can be utilized easily in conjunction with all of these techniques.

Imaginal exposure. Imagery is used by many CBT clinicians to facilitate anxiety reduction. The purposes of imagery are twofold: first, it can be utilized to induce relaxation by suggesting soothing and relaxing images to the patient. Secondly, imagery can be helpful for imaginal exposures, which is what is used to treat anxiety-provoking memories, images or thoughts. It consists of eliciting the patients to imagine their most feared memories or worst imagined outcome of feared situations and then to make them realize that their anxiety subsides even though they still think of the situation. By definition, hypnosis is an intense absorption into internal experiences that has the ability to create vivid images through increased body awareness, heightened suggestibility and a relaxed state [16, 21]. Also, suggestions under hypnosis can touch many aspects such as cognition, physical sensations and emotions [16]. Hypnosis can thus greatly enhance the emotional engagement of patients during exposure as well as make people experience their fears more intensely than with relaxation, which in turn could improve its efficacy [16, 21]. Hypnosis could also be used in the context of imagery rescripting therapy (IRT;23). As an imagery-based cognitive treatment, IRT employs exposure not for habituation but rather as a way for activating images, emotions, and beliefs associated with traumatic memories. Through the process of activation, the goal of this therapy is to modify and restructure the traumatic images, dysfunctional beliefs, attributions and schemas. Alladins' IRT [23] is comprised of four components: imaginal exposure, imaginal restructuring, self-calming and self-nurturing, and emotional linguistic processing. Within each of these components, well-known hypnotic techniques such as the *bubble technique* and the *comforting the child technique* can be used. For example, during the imaginal rescripting phase, the patient creates a mastery image during which the "survivor self" enters the traumatic scene to assist the "traumatized self". The integration of the *split screen technique*[6] can be used to render the traumatic event more bearable. Finally, in addition to augmenting imagination, hypnosis facilitates both non-conscious and non-linguistic information processing that are often part of traumas [23].

In vivo-exposure. In-vivo exposure is an important element of therapy for all anxiety disorders; however, this experience can be very distressing and disorienting for certain patients, and can even lead to early dropouts [80, 100]. Moreover, with patients suffering from a trauma, a degree of symptom stability, ego-strengthening and the capacity to tolerate emotionally charged imageries are required before beginning exposure therapy [17, 115]. Hypnosis can thus be used as an effective preparation tool for the expositions [17]. Indeed, hypnosis can help control and modulate the experience of patients and give them adequate tools to feel more secure and calm [100, 119]. For example, patients can learn, through self-hypnosis, to imagine a comforting and secure place in order to render their experience less distressing [17]. In addition, a patient who suffers from OCD can be instructed to touch objects which the person feels are contaminated while the hypnotherapist provides suggestions that "no harm will come to him" [132]. Through many imagined rehearsals of coping, resistant patients may become more confident in their ability to face in-vivo exposures. During exposure in PTSD, clinical psychologists must be careful not to re-traumatize the clients.

---

6 In the treatment of PTSD, for example, this technique involves the projection of different images of memories of the trauma on one side of an imagined screen, and on the other side something that comfort the person [23].

Hypnosis can therefore help to prevent unnecessary exposure to too many traumatic events [119]. Indeed, indirect hypnotic safeguards such as ideomotor signalling for answering specific questions (e.g. Do you feel ready to regress to the past and address some event that is necessary for healing and which you feel able to cope with at present with help?) provide the hypnotherapist with the confirmation that the patient is able to embark on age-regression of the traumatic events [119].

Cognitive restructuring. Some of the early hypnotherapists already recognized the usefulness of hypnosis for cognitive restructuring [6]. Indeed, one important part of therapy is to teach patients to monitor and recognize their maladaptive thoughts. The increased suggestibility and reduced cognitive processing that accompany hypnosis make it a tool for rapid cognitive changes [133]. Hypnotherapy can be used to teach patients to replace their negative self-suggestions (e.g." I'm not good enough to make a good presentation") with hypnotic suggestions ("I've done many of them and I've always had good feedback") that reduce their anxiety [6]. These suggestions also can be applied during self-hypnosis [6]. Hypnotic interventions also can help to strengthen patients' flexible thinking styles [134]. For example, it can help facilitate cognitive restructuring and re-appraisal of traumas; for example, through dissociation and self-distancing techniques, such as the split-screen technique, the imagination of a safe place, and the use of the "older" or "compassionate" self [17, 119]. A self-distance perspective is thought to promote insight and closure, as well as a reduction in rumination and distress [17]. With a self-distance perspective, people can come to see the situation from a different angle, which was impossible for them before as they focused on simply recounting their experience (and creating a whole lot of distressing symptoms). For example, with the use of the "compassionate self', a guilty PTSD patient can realize that he/she could not have done more and that the situation in question was out of his or her control. Another use of hypnosis is as a tool for memory integration, which can help promote cognitive restructuring [118].

Building coping skills. An important aspect of anxiety is its physical symptoms. For example, according to the DSM-IV [63], GAD is characterized by somatic symptoms such as muscle tension, irritability, insomnia and restlessness [135]. Moreover, according to cognitive-behavioural theories, PD/A is based on the acquisition of the fear of physical sensations, especially those associated with the autonomic nervous system [136]. When PDA patients feel anxious, physical symptoms such as heart palpitations, headaches, and difficulty breathing can arise [18]. Building coping skills and self-efficacy under hypnosis is an effective way to control these symptoms [18]. Recently, autogenic training was found to produce significant reductions in blood pressure and pulse rate, which are often symptoms of anxiety [137]. According to Hammond [138], autogenic training is like a "structured German form of self-hypnosis" (p.264). Hypnosis also can be utilized to help patients manage their physical responses to anxiety provoking stimuli so that they can dissociate somatic responses to psychological distress [135].

Another coping skill that patients can acquire is to learn to redirect their attention away from distressing cues. For example, in PTSD, arousal and avoidant symptoms are triggered by both internal and external cues associated with the memories of the trauma. Unfortunately, PTSD patients seem to be particularly distractible to these cues and the result is that their condition cannot improve. Lynn et al. [17] propose that hypnosis can facilitate attention control in these patients so that they can stop being absorbed by cues of traumatic memories. Indeed, they propose that if it is possible to suggest to a patient to enter a state of hypnosis, it is possible to suggest that this same patient experiences enhanced attention and concentration (p.322). Thus, people under hypnosis can learn not only how to focus their attention in the moment, but also how to switch their attention away from increasingly distracting cues [17]. The latter hypnotic attentional control learning can also be useful to help patients contend with their flashbacks [17]. However, Lynn et al. [17] also propose that this technique should also be accompanied with suggestions for increased tolerance to disturbing flashbacks.

Building of social skills. Anxiety disorders can create disturbances in interpersonal relationships or even be exacerbated by a lack of social competence [133]. The teaching of social skills is thus a common component of CBT protocols. With hypnosis, the patients can practice their new social skills in imaginal rehearsals [133]. On a different level, as explained by Alladin [23], early traumas created by abuse and neglect, for example, can affect people's internal working models or relational schemas. Moreover, these core relational schemas are sometimes relatively unresponsive to verbal information or the views expressed by the patients' relatives so that when different opinions are uttered, the patient will not believe them. In conjunction with a hypnotic technique such as age regression, reframing work can be done to change some of these core beliefs.

Overcoming resistance. According to Kraft [139], hypnosis can be used as a technique to counteract resistance to therapy and exposure that is sometimes found in agoraphobics, for example. Moreover, hypnotists can resort to indirect hypnotic suggestions to counteract patients' resistance to suggestions. For example, they can paradoxically instruct a patient to continue to resist to a given suggestion in order for this individual to get some control in the decision-making during the psychological intervention. The objective is to ultimately elicit compliance [23].

Behavioural modification. Another way that hypnosis can be useful is through the administration of post-hypnotic suggestions, which works by shaping the patients' behaviours and experiences after therapy [16]. Post-hypnotic suggestions are defined as instructions to a hypnotised person to show certain behaviours or have certain experiences after hypnosis [32]. For anxious individuals, suggestions can include to experience less anxiety during their daily routines, comply with therapy homework, employ coping strategies when faced with distressing situations or stimuli, and become aware of adaptive appraisals made during times of anxiety [16]. Furthermore, the hypnotherapist can make post-hypnotic suggestions that the patient will be able to deal with adverse situations with greater confidence [17]. According to Yapko [70], post-hypnotic suggestions are widely used in hypnotherapy. So far, there is little yet increasing empirical evidence of the efficacy of post-hypnotic suggestions. For instance, recently it was discovered that post-hypnotic suggestions were capable of simulating several clinical conditions such as blindness, amnesia, auditory hallucinations, conversion disorder paralysis, selected delusions, [31, 140] and neglect-like visual behaviours in healthy patients [141]. Moreover, with highly hypnotisable participants, post-hypnotic suggestions were used to reduce the automatic tendency to read printed words in a Stroop task [142, 143], and to reduce the Simon effect, which is the facilitation of lateralized responses, when they are executed in the same side of space as that of the stimulus [144]. The latter demonstrations thus support the clinical use of post-hypnotic suggestions to extend the achievements made during therapy.

Power of treatment. Finally, recent studies show that when used properly, hypnosis adds leverage to treatment and accelerates the recovery processes [18, 23, 27, 103]. According to Alladin [23], this is due to the fact that "hypnosis produces a syncretic cognition, which consists of a matrix of cognitive, somatic, perceptual, physiological, visceral, and kinaesthetic changes" (p.104).

5.2. Hypnotisability assessment

Different opinions remain as to whether or not levels of hypnotisability should be assessed before undergoing hypnotherapy [145]. These divergent opinions are based among other things, by the fact that some studies do report a link between levels of hypnotisability and treatment gains [102, 103] while others do not [121, 146, 147]. Moreover, researchers are facing some difficulties when trying to link hypnotisability with treatment outcomes. Indeed, one problem lies in the timing of the assessment [56]. When participants undergo a standard test of hypnotisability prior to their treatment, they are likely to infer conclusions about their own susceptibility to hypnosis. This could, in turn, influence their expectations toward the success of the treatment, which could ultimately affect their treatment outcome [56]. On the other hand, when hypnotisability levels are assessed after the treatment, the participants' experience during the treatment might then have an influence on subsequent levels of responsiveness under hypnosis [56]. On a more positive note, Lynn and Shindler [145] state that modern evaluation techniques have rendered possible the use of a good hypnotisability assessment. They also present the advantage of being able to evaluate a variety of factors (attitudes, beliefs, rapport with therapist, motivation to respond) that could influence the response to hypnosis, and to model the hypnotherapy techniques around it in order to augment the efficacy of the treatment [145]. Indeed, as it was stated before, considering participants' attitudes and expectations of hypnosis is crucial, as expectation of positive therapeutic outcome is more often than not predictive of improvement in treatment [148]. In term of hypnotisability levels displayed by participants, expectancies have also been demonstrated to play a major role [149]. Moreover, a good assessment is imperative to remove clients who are unsuitable candidates for hypnotherapy due to their conditions (e.g. patients who are more prone to psychotic decompensation, those with a paranoid level of resistance to being controlled) [145]. Needless to say, this evaluation goes beyond the simple use of formal scales of hypnotisability [145]. For guidelines on how to assess patients' level of hypnotisability, refer to Lynn and Shindler [145].

5.3. Research on hypnosis

There remains a long way to go before hypnosis as an adjunct to the treatment of anxiety disorders is considered a first-line treatment. Future research will need to conduct good quality randomized controlled trials for each of the anxiety disorders. Well-conducted multiple case studies from independent researchers also must be done to establish the validity of hypnosis as an adjunct to CBT. Studies must have adequate sample sizes so that good power can be achieved, and provide an intent-to-treat analysis in order to have better chances of finding conclusive results. They also need to have a clear detailed protocol for the hypnotic techniques used, for replication purposes. Moreover, as suggested by Lynn et al. [43], good descriptions of the population at hand permit replication and help in assessing the external validity of the results. Such descriptions should include the diagnostic procedures, patients' demographic and treatment history, use of medication, comorbid diagnoses, and tests administered [43]. According to Schoengerber [56], despite the difficulties met while assessing hypnotisability levels, good attempts should be made to do so. For example, the Stanford Hypnotic Susceptibility Scale-Form C (SHSSC) is considered a gold standard measure and a good individual measure, and the Waterloo adaptation of this scale, the WGSC, is good for group administration [62]. Furthermore, in order to avoid the possibility that disproportionate numbers of high hypnotisable participants end up in one group compared to another, researchers could randomly match or stratify participants in terms of their hypnotisability scores or at least report the hypnotic suggestibility of each group in terms of scores. These scores could then be used as covariates in statistical analyses if groups differ considerably on this variable [43]. As some studies seemed to indicate that the effect of adding hypnosis appeared or persisted in the long-term [15, 126], studies should include follow-up measures. In conclusion, in accordance with the Society for Clinical and Experimental Hypnosis, this chapter argues that hypnosis is a technique and not a type of therapy and that it should be used as a tool to augment the efficacy as well as the patients' understanding of CBT principles [43, 134].

6. Conclusion

Clinical hypnosis is a flourishing area of research that has so far demonstrated the usefulness of hypnosis in many domains, especially in the treatment of pain in the medical environment and during medical procedures [55]. According to Bryant [16], there is no doubt that hypnosis can ameliorate established means of treating anxiety disorders. However, more research needs to be conducted in order to provide the information necessary to establish hypnosis (added to CBT) as an empirically supported treatment for anxiety disorders. The lack of adequate studies on this topic points to the need for more rigorous randomized controlled investigations on the use of hypnosis for anxiety disorders. This chapter, as well as many other books and articles [16, 23, 94, 150] present many ways in which hypnosis can be added to CBT. Researchers who wish to study hypnosis can refer to these as guidelines.

William [6] pointed out that hypnotherapy does not need to prove that it is superior to other forms of treatment in order to have clinical value. Indeed, the goal of clinical psychology is to determine what treatments are working for which patients with which problems, and under what conditions (Lazarus, 1973; cited in 6). Moreover, as stated before, hypnosis is a very cost-effective method [43] that could represent in some cases, a rapid, non-addictive and safe substitute to the use of medication, which is particularly important given the current increase in health care costs and adverse economic conditions [138]. Another advantage of hypnotherapy is that it can be used easily outside the clinic under the form of self-hypnosis. Self-hypnosis is defined as the employment of hypnotic suggestions through self-talk or listening to a recording of hypnotic suggestions [16]. Contrary to popular belief, how intensely someone responds to hypnosis resides in the ability of the individual, rather than in the special skills of the hypnotist [16]. Thus, self-hypnosis is a viable solution to help maintain the skills that were acquired during therapy. Consequently, hypnosis seems to respect the principle of parsimony, one of the most popular principles of clinical psychology, by creating more rapid gains and enhancing the efficacy of CBT interventions. Indeed, clinical psychologists should always try to utilize the least complex and most efficacious mode of treatment first [138].

This chapter focused on the use of hypnosis in the treatment of adult anxiety disorders. It is important to note that hypnosis is a therapeutic tool that is suitable for child and adolescent therapy. Indeed, although most research on hypnosis focus on adults, the popularity of complementary and alternative forms of therapies has started to attract parents of children with different problems [151]. According to Saadat and Kain [151], hypnosis is a suitable therapy for children because in general, they are more hypnotisable than adults. This is thought to be due to their increased capacity and willingness to become absorbed in fantasy, play, and imagination [151]. Moreover, psychologists can easily design specific hypnosis goals and suggestions that are individualized to the child and respect a developmental psychopathology perspective [152]. As for adults, meta-analyses and overviews have demonstrated the efficacy of hypnotherapy in treating children medical conditions such as asthma, chronic and acute pain, along with procedure-related distress for cancer patients [3]. Hypnosis also has improved child behavioural conditions such as trichotillomania, thumb-sucking, enuresis, dysphasia and chronic dyspnea [151]. However, Huynh et al's. [3] review of the literature revealed no randomised or controlled trials on the use of hypnotherapy for children with psychiatric disorders. Still, a high number of case reports indicated that hypnotherapy can be useful in treating children with PDA, social and specific phobias, OCD, GAD, and PTSD [3]. However, as is the case for adult anxiety disorders, the addition of hypnosis to clinical practice for children and adolescents needs to be developed and studied further before it is recognized as an empirically supported treatment.

Author details

Catherine Fredette[1], Ghassan El-Baalbaki[1,2], Sylvain Neron[2] and Veronique Palardy[1]

1 University of Quebec at Montreal, Quebec, Canada

2 Mcgill University, Quebec, Canada

References

[1] Chambless D, L., , Baker M, J., , Baucom H, D., , Beutler L, E , Calhoun K, S, Crits-Christoph P, et al. Update on Empirically Validated Therapies, II. The Clinical Psychologist. 1998;51(1):3-16.

[2] Hofmann SG, Smits JA. Cognitive-behavioral therapy for adult anxiety disorders: a meta-analysis of randomized placebo-controlled trials. J Clin Psychiatry. 2008;69(4): 621-32. Epub 2008/03/28.

[3] Huynh ME, Vandvik IH, Diseth TH. Hypnotherapy in child psychiatry: The state of the art. Clinical Child Psychology and Psychiatry. 2008;13(3):377-93.

[4] Kirsch I, Lynn SJ, Rhue JW. Introduction to clinical hypnosis. In: troduction to clinical hypnosis JWR, Lynn SJ, Kirsch I, editors. Handbook of clinical hypnosis. Washington, DC, US: American Psychological Association; 1993. p. 3-22.

[5] Schoenberger NE. Cognitive-Behavioral Hypnotherapy for Phobic Anxiety. Casebook of clinical hypnosis. Washington, DC, US: American Psychological Association; 1996. p. 33-49.

[6] William L, Golden. Cognitive hypnotherapy for anxiety disorders. American Journal of Clinical Hypnosis. 2012;54(4):263-74.

[7] Alladin A. Handbook of cognitive hypnotherapy for depression : an evidence-based approach. Philadelphia: Wolters Kluwer Health/Lippincott Williams & Wilkins; 2007.

[8] Ambrose G, & Newbold, G. A handbook of medical hypnosis; an introduction for practitioners and students (3d ed.). Baltimore: Williams and Wilkins Co.; 1968.

[9] Brann L, Owens J, Williamson A. The handbook of contemporary clinical hypnosis : theory and practice. Chichester, West Sussex, UK: John Wiley & Sons; 2011.

[10] Burrows GD, Dennerstein L. Handbook of hypnosis and psychosomatic medicine. New-York1988.

[11] Lynn SJ, Kirsch I, Rhue JW. An introduction to clinical hypnosis. In: Lynn SJ, Rhue JW, Kirsch I, editors. Handbook of clinical hypnosis (2nd ed). Washington, DC, US: American Psychological Association; 2010. p. 3-18.

[12] Nash M, R, Barnier A, J. The Oxford handbook of hypnosis: Theory, research, and practice. New-York, NY, US: Oxford University Press; 2008.

[13] Van Pelt SJ. Medical hypnosis handbook. Hollywood, California: Wilshire Book Co; 1957.

[14] Coelho HF, Canter PH, Ernst E. The effectiveness of hypnosis for the treatment of anxiety: A systematic review. Primary Care & Community Psychiatry. 2008;12(2): 49-63.

[15] Kirsch I, Montgomery G, Sapirstein G. Hypnosis as an adjunct to cognitive-behavioral psychotherapy: A meta-analysis. Journal of Consulting and Clinical Psychology. 1995;63(2):214-20.

[16] Bryant RA. Hypnosis and anxiety: Early interventions. The Oxford handbook of hypnosis: Theory, research, and practice. New York, NY, US: Oxford University Press; 2008. p. 535-47.

[17] Lynn SJ, Malakataris A, Condon L, Maxwell R, Cleere C. Post-traumatic Stress Disorder: Cognitive Hypnotherapy, Mindfulness, and Acceptance-Based Treatment Approaches. American Journal of Clinical Hypnosis. 2012;54(4):311-30.

[18] Nolan M. Hypnosis to enhance time limited cognitive-behaviour therapy for anxiety. Australian Journal of Clinical & Experimental Hypnosis. 2008;36(1):30-40.

[19] Haque A. Psychology from Islamic Perspective: Contributions of Early Muslim Scholars and Challenges to Contemporary Muslim Psychologists. Journal of Religion and Health. 2004;43(4):357-77.

[20] Sina I. Kitab ash-Shifa (book of Healing). Jan Bakos ed. Prague: http://www.muslim-philosophy.com/books/shifa2.pdf; 1027 1956.

[21] Llobet P. Group hypnotherapy in the treatment of specific phobias: An exploratory study [3324378]. United States -- California: Alliant International University, San Diego; 2008.

[22] Barnier A, J., Nash M, R. Introduction: a roadmap for explanation, a working definition. In: Nash M, R and Barnier, A, J, editor. The oxford handbook of hypnosis: theory, research, and practice. New-York: Oxford University Press; 2008. p. 1-20.

[23] Alladin A. Cogntive hypnotherapy: An integrated approach to the treatment of emotional disorders. Chichester, England: John Wiley & Sons, Ltd.; 2008.

[24] Lynn S, J, Green JP. The Sociocognitive and Dissociation Theories of Hypnosis: Toward a Rapprochement. International Journal of Clinical and Experimental Hypnosis. 2011;59(3):277-93.

[25] Lynn SJ, Green JP. The sociocognitive and dissociation theories of hypnosis: Toward a rapprochement. International Journal of Clinical and Experimental Hypnosis. 2011;59(3):277-93.

[26] Burrows GD, Stanley R, Bloom PB. International handbook of clinical hypnosis. Chichester, New-York: Wiley; 2001.

[27] Huston TR. The effects of using hypnosis for treating anxiety in outpatients diagnosed with generalized anxiety disorder. US: ProQuest Information & Learning; 2011.

[28] Kirsch I, Lynn SJ. Dissociation theories of hypnosis. Psychological Bulletin. 1998;123(1):100-15.

[29] Hilgard ER. The domain of hypnosis: With some comments on alternative paradigms. American Psychologist. 1973;28(11):972-82.

[30] Kihlstrom J, F. The domain of hypnosis, revisited. In: Press OU, editor. The oxford handbook of hypnosis: theory, research and practice. New-York, N-Y, US2008.

[31] Oakley DA, Halligan PW. Hypnotic suggestion and cognitive neuroscience. Trends in Cognitive Sciences. 2009;13(6):264-70.

[32] McConkey KM. Generations and landscapes of hypnosis: Questions we've asked, questions we should ask. In: Barnier MRNAJ, editor. The Oxford handbook of hypnosis: Theory, research, and practice. New York, NY, US: Oxford University Press; 2008. p. 53-77.

[33] Wilson SC, Barber TX. The fantasy-prone personality: Implications for understanding imagery, hypnosis, and parapsychological phenomena. PSI Research. 1982;1(3): 94-116.

[34] Aikins D, Ray WJ. Frontal lobe contributions to hypnotic susceptibility: A neuropsychological screening of executive functioning. International Journal of Clinical and Experimental Hypnosis. 2001;49(4):320-9.

[35] Spanos NP, et al. The Carleton University Responsiveness to Suggestion Scale: Relationship with other measures of hypnotic susceptibility, expectancies, and absorption. Psychological Reports. 1983;53(3, Pt 1):723-34.

[36] Lynn SJ, Rhue JW. The fantasy-prone person: Hypnosis, imagination, and creativity. Journal of Personality and Social Psychology. 1986;51(2):404-8.

[37] Dienes Z, Perner J. Executive control without conscious awareness: The cold control theory of hypnosis. Hypnosis and conscious states: The cognitive neuroscience perspective. New York, NY, US: Oxford University Press; 2007. p. 293-314.

[38] Barnier A, J,, Mitchell C, J. Looking for the fundamental effects of hypnosis: . 35th Annual Congress of the Australian Society of Hypnosis (Scientific Program); Sydney, Australia2005.

[39] Woody EZ, Sadler P. Dissociation theories of hypnosis. In: Barnier MRNAJ, editor. The Oxford handbook of hypnosis: Theory, research, and practice. New York, NY, US: Oxford University Press; 2008. p. 81-110.

[40] Hilgard ER. Divided consciousness: Multiple controls in human thought and action. New-York: Wiley; 1986.

[41] Lynn SJ, O'Hagen S. The sociocognitive and conditioning and inhibition theories of hypnosis. Contemporary Hypnosis. 2009;26(2):121-5.

[42] Lynn SJ, Kirsch I, Hallquist MN. Social cognitive theories of hypnosis. In: Barnier MRNAJ, editor. The Oxford handbook of hypnosis: Theory, research, and practice. New York, NY, US: Oxford University Press; 2008. p. 111-39.

[43] Lynn SJ, Kirsch I, Barabasz A, Carden~a E, Patterson D. Hypnosis as an empirically supported clinical intervention: The state of the evidence and a look to the future. International Journal of Clinical and Experimental Hypnosis. 2000;48(2):239-59.

[44] Montgomery GH, DuHamel KN, Redd WH. A meta-analysis of hypnotically induced analgesia: How effective is hypnosis? International Journal of Clinical and Experimental Hypnosis. 2000;48(2):138-53.

[45] Néron S, Stephenson R. Effectiveness of Hypnotherapy with Cancer Patients' Trajectory: Emesis, Acute Pain, and Analgesia and Anxiolysis in Procedures. International Journal of Clinical and Experimental Hypnosis. 2007;55(3):336-54.

[46] Montgomery GH, Bovbjerg DH, Schnur JB, David D, Goldfarb A, Weltz CR, et al. A Randomized Clinical Trial of a Brief Hypnosis Intervention to Control Side Effects in Breast Surgery Patients. Journal of the National Cancer Institute. 2007;99(17):1304-12.

[47] Snow A, Dorfman D, Warbet R, Cammarata M, Eisenman S, Zilberfein F, et al. A randomized trial of hypnosis for relief of pain and anxiety in adult cancer patients undergoing bone marrow procedures. Journal of Psychosocial Oncology. 2012;30(3): 281-93.

[48] Lang EV, Berbaum KS, Faintuch S, Hatsiopoulou O, Halsey N, Li X, et al. Adjunctive self-hypnotic relaxation for outpatient medical procedures: A prospective randomized trial with women undergoing large core breast biopsy. Pain. 2006;126(1-3): 155-64.

[49] Jensen MP, Gralow JR, Braden A, Gertz KJ, Fann JR, Syrjala KL. Hypnosis for symptom management in women with breast cancer: A pilot study. International Journal of Clinical and Experimental Hypnosis. 2012;60(2):135-59.

[50] Faymonville ME, Mambourg PH, Joris J, Vrigens B, Fissette J, Albert A, et al. Psychological approaches during conscious sedation. Hypnosis versus stress reducing strategies: A prospective randomized study. Pain. 1997;73(3):361-7.

[51] Harandi AA, Esfandani A, Shakibaei F. The effect of hypnotherapy on procedural pain and state anxiety related to physiotherapy in women hospitalized in a burn unit. Contemporary Hypnosis. 2004;21(1):28-34.

[52] Landolt AS, Milling LS. The efficacy of hypnosis as an intervention for labor and delivery pain: A comprehensive methodological review. Clinical Psychology Review. 2011;31(6):1022-31.

[53] Montgomery GH, Weltz CR, Seltz M, Bovbjerg DH. Brief presurgery hypnosis reduces distress and pain in excisional breast biopsy patients. The International journal of clinical and experimental hypnosis. 2002;50(1):17-32. Epub 2002/01/10.

[54] Mackey EF. Effects of Hypnosis as an Adjunct to Intravenous Sedation for Third Molar Extraction: A Randomized, Blind, Controlled Study. International Journal of Clinical and Experimental Hypnosis. 2009;58(1):21-38.

[55] Flory N, Lang E. Practical Hypnotic Interventions During Invasive Cancer Diagnosis and Treatment. Hematology/Oncology Clinics of North America. 2008;22(4):709-25.

[56] Schoenberger NE. Research on hypnosis as an adjunct to cognitive-behavioral psychotherapy. International Journal of Clinical and Experimental Hypnosis. 2000;48(2): 154-69.

[57] Chambless D, L., , Ollendick T, H. . Empirically supported psychological interventions: Controversies and evidence. Annual Review of Psychology. 2001;52.

[58] Elkins G, Johnson A, Fisher W. Cognitive hypnotherapy for pain management. American Journal of Clinical Hypnosis. 2012;54(4):294-310.

[59] Green JP. Hypnosis and the treatment of smoking cessation and weight loss. In: Kirsch I, Capafons A, Cardeña-Buelna E, Amigó S, editors. Clinical hypnosis and self-regulation: Cognitive-behavioral perspectives. Washington, DC, US: American Psychological Association; 1999. p. 249-76.

[60] Carmody TP, Duncan C, Simon JA, Solkowitz S, Huggins J, Lee S, et al. Hypnosis for smoking cessation: A randomized trial. Nicotine & Tobacco Research. 2008;10(5): 811-8.

[61] Elkins G, Marcus J, Bates J, Rajab MH, Cook T. Intensive Hypnotherapy for Smoking Cessation: A Prospective Study. International Journal of Clinical and Experimental Hypnosis. 2006;54(3):303-15.

[62] Schoenberger NE. Hypnosis in the treatment of women with anxiety disorders. Healing from within: The use of hypnosis in women's health care. Washington, DC, US: American Psychological Association; 2000. p. 45-64.

[63] APA. DSM-IV-TR. Washington, DC: American Psychiatric Association; 2000.

[64] Rodebaugh TL, Holaway RM, Heimberg RG. The treatment of social anxiety disorder. Clinical Psychology Review. 2004;24(7):883-908.

[65] Stanton HE. A comparison of the effects of an hypnotic procedure and music on anxiety level. Australian Journal of Clinical & Experimental Hypnosis. 1984;12(2): 127-32.

[66] Rogers J. Hypnosis in the treatment of social phobia. Australian Journal of Clinical & Experimental Hypnosis. 2008;36(1):64-8.

[67] Schoenberger NE, Kirsch I, Gearan P, Montgomery G, Pastyrnak SL. Hypnotic enhancement of a cognitive behavioral treatment for public speaking anxiety. Behavior Therapy. 1997;28(1):127-40.

[68] Barlow DH, Allen LB, Basden SL. Psychological treatments for panic disorders, phobias, and generalized anxiety disorder. In: Gorman PENJM, editor. A guide to treatments that work (3rd ed). New York, NY, US: Oxford University Press; 2007. p. 351-94.

[69] Hammarstrand G, Berggren U, Hakeberg M. Psychophysiological therapy vs. hypnotherapy in the treatment of patients with dental phobia. European Journal of Oral Sciences. 1995;103(6):399-404.

[70] Yapko MD. Trancework: An introduction to the practice of clinical hypnosis (3th Ed.). New York, NY, US: Routledge/Taylor & Francis Group; 2003. 528 p.

[71] Forbes S. Relative effectiveness of imaginal exposure with and without hypnosis in the treatment of specific animal phobias. [Dissertation]. London: University College; 2007.

[72] Hill R, & Bannon-Ryder, G. The use of hypnosis in the treatment of driving phobia. Contemporary Hypnosis. 2005;22:99-103.

[73] Kraft D, Kraft T. Use of in vivo and in vitro desensitization in the treatment of mouse phobia: Review and case study. Contemporary Hypnosis. 2010;27(3):184-94.

[74] Volpe G, E., & Nash, R, M. The use of Hypnosis for Airplane Phobia With an Obsessive Character: a Case Study. Clinical Cases Studies. 2012;11(1):1-15.

[75] Stein MB, Roy-Byrne PP, Craske MG, Bystritsky A, Sullivan G, Pyne JM, et al. Functional Impact and Health Utility of Anxiety Disorders in Primary Care Outpatients. Medical Care. 2005;43(12):1164-70.

[76] McCabe RE, Gifford S. Psychological treatment of panic disorder and agoraphobia. In: Stein MMAMB, editor. Oxford handbook of anxiety and related disorders. New York, NY, US: Oxford University Press; 2009. p. 308-20.

[77] DelMonte MM. The use of hypnotic regression with panic disorder: A case report. Australian Journal of Clinical Hypnotherapy and Hypnosis. 1996;17(1):1-5.

[78] Iglesias A, Iglesias A. Awake-Alert Hypnosis in the Treatment of Panic Disorder: A Case Report. American Journal of Clinical Hypnosis. 2005;47(4):249-57.

[79] Wild AJ. Hypnosis as an adjunct in the treatment of panic disorder. Australian Journal of Clinical & Experimental Hypnosis. 1994;22(2):109-17.

[80] Dyck RV, Spinhoven P. Does preference for treatment matter? A study of exposure in vivo with or without hypnosis in the treatment of panic disorder with agoraphobia. Behavior Modification. 1997;21(2):172-86.

[81] Stafrace S. Hypnosis in the treatment of panic disorder with agoraphobia. Australian Journal of Clinical & Experimental Hypnosis. 1994;22(1):73-86.

[82] Singh AR, Banerjee KR. Treating panic attack with hypnosis in combination with rational emotive therapy--A case report. Journal of Projective Psychology & Mental Health. 2002;9(2):105-8.

[83] Fisher PL. The Efficacy of Psychological Treatments for Generalised Anxiety Disorder? Worry and its psychological disorders: Theory, assessment and treatment. Hoboken, NJ, US: Wiley Publishing; 2006. p. 359-77.

[84] Allen BT. A design of a combined cognitive-behavioral, biofeedback, and hypnosis training protocol for the reduction of generalized anxiety disorder. US: ProQuest Information & Learning; 1998.

[85] Baker H. Hypnosis for anxiety reduction and ego-enhancement. Australian Journal of Clinical & Experimental Hypnosis. 2001;29(2):147-51.

[86] Podea D, Suciu R, Suciu C, Ardelean M. An update on the cognitive behavior therapy of obsessive compulsive disorder in adults. Journal of Cognitive and Behavioral Psychotherapies. 2009;9(2):221-33.

[87] Meyerson J, Konichezky A. Hypnotically induced dissociation (HID) as a strategic intervention for enhancing OCD treatment. American Journal of Clinical Hypnosis. 2011;53(3):169-81.

[88] Frederick C. Review of Hypnotically facilitated treatment of obsessive compulsive disorder: Can it be evidence-based? American Journal of Clinical Hypnosis. 2007;50(1):97.

[89] Moore KA, Burrows GD. Hypnosis in the treatment of obsessive-compulsive disorder. Australian Journal of Clinical & Experimental Hypnosis. 1991;19(2):63-75.

[90] Proescher EJ. Hypnotically facilitated exposure response prevention therapy for an OIF veteran with OCD. American Journal of Clinical Hypnosis. 2010;53(1):19-26.

[91] Scrignar CB. Rapid treatment of contamination phobia with hand-washing compulsion by flooding with hypnosis. American Journal of Clinical Hypnosis. 1981;23(4): 252-7.

[92] Kroger WS, Fezler WD. Hypnosis and behavior modification: Imagery conditioning. Oxford, England: J. B. Lippincott; 1976. xxv, 426 p.

[93] Yapko MD. Essentials of hypnosis. Philadelphia, PA, US: Brunner/Mazel; 1995. xv, 185 p.

[94] Lynn SJ, Cardeña E. Hypnosis and the Treatment of Posttraumatic Conditions: An Evidence-Based Approach. International Journal of Clinical and Experimental Hypnosis. 2007;55(2):167-88.

[95] Bomyea J, Lang AJ. Emerging interventions for PTSD: Future directions for clinical care and research. Neuropharmacology. 2012;62(2):607-16.

[96] Bryant RA, Guthrie RM, Moulds ML. Hypnotizability in acute stress disorder. The American Journal of Psychiatry. 2001;158(4):600-4.

[97] Spiegel D, Hunt T, Dondershine HE. Dissociation and hypnotizability in posttraumatic stress disorder. The American Journal of Psychiatry. 1988;145(3):301-5.

[98] Stutman RK, Bliss EL. Posttraumatic stress disorder, hypnotizability, and imagery. The American Journal of Psychiatry. 1985;142(6):741-3.

[99] Butler LD, Duran REF, Jasiukaitis P, Koopman C, et al. Hypnotizability and traumatic experience: A diathesis-stress model of dissociative symptomatology. The American Journal of Psychiatry. 1996;153(Suppl):42-63.

[100] Carden~a E. Hypnosis in the treatment of trauma: A promising, but not fully supported, efficacious intervention. International Journal of Clinical and Experimental Hypnosis. 2000;48(2):225-38.

[101] Poon MW-L. Using hypnosis with a battered women with post-traumatic stress disorder. Australian Journal of Clinical & Experimental Hypnosis. 2007;35(1):63-74.

[102] Abramowitz E, G., Lichtengerb P. A New Hypnotic Technique for Treating Combat-Related Posttraumatic Stress Disorder: A Prospective Open Study International Journal of Clinical and Experimental Hypnosis 2010;58(3):316-28.

[103] Auringer ML. Clinical efficacy of a brief hypnotic intervention for hyperarousal symptoms in sexual trauma. US: ProQuest Information & Learning; 2011.

[104] Stanton HE. Hypnotic relaxation and the reduction of sleep onset insomnia. International Journal of Psychosomatics. 1989;36(1-4):64-8.

[105] Stanton HE. Hypnotic relaxation and insomnia: A simple solution? Sleep and Hypnosis. 1999;1(1):64-7.

[106] Morin CM, Culbert JP, Schwartz SM. Nonpharmacological interventions for insomnia: A meta-analysis of treatment efficacy. The American Journal of Psychiatry. 1994;151(8):1172-80.

[107] Abramowitz EG, Barak Y, Ben-Avi I, Knobler HY. Hypnotherapy in the Treatment of Chronic Combat-Related PTSD Patients Suffering From Insomnia: A Randomized, Zolpidem-Controlled Clinical Trial. International Journal of Clinical and Experimental Hypnosis. 2008;56(3):270-80.

[108] Carter C. The Use of Hypnosis in the Treatment of PTSD. Australian Journal of Clinical & Experimental Hypnosis. 2005;33(1):82-92.

[109] Jiranek D. Use of hypnosis in pain management and post-traumatic stress disorder. Australian Journal of Clinical & Experimental Hypnosis. 2000;28(2):176-87.

[110] Willshire D. Trauma and treatment with hypnosis. Australian Journal of Clinical & Experimental Hypnosis. 1996;24(2):125-36.

[111] Chan R. A case study of chronic post-traumatic stress and grief: Hypnosis as an integral part of cognitive-behaviour therapy. Australian Journal of Clinical & Experimental Hypnosis. 2008;36(1):13-22.

[112] Desland M. Post-traumatic stress disorder. Australian Journal of Clinical & Experimental Hypnosis. 1997;25(1):61-73.

[113] Ebert BW. Hypnosis and rape victims. American Journal of Clinical Hypnosis. 1988;31(1):50-6.

[114] Poon MW-l. Hypnosis for complex trauma survivors: Four case studies. American Journal of Clinical Hypnosis. 2009;51(3):263-71.

[115] Kwan PSK. Phase-oriented hypnotherapy for complex PTSD in battered women: An overview and case studies from Hong Kong. Australian Journal of Clinical & Experimental Hypnosis. 2009;37(1):49-59.

[116] Kwan P, S, K. Hypnosis in complex trauma and breast cancer pain: a single case study Contemporary Hypnosis. 2007;24(2):86-96.

[117] Moore M. Hypnosis and post-traumatic stress disorder. Australian Journal of Clinical & Experimental Hypnosis. 2001;29(2):93-106.

[118] Degun-Mather M. The value of hypnosis in the treatment of chronic PTSD with dissociative fugues in a war veteran. Contemporary Hypnosis. 2001;18(1):4-13.

[119] Degun-Mather MD. The use of hypnosis in the treatment of post-traumatic stress disorder in a survivor of multiple childhood trauma. Contemporary Hypnosis. 1997;14(2):100-4.

[120] Brom D, Kleber RJ, Defares PB. Brief psychotherapy for posttraumatic stress disorders. Journal of Consulting and Clinical Psychology. 1989;57(5):607-12.

[121] Bryant RA, Moulds ML, Nixon RDV, Mastrodomenico J, Felmingham K, Hopwood S. Hypnotherapy and cognitive behaviour therapy of acute stress disorder: A 3-year follow-up. Behaviour Research and Therapy. 2006;44(9):1331-5.

[122] Abramowitz EG, Lichtenberg P. Hypnotherapeutic olfactory conditioning (HOC): Case studies of needle phobia, panic disorder, and combat-induced PTSD. International Journal of Clinical and Experimental Hypnosis. 2009;57(2):184-97.

[123] Benson H, et al. Treatment of anxiety: A comparison of the usefulness of self-hypnosis and a meditational relaxation technique: An overview. Psychotherapy and Psychosomatics. 1978;30(3-4):229-42.

[124] Stanton HE. Self-hypnosis: One path to reduced test anxiety. Contemporary Hypnosis. 1994;11(1):14-8.

[125] O'Neill LM, Barnier AJ, McConkey K. Treating anxiety with self-hypnosis and relaxation. Contemporary Hypnosis. 1999;16(2):68-80.

[126] Hyman BH. Hypnotic treatment of test anxiety. US: ProQuest Information & Learning; 2005.

[127] Boutin GE, Tosi DJ. Modification of irrational ideas and test anxiety through rational stage directed hypnotherapy [RSDH]. Journal of Clinical Psychology. 1983;39(3): 382-91.

[128] Mellinger DI. The role of hypnosis and imagery techniques in the treatment of agoraphobia: A case study. Contemporary Hypnosis. 1992;9(1):57-61.

[129] Dent T. Hypnotherapy for anxiety disorders. Southampton: 2003.

[130] Godoy PHT, Araoz DL. The use of hypnosis in posttraumatic stress disorders, eating disorders, sexual disorders, addictions, depression and psychosis: An eight-year review (part two). Australian Journal of Clinical Hypnotherapy and Hypnosis. 1999;20(2):73-85.

[131] Weems CF, Varela RE. Generalized anxiety disorder. In: Storch DMEA, editor. Handbook of child and adolescent anxiety disorders. New York, NY, US: Springer Science + Business Media; 2011. p. 261-74.

[132] Kraft T, Kraft D. The place of hypnosis in psychiatry: Its applications in treating anxiety disorders and sleep disturbances. Australian Journal of Clinical & Experimental Hypnosis. 2006;34(2):187-203.

[133] Evans BJ, Coman GJ. Hypnosis with treatment for the anxiety disorders. Australian Journal of Clinical & Experimental Hypnosis. 2003;31(1):1-31.

[134] Kellis E. Clinical hypnosis and cognitive-behaviour therapy in the treatment of a young woman with anxiety, depression, and self-esteem issues. Australian Journal of Clinical & Experimental Hypnosis. 2011;38(2):155-65.

[135] Nanda R, Singh B. Hypnotherapy in management of generalized anxiety disorder. In: Sharma R, Palan BM, editors. Hypnosis: Psycho-philosophical Perspectives and Therapeutic Relevance: Concept Publishing Compagny; 2011.

[136] Barlow DH. Clinical Handbook of Psychological Disorders: A Step-By-Step Treatment Manual: Guilford Press; 2007.

[137] Kanji N, White A, Ernst E. Autogenic training to reduce anxiety in nursing students: Randomized controlled trial. Journal of Advanced Nursing. 2006;53(6):729-35.

[138] Hammond DC. Hypnosis in the treatment of anxiety- and stress-related disorders. Expert Review of Neurotherapeutics. 2010;10(2):263-73.

[139] Kraft D. Counteracting resistance in agoraphobia using hypnosis. Contemporary Hypnosis & Integrative Therapy. 2011;28(3):235-48.

[140] Oakley DA. Hypnosis as a tool in research: experimental psychopathology. Contemporary Hypnosis. 2006;23(1):3-14.

[141] Priftis K, Schiff S, Tikhonoff V, Giordano N, Amodio P, Umiltà C, et al. Hypnosis meets neuropsychology: Simulating visuospatial neglect in healthy participants. Neuropsychologia. 2011;49(12):3346-50.

[142] Raz A, Kirsch I, Pollard J, Nitkin-Kaner Y. Suggestion Reduces the Stroop Effect. Psychological Science. 2006;17(2):91-5.

[143] Raz A, Fan J, Posner MI. Hypnotic suggestion reduces conflict in the human brain. Proceedings of the National Academy of Sciences of the United States of America. 2005;102(28):9978-83. Epub 2005/07/05.

[144] Iani C, Ricci F, Baroni G, Rubichi S. Attention control and susceptibility to hypnosis. Consciousness and Cognition: An International Journal. 2009;18(4):856-63.

[145] Lynn SJ, Shindler K. The Role of Hypnotizability Assessment in Treatment. American Journal of Clinical Hypnosis. 2002;44(3-4):185-97.

[146] Bryant RA, Moulds ML, Guthrie RM, Nixon RDV. The Additive Benefit of Hypnosis and Cognitive-Behavioral Therapy in Treating Acute Stress Disorder. Journal of Consulting and Clinical Psychology. 2005;73(2):334-40.

[147] Wadden TA, Anderton CH. The clinical use of hypnosis. Psychological Bulletin. 1982;91(2):215-43.

[148] Kirsch I. Changing expectations: A key to effective psychotherapy. Belmont, CA, US: Thomson Brooks/Cole Publishing Co; 1990. xviii, 231 p.

[149] Barnier AJ, Dienes Z, Mitchell CJ. How hypnosis happens: New cognitive theories of hypnotic responding. In: Barnier MRNAJ, editor. The Oxford handbook of hypnosis: Theory, research, and practice. New York, NY, US: Oxford University Press; 2008. p. 141-77.

[150] Zahi A, Meyerson J. Application of hypnotic strategies sustained by a positive psychology orientation in treating OCD patients. Contemporary Hypnosis. 2010;27(3): 177-83.

[151] Saadat H, Kain ZN. Hypnosis as a therapeutic tool in pediatrics. Pediatrics. 2007;120(1):179-81.

[152] Kaiser P. Childhood anxiety, worry, and fear: Individualizing hypnosis goals and suggestions for self-regulation. American Journal of Clinical Hypnosis. 2011;54(1): 16-31.

Chapter 8

Treatment of Generalized Anxiety Disorders: Unmet Needs

Nesrin Dilbaz and Aslı Enez Darcin

Additional information is available at the end of the chapter

1. Introduction

Generalized anxiety disorder (GAD) is defined in the Diagnostic and Statistical Manual of Mental Disorders, Fourth Edition (DSM-IV) as the presence of persistent, excessive anxiety and worry about a number of events and activities occurring on most of the days for at least 6 months. The patient must also experience at least three of the following six symptoms: restlessness or feeling keyed up or on edge, being easily fatigued, difficulty concentrating or mind going blank, irritability, muscle tension, and sleep disturbance.

GAD has a 12-month prevalence of 1% – 2.1% and a lifetime prevalence of 2.8% – 4.1% in Europe and in the US (Grant et al., 2005), often occurs early in life with twice the number of women suffering from it compared to men (ESEMeD/MHEDEA Investigators, 2000). GAD is chronic and disabling, and is associated with high rates of psychiatric comorbidity and substantial personal, social and economic costs (Wittchen et al., 1994; Ballenger et al., 2001; Wittchen, 2002). Evidence shows GAD's impact on social functioning, distress levels, and utilization of medical care is equivalent to those of other major psychiatric disorders (Mennin et al. 2004). In the National Comorbidity Survey, Wittchen and colleagues found that ~38% of patients with GAD may have another anxiety disorder and 48% may have major depression in addition to GAD (Wittchen et al., 1994). In addition to psychiatric comorbidities, patients with anxiety disorders have a higher risk for developing medical diseases in the areas of cardiovascular, gastrointestinal and respiratory as compared with control groups (Bowen et al., 2000).

Remission criteria defined by Ballenger include no or minimal symptoms of anxiety (Hamilton Anxiety Scale score ≤7-10), no functional impairment (Sheehan Disability Scale score ≤1 on each item) and no or minimal symptoms of depression (Hamilton Depression Scale score ≤7) for generalized anxiety disorder (Ballenger, 1999). Remission rates are considerably low in generalised anxiety disorder. Yonkers and colleagues have shown that the remission rates are only 15% and 25% among 164 patients after one and two years respectively (Yonkers et al., 1996). The probability of remission of GAD is only 38% at 5 years, and the probability of relapse after remission is 27-39% by 3 years (Yonkers et al., 2000).

GAD is often unrecognized or misdiagnosed as a physical condition due to the range of clinical presentations, including somatic symptoms, and the frequent occurrence of comorbid conditions. The main treatment approaches for GAD comprise pharmacotherapy or psychotherapy or a combination of both. The chronic and disabling nature of GAD often means that some individuals may fail to respond fully to first-line treatment (Bandelow et al., 2008; Goodwin et al., 2002; Altamura et al., 2008; Allgulander et al., 2002; Baldwin et al; 2005). Patients may therefore require a sequential trial of treatments or possibly a combination therapy (Davidson et al; 2010).

Research in the treatment of GAD has primarily focused on the efficacy of pharmacotherapy. Antidepressant and anxiolytic drugs are the two most commonly used pharmacological treatments for anxiety disorders. Newer anticonvulsant and sometimes antipsychotic drugs are also used in the treatment of some anxiety disorders including generalized anxiety disorder. More recently, there has been an increasing interest in the efficacy of psychotherapy. Of all the therapies, cognitive behavioral therapy (CBT) has established the most empirical support as an effective treatment for GAD (Gould et al. 2004).

In recent years, GAD-related disability (Wittchen, 2002) as well as impairment in quality of life and functioning has gain importance. Anxiety disorders result in considerable economic loss both decreasing working performance and increasing the number of applications for health care services (Wittchen, 2002; DuPont et al., 1996; Greenberg et al., 1999). GAD poses both personal and public substantial economic and social burden (Pollack et al., 2009).

According to the preliminary findings of our ongoing study on the evaluation of patient burden due to wrong diagnosis and treatment in patients with generalized anxiety disorder (GAD), the mean duration of GAD was 5.6±6.1 years, and the patients received initial treatment for their GAD 27.6±36.7 for months ago. It was noted that GAD was mostly accompanied by major depression (60.5%), followed by other anxiety disorders (31.6%). Of the patients diagnosed with GAD, 86.4% were using medication for GAD and 40.9% were admitted to an emergency service for any reason within the last 6 months. The mean number of emergency admissions was 3.1±3.7. Of the patients admitted to emergency services, 51.9% underwent analyses such as blood analysis, radiological examination, electrocardiography (ECG) and ultrasonography (USG), and 48.5% were referred to another specialist for consultation. The preliminary findings of the present study indicate that admissions of GAD patients to emergency services due to various complaints continue when these patients are not treated adequately and sufficiently, and that financial burden of this disorder increases incrementally due to laboratory analyses and imaging techniques, consultations and additional therapies performed during these admissions (Dilbaz and Karamustafalıoğlu 2012a).

This chapter presents the unmet needs in the treatment of generalised anxiety disorders and new strategies in treatment for GAD.

2. Treatment

The primary goal of treatment of GAD is to alleviate psychic and somatic complaints, promote sleep, improve patient's functioning and enhance patient quality of life. Besides, treating other concomitant medical conditions (psychiatric and/or medical co-morbidity) and consequently providing remission and preventing relapses are also aimed. The important requirements for the therapy drug include rapid action, broad spectrum, increasing remission rates, preventing relapses, absence of symptoms due to discontinuation of drug, minimum interaction with other drugs, and safety for elderly and children (Dilbaz et al., 2011; Davidson et al., 2010). Treatment of GAD comprises drug therapy together with behavioral therapy and psychotherapy. Characteristics and severity of symptoms, co-morbidities, presence of substance addiction and risk for suicide, results of previous therapies, costs, availability of drug and patient preference should be considered while planning GAD treatment (Davidson et al., 2010).

2.1. Pharmacological strategies

2.1.1. Benzodiazepines

Many randomized, double-blind trials have demonstrated the efficacy of benzodiazepines in the acute treatment of GAD (Greenblatt et al., 1983; Rickels et al., 1987; Hollister et al., 1993). However, there is evidence that more than a third of patients will not meet remission criteria in the treatments with benzodiazepines (Shader and Greenblatt, 1983).

The risks and benefits of using benzodiazepines should be carefully considered in each patient. Benzodiazepines have rapid onset, relatively low toxicity, and anxiolytic potency but these benefits should be weighed against for potential motor impairment, dependence and withdrawal symptoms esspecially when prescribed for >4 weeks (Rynn and Brawman-Mintzer, 2004).

Particularly in older people, benzodiazepine use can be problematic due to side effects such as falls, memory impairment, incoordination, drowsiness, and confusion (Petrovic et al., 2003). They can also disrupt sleep architecture, and rebound insomnia may occur after stopping treatment (Longo and Johnson, 2000).

2.1.2. Antidepressants

Selective serotonin reuptake inhibitors (SSRIs), serotonin noradrenalin reuptake inhibitors (SNRIs), tricyclic antidepressants (TCAs, particularly imipramine), and, in a single controlled trial, trazodone have demonstrated efficacy in treatment of GAD compared to placebo (Rickels et al., 1993). Several analyses have shown similar efficacy among antidepressant agents in the management of GAD (Kapczinski et al, 2003).

2.1.2.1. SSRIs and SNRIs

Of these, SSRIs and SNRIs are the recommended first-line drugs for treatment of anxiety based on strength of evidence and acceptable tolerability. Antidepressants, particularly SSRI, may be associated with an initial worsening of anxiety symptoms in some patients. A retrospective cohort study defined characteristics of patients which developed emergent anxiety following an antidepressant intiation as young age, white and women sex (Li et al., 2011). Li et al. also found that receiving bupropion, fluoxetine or sertraline had lower risk of anxiety development than citalopram, paroxetine, venlafaxine and mirtazapine (Li et al, 2009). It is recommended to start on low doses and slowly titrate up to a therapeutic dose to reduce these "activation" symptoms (Sinclair et al., 2009). Patients should be advised of the potential for initial increase/worsening of symptoms and the likely delay of clinical effect (some response often seen by 4 weeks). Patient awareness of these factors when commencing SSRI treatment assists in reducing early discontinuation of treatment. Concomitant use of benzodiazepines during early treatment with SSRI may be useful in moderating these "activation effects" of SSRI early in treatment, although the potential for dependence must be considered. SSRI need to be taken for up to 12 weeks in order to assess a patient's response to treatment. Dosing requirements (like initiation in lower doses and reaching optimal doses by weekly increments) for antidepressants differ to that needed in the treatment of depression. All patients being treated with antidepressants (irrespective of diagnosis) should be monitored for worsening of their clinical condition and the emergence of suicidal ideation (Anxiety Disorders – Drug Treatment Guidelines, 2008)

According to Western Australian Psychotropic Drugs Committee; sertralin, escitalopram and venlafaxin have second line of evidence in treatment of generalized anxiety disorders whereas paroxetine has first line evidence (Hidalgo et al., 2007; Kapczinski et al., 2003; Anxiety Disorders – Drug Treatment Guidelines, 2008). There was a small statistically significance in favour of escitalopram compared with paroxetine based on a reduction in HAM-A scores. In addition, there was a 40% reduction in risk of non-response and lower risk (although not statistically significant) of discontinuation of treatment due to adverse events for escitalopram compared with paroxetine (Baldwin et al., 2006). There were no statistically significant differences found between paroxetine and sertraline on any outcomes (Ball et al., 2005).

There were no differences found on reduction of anxiety symptoms between escitalopram and venlafaxine while venlafaxine was associated with a greater risk of discontinuation (although this was not statistically significant) (Bose et al., 2008). Duloxetine was found to be effective in 60-120 mg/d doses in treatment of generalised anxiety disorder when compared to placebo (Rynn et al., 2008; Hartford et al., 2007). No difference was found between duloxetine and venlafaxine for reduction in anxiety and discontinuation due to adverse events (Nicolini et al; 2009).

2.1.2.2. Bupropion

Bystritsky and colleagues compared bupropion XL and escitalopram in 24 patients with generalised anxiety disorder in a 12-week, double-blind, randomized controlled trial and reported comparable efficacy between bupropion and escitalopram (2008).

2.1.2.3. Agomelatine

The efficacy of 25 to 50 mg/day agomelatine in generalised anxiety disorder (GAD) was assessed in a 12-week double-blind, placebo-controlled study of 121 patients with no comorbid disorders (Stein et al., 2008). Agomelatine was found more effective than placebo at
reducing anxiety (based on Hamilton rating scale for Anxiety; p=0.04). Agomelatine also improved sleep symptoms, sleep latency (p≤0.001), quality of sleep (p=0.002) and awakenings
(p≤0.0001).

2.1.3. Anticonvulsants

2.1.3.1. Valproate

Valproate has been investigated for the management of GAD in a double-blind, placebo-
controlled randomized trial involving 80 male patients with GAD in a double-blind placebo-
controlled design (Aliyev and Aliyev, 2008). 40 patients randomized to receive 500 mg
valproate three times per day and 40 patients received mathed plasebo. At week 4, valproate
separated from placebo by mean total HARS score, and at 6 weeks, the mean change in
HARS score reached significance. The most common side effects in the valproate group
were dizziness and nausea and further investigation is recommended.

2.1.3.2. Gabapentine

Pollack and colleagues reported two cases documenting improvements in patients with
GAD, following addition of gabapentin to their treatment (Pollack et al., 1998).

2.1.3.3. Tiagabine

There are case series documenting patients with generalised anxiety disorder treated with
tiagabine successfully (Schwarts, 2002; Crane et al., 2003; Schaller et al., 2004). Schwartz et al
followed up 17 patients with GAD in an 8-week, open-label trial of tiagabine (mean dose 13
mg/d) augmentation to SSRIs or benzodiazepines. 76% of patients responded [≥ 50% reduction in anxiety symptoms (HARS)] and 59% achieved remission (HARS score ≤ 7) (Schwartz
et al., 2005).

Pollack et al reported on 3 large 10-week, randomized, double-blind, placebo-controlled,
parallel-group studies. In the fixed-dose study, 910 patients received 4, 8, or 12 mg/d of tiagabine and in two flexible-dose studies, a total of 920 participants were enrolled. The mean
doses of tiagabine were 8.9 and 9.2 mg/d. Neither study found significant differences in
anxiety symptoms (HARS used) when compared to placebo and investigators concluded
that these studies do not support the efficacy of tiagabine in adult patients with GAD (Pollack et al., 2008).

2.1.3.4. Pregabaline

There have been several industry-sponsored, multicenter, outpatient, prospective, randomized, double-blind, placebo-controlled studies. Pande et al. showed a significant improvement with pregabalin compared to placebo, but no significant differences in response were observed when comparing pregabalin 50 mg tid to pregabalin 200 mg tid or lorazepam to pregabalin 200 mg tid. The most commonly associated adverse events with pregabalin were dizziness, somnolence, and headache (Pande et al., 2003). Feltner and colleagues also compared pregabalin (in different doses), lorazepam 2 mg tid, or placebo. They also found pregabalin 200 mg tid effective in treatment of GAD, however, pregabalin 50 mg tid wasn't effective and 200 mg tid was not significantly different from lorazepam (Feltner et al., 2003). Pohl et al. found pregabalin in 100 mg bid, 200 mg bid, and 150 mg tid doses significantly effective than in reducing anxiety symptoms (Pohl et al., 2005).

In another large study of 454 participants with GAD, Rickels et al. compared pregabaline (in different doses) with alprazolam and placebo. Investigators reported that of the 5 treatment groups, the 300-mg pregabalin group was the only medication group that differed statistically in global improvement at treatment end point not only from the placebo group but also from the alprazolam group (Rickels et al., 2005). Another study found pregabaline (400-600 mg/day) effective in treatment of GAD compared to placebo and safer than venlafaxine (Montgomery et al., 2006).

Lydiard et al combined data from 6 short-term, double-blind, placebo-controlled, fixed-dose trials of pregabalin for the treatment of GAD. They concluded that pregabalin had significant efficacy in treating both HARS psychic and somatic anxiety measures. Furthermore, they indicated that a dose-response effect was evident for pregabalin that appeared to reach a plateau at a dose of 300 mg/d (Lydiard et al., 2010).

Pregabalin is promising in both add-on and switch therapies in treatment-resistant GAD cases. Pregabalin rapidly (within days) relieves anxiety symptoms providing substantial advantage over SSRI and SNRIs (Dilbaz and Karamustafalıoğlu, 2012a).

2.1.3.5. Levetiracetam

One case with GAD reported by Pollack, had improved with levetiracetam 250 mg/d added to citalopram treatment (Pollack, 2002).

2.1.4. Atypical antipsychotics

Some first-generation antipsychotics were approved for a condition similar to GAD, and recent studies have suggested that atypical antipsychotics may also have a role in GAD. A Cochrane metaanalysis reported that nine studies investigated the effects of second-generation antipsychotics in generalised anxiety disorder. Seven of them investigated the effects of quetiapine. Participants with generalised anxiety disorder responded significantly better to quetiapine than to placebo (4 RCTs, N = 2265, OR = 2.21, 95% CI 1.10 to 4.45). However, patients on quetiapine arm were more likely to drop out due to adverse events, like gain weight or sedation. When quetiapine was compared with antidepressants in GAD, there was no significant difference in efficacy-related outcomes, but more participants in the quetiapine groups dropped out due to adverse events.

2.1.4.1. Quetiapine

Several preliminary reports of monotherapy trials of quetiapine versus placebo have described efficacy at doses in the range of 50–150 mg/d (Chouinard et al., 2008; Khan et al., 2008; Joyce et al., 2008; Bandelow et al., 2009), but quetiapine cannot yet be recommended as a routine GAD treatment until a full description of efficacy and safety from these studies have been published. However, the use of quetiapine could be considered after other classes of drugs have proved ineffective or when certain types of symptoms are present like insomnia.

2.1.4.2. Olanzapine

Pollack investigated olanzapine augmentation to fluoxetine at a mean dose of 8.7 mg daily and reported that olanzapine may be helpful for patients who fail to respond to SSRIs alone, considering the advers events like wight gain (Pollack et al., 2006).

2.1.4.3. Aripiprazole

Two studies demonstrate that aripiprazole has promise in augmentation at dosages starting at 10 mg daily (Menza et al., 2007; Hoge et al., 2008).

2.1.4.4. Risperidone

Adjunctive risperidone could be tried in patients with poor response at titrated doses up to 3 mg daily (Brawman-Mintzer et al., 2005; Simon et al., 2006).

2.1.4.5. Ziprasidone

Ziprasidone at a daily dose range of 20 to 80 mg may be helpful for patients with GAD who did not have an adequate response to other medication treatment (Snyderman et al., 2005).

2.1.5. Other drugs

2.1.5.1. Azapirones

Buspirone was approved for the treatment of GAD more than 20 years ago. In recent years, multiple members of the azapirone class, which comprises the partial or full 5-HTIA agonists gepirone, zalospirone, and ipsapirone, have been studied. These molecules show anxiolytic properties but have limitations in terms of tolerability. In a recent brief report, Mathew *et al.* tested the short-term tolerability and efficacy of PRX-00023, a nonazapirone 5-HTIA selective partial agonist, in 23 outpatients with GAD (Mathew et al., 2008). This preliminary study indicated that PRX-00023 appeared to be generally well tolerated in patients with GAD. But further investigations needed.

2.1.5.2. Riluzole

Although double-blind, placebo-controlled trials are lacking, several open label trials have suggested that riluzole, either as monotherapy or as augmentation of standard therapy, reduces symptoms of some psychiatric disorders including generalized anxiety disorder (Grant et al., 2007; Mathew et al., 2005).

Mathew et al.,investigated the efficacy and safety of treatment with riluzole (100 mg/day): of the 15 patients who completed the trial, 12 had a rapid improvement of anxiety symptomatology (Mathew et al., 2005). Recently, Mathew et al. (2008), in an open-label trial, used proton magnetic resonance spectroscopic imaging (1H MRSI) to examine the effects of the glutamate-release inhibitor riluzole on hippocampal N-acetylaspartate (NAA), a neuronal marker, in 14 patients with GAD. Investigators demonstrated a relationship between hippocampal NAA and symptom alleviation after the administration of riluzole in patients for 8 weeks; this result suggested that riluzole might be efficacious for GAD (and subtypes of mood disorders) in part because of reduced glutamate excitotoxicity and enhancement of hippocampal neuroplasticity. In studies of psychiatrically ill patients conducted to date, the drug has been quite well tolerated; common adverse effects include nausea and sedation. Elevation of liver function tests is common and necessitates periodic monitoring. Riluzole may hold promise for the treatment of several psychiatric conditions, possibly through its ability to modulate pathologically dysregulated glutamate levels, and merits further investigation (Pittenger et al., 2008).

2.2. Nonpharmacological strategies; Psychotherapy

2.2.1. Cognitive behavioral therapy

One of the most successful psychosocial treatments for the treatment of GAD is cognitive-behavioral therapy (CBT). The components of this therapy may vary to include the following: education about the symptoms and causes of anxiety, cognitive restructuring, applied relaxation, increasing awareness, learning to monitor of anxious symptoms presenting as physical symptoms, and the automatic thoughts of worry created from situational and behavioral cues. Patients are taught to manage these symptoms through training in arousal reduction techniques such as pleasant imagery and diaphragmatic breathing; and imaginal and in vivo exposure to anxiety cues coupled with copings skill rehearsal (Roemer et al; 2002).

A Cochrane collaboration review concluded that current evidence demonstrates that CBT is effective for the short-term management of GAD relative to wait-list control but not active supportive therapy or supportive treatment (ie, active supportive therapies underpinned by humanistic principals). The most successful CBT treatment protocols have included motivational therapy, interpersonal psychotherapy, integrative CBT (ICBT) to treat GAD (Baer, 2003). Although CBT is the most effective of the psychological treatments available for GAD, available data indicate that a clinical response occurs in less than 50% of people receiving CBT, so unmet needs still remain (Hunot et al., 2007).

One promising form of psychotherapy emphasizes the promotion of positive emotional states and active coping behaviors, rather than focusing on how to reduce symptoms. This resilience-building treatment is referred to as "well-being therapy" and appears to be superior to CBT on some measures in treatment-resistant GAD and other forms of anxiety (Fava et al., 2005).

2.2.2. Mindfulness based cognitive therapy

A number of approaches have integrated features of Buddhist mindfulness practices with CBT to treat a number of psychiatric disorders including GAD (Baer 2003). Mindfulness was conceptualized as being a set of skills that can be learned independently of any spiritual or cultural tradition and then applied to help manage psychiatric symptoms. These approaches have included mindfulness based stress reduction (MBSR) (Kabat-Zinn 1982, 2003), mindfulness based cognitive therapy (MBCT) (Segal et al. 2002), dialectical behavior therapy (DBT) for borderline personality disorders (Linehan 1993a, b), and acceptance and commitment therapy (ACT) mostly for anxiety and major mood disorders (Hayes et al. 1999).

There are two objectives associated with classical mindfulness (CM) skill training for treating GAD: (1) to achieve a level of sustained, detailed, non-conceptual divided attention and awareness (also known as bare attention or direct experience), and (2) develop the ability to carry out experiential based insight based on the way of experiencing as described in (1). These two objectives clearly imply that there are two major stages of mindfulness practice. The first stage is training in sustaining, detailed, nonconceptual divided attention and awareness which needs to be distinguished as significantly different from MBSR practice of mindfulness. The second stage involves the reinstatement of gradual application of discriminative processes informed by direct experience in order to enrich the process of knowing (Rapgay et al., 2011).

MBCT may be an acceptable and potentially effective treatment for reducing anxiety and mood symptoms and increasing awareness of everyday experiences in patients with GAD. Future directions include development of a randomized clinical trial of MBCT for GAD (Evans et al., 2008).

2.3. Combination strategies

CBT in combination with a sub-therapeutic dose of diazepam produces a greater effect than the same dose of diazepam alone (Power, et al., 1989). Given that GAD has a chronic course and is often comorbid with depression it may be that the combined treatment of medication and psychotherapy may provide an important treatment option that could lead to improved outcomes beyond monotherapy (Barlow, 2002). Unfortunately, at this time there is no data to support this conclusion.

3. Conclusion

GAD is a prevalent and disabling disorder that may appear with physical and psychiatric comorbitidies. SSRIs and SNRIs defined as first line treatment options in GAD, and there is increasing interest in enhancement new strategies to deal with the disorder. Novel antidepressants agomelatine and bupropion, atypical antipsychotics and anticonvulsants are promising in the treatment of GAD but still far from expectations because the necessity of close monitoring and some adverse events. Pharmacological interventions are still the most effective interventions to manage the disorder while augmentation strategies promising. However clinicians still in need of more effective treatment options that have rapid effect and safe.

Author details

Nesrin Dilbaz and Aslı Enez Darcin

Üsküdar University, Neuropsychiatry (NP) Hospital. Istanbul, Turkey

References

[1] Aliyev NA, Aliyev ZN. Valproate (depakine-chrono) in the acute treatment of outpatients with generalized anxiety disorder without psychiatric comorbidity: randomized, double blind placebo-controlled study. *Eur Psychiatry* 2008;23:109-14.

[2] Allgulander C, Hirschfeld RM, Nutt DJ. Long-term treatment strategies in anxiety disorders. *Psychopharmacol Bull.* 2002;36(suppl 2):79–92.

[3] Altamura AC, Dell'osso B, D'Urso N, et al. Duration of untreated illness as a predictor of treatment response and clinical course in generalized anxiety disorder. *CNS Spectr.* 2008;13(5):415–422.

[4] *Anxiety Disorders – Drug Treatment Guidelines (August 2008)*. Western Australian Therapeutics Advisory Group. Psychotropic Drugs Committee. http://www.watag.org.au/wapdc/guidelines.cfm#Anxiety

[5] Baer RA. Mindfulness training as a clinical intervention: A conceptual and empirical review. Clinical Psychology: Science and Practice 2003; 10(2), 125–143.

[6] Baldwin DS, Anderson IM, Nutt DJ, et al. Evidence-based guidelines for the pharmacological treatment of anxiety disorders: recommendations from the British Association for Psychopharmacology. *J Psychopharmacol.* 2005;19(6):567–596.

[7] Baldwin DS, Huusom, A K T and Maehlum E. Escitalopram and paroxetine in the treatment of generalised anxiety disorder: randomised, placebo controlled, double-blind study. British Journal of Psychiatry, 2006;189, 264–272.

[8] Ball S, Kuhn A, Wall D et al. Selective serotonin reuptake inhibitor treatment for generalized anxiety disorder: a double-blind, prospective comparison between paroxetine and sertraline. Journal of Clinical Psychiatry, 2005;66, 94–99.

[9]   Ballenger JC. Clinical guidelines for establishing remission in patients with depression and anxiety. J Clin Psychiatry 1999;60(suppl 22):29–34

[10] Ballenger JC, Davidson JR, Lecrubier Y, et al. Consensus statement on depression, anxiety, and oncology. J Clin Psychiatry 2001;62:64–67.

[11] Bandelow B, Chouinard G, Bobes J, et al. Extended-release quetiapine fumarate (quetiapine XR): a once-daily monotherapy effective in generalized anxiety disorder. Data from a randomized, double-blind, placebo- and active-controlled study. Int J Neuropsychopharmacol. 2009:1- 16.19691907

[12] Bandelow B, Zohar J, Hollander E, et al. World Federation of Societies of Biological Psychiatry (WFSBP) Guidelines for the Pharmacological Treatment of Anxiety, Obsessive-Compulsive and Post-Traumatic Stress Disorders: First Revision. *World J Biol Psychiatry.* 2008;9(4):248–312.

[13] Barlow DH. Anxiety and Its Disorders. 2nd ed. New York, NY: Guilford; 2002.

[14] Bose A, Korotzer A, Gommoll C et al. Randomized placebo-controlled trial of escitalopram and venlafaxine XR in the treatment of generalized anxiety disorder. Depression and Anxiety, 2008; 25, 854–861.

[15] Bowen RC, Senthilselvan A, Barale A. Physical illness as an outcome of chronic anxiety disorders. Can J Psychiatry. 2000;45:459-464.

[16] Brawman-Mintzer O, Knapp RG, Nietert PJ. Adjunctive risperidone in generalized anxiety disorder: a double-blind, placebo-controlled study. J Clin Psychiatry. 2005;66(10):1321–1325.

[17] Bystritsky A, Kerwin L, Feusner JD, Vapnik T. A pilot controlled trial of bupropion XL versus escitalopram in generalized anxiety disorder. Psychopharmacol Bull. 2008;41(1):46-51.

[18] Chambless DL and Gillis MM. Cognitive therapy for anxiety disorders. Journal of Consulting and Clinical Psychology, 1993;61, 248–260.

[19] Chouinard G, Ahokas A, Bandelow B, et al. St Louis, MO: Extended release quetiapine fumarate (quetiapine XR) once-daily monotherapy in generalized anxiety disorder (GAD) Presented at the 27th Annual Meeting of the Anxiety Disorders Association of America; March 6–9, 2008.

[20] Crane D. Tiagabine for the treatment of anxiety. Depress Anxiety. 2003;18(1):51–52.

[21] Davidson JR, Feltner DE, Dugar A. Management of generalized anxiety disorder in primary care: identifying the challenges and unmet needs. Prim Care Companion J Clin Psychiatry. 2010;12(2):772.

[22] Diagnostic and Statistical Manual of Mental Disorders. 4th ed. Washington DC, American Psychiatric Association; 1994.

[23] Dilbaz N, Yalcın Cavus S, Enez Darcin A. Treatment resistant generalized anxiety disorder. Selek S (ed), Different Views of Anxiety Disorders. InTech open access book, 2011, p.219-232.

[24] Dilbaz N, Karamustafalıoğlu KO. Unmet needs in the generalized anxiety disorder: pregabalin as a new option. Anatolia Journal Psychitary, 2012; 13(3): 232-238.

[25] Dilbaz N, Karamustafalıoğlu O. Burden due to misdiagnosis and mistreated patients with generalized anxiety disorder; preliminary findings (Anatolian Jounal of Psychiatry, 2012a)

[26] DuPont RL, Rice DP, Miller LS, Shiraki SS, Rowland CR, Harwood HJ. Economic costs of anxiety disorders. Anxiety 1996; 2:167-172.

[27] ESEMeD/MHEDEA 2000 Investigators. Prevalence of mental disorders in Europe: Results from the European Study of the Epidemiology of Mental Disorders (ESEMeD) project. Acta Psychiatr Scand 2004;109:21–27.

[28] Evans S, Ferrando S, Findler M, Stowell C, Smart C, Haglin D. Mindfulness-based cognitive therapy for generalized anxiety disorder. J Anxiety Disord. 2008;22(4): 716-21.

[29] Fava GA, Ruini C, Rafanelli C, et al. Well-being therapy of generalized anxiety disorder. Psychother Psychosom. 2005;74(1):26–30.

[30] Feltner DE, Crockatt JG, Dubovsky SJ, et al. A randomized, double-blind, placebo-controlled, fixed-dose, multicenter study of pregabalin in patients with generalized anxiety disorder. J Clin Psychopharmacol. 2003;23(3):240–249.

[31] Goodwin RD, Gorman JM. Psychopharmacologic treatment of generalized anxiety disorder and the risk of major depression. Am J Psychiatry. 2002;159(11):1935–1937.

[32] Gould RA, Safren SA, Washington D and Otto MW. A meta-analytic review of cognitive behavioral treatments. In RG Heimberg, CL Turk, & DS Mennin (Eds.), Generalized anxiety disorder: Advances in research and practice. New York: The Guilford Press 2004.

[33] Grant BF, Hasin DS, Stinson FS, et al. Prevalence, correlates, co-morbidity, and comparative disability of DSM-IV generalized anxiety disorder in the USA: results from the National Epidemiologic Survey on Alcohol and Related Conditions. Psychol Med 2005;35:1747–1759.

[34] Grant P, Lougee L, Hirschtritt M, et al. An open-label trial of riluzole, a glutamate antagonist, in children with treatment- resistant obsessive-compulsive disorder. J Child Adolesc Psychopharmacol 2007; 17: 761-7

[35] Greenberg PE, Sisitsky T, Kessler RC, Finkelstein SN, Berndt ER, Davidson JR, et al. The economic burden of anxiety disorders in the 1990s. J Clin Psychiatry 1999; 60:427-435.

[36] Greenblatt DJ, Shader RI, Abernethy DR. Drug therapy. Current status of benzodia-zepines. New Eng J Med. 1983;309:354-358.

[37] Hartford J. Komstein S. Liebowitz M, et al. Duloxetine as an SNRI treatment for gen-eralized anxiety disorder: results from a placebo and active-controlled trial. Int Clin Psvchopharmacol 2007; 22 (3): 167-74.

[38] Hayes SC, Strosahl KD and Wilson KG. Acceptance and commitment therapy: An ex-periential approach to behavior change, 1999. New York: Guilford.

[39] Hidalgo RB, Tupler LA, Davidson JR. An effect-size analysis of pharmacologic treat-ments for generalized anxiety disorder. J Psychopharmacol 2007; 21(8):864-872.

[40] Hoge EA, Worthington JJ, 3rd, Kaufman RE, et al. Aripiprazole as augmentation treatment of refractory generalized anxiety disorder and panic disorder. CNS Spectr. 2008;13(6):522–527.

[41] Hollister LE, Muller-Oerlinghausen B, Rickels K, Shader RI. Clinical uses of benzo-diazepines. J Clin Psychopharmacol. 1993;13(6 suppl 1):1S-169S.

[42] Hunot V, Churchill R, Silva de Lima M, et al. Psychological therapies for generalised anxiety disorder. Cochrane Database Syst Rev. 2007;(1):CD001848.

[43] Joyce M, Khan A, Eggens I, et al. Efficacy and safety of extended release quetiapine fumarate (quetiapine XR) monotherapy in patients with generalized anxiety disorder (GAD). Poster presented at the 161st annual meeting of the American Psychiatric As-sociation. May 3-8, 2008.

[44] Kabat-Zinn J. An outpatient program in behavioral medicine for chronic pain pa-tients based on the practice of mindfulness meditation: Theoretical considerations and preliminary results. General Hospital Psychiatry,1982;4, 33–47.

[45] Kabat-Zinn J. Mindfulness-based interventions in context: Past, present, and future. Clinical Psychology: Science and Practice 2003;10, 144–156.

[46] Kapczinski F, Lima MS, Souza JS, Schmitt R. Antidepressants for generalized anxiety disorder. Cochrane Database Syst Rev 2003;(2):CD003592.

[47] Khan A, Joyce M, Eggens I, et al. St Louis, MO: Extended release quetiapine fumarate (quetiapine XR) monotherapy in the treatment of generalized anxiety disorder (GAD) Presented at the 27th Annual Meeting of the Anxiety Disorders Association of America; March 6–9, 2008.

[48] Li Z, Pfeiffer PN, Hoggatt KJ, Zivin K, Downing K, Ganoczy D, Valenstein M. Emer-gent anxiety after antidepressant initiation: a retrospective cohort study of Veterans Affairs Health System patients with depression. Clin Ther. 2011;33(12):1985-92.

[49] Li Z, Hoggatt K, Pfeiffer PN, Downing K, Kim HM, Zivin K, Valenstein M. Develop-ment of anxiety after antidepressant usage among depressed veterans. Annual Albert J. Silverman Conference, Ann Arbor, MI, June 2009.

[50] Linehan MM. Cognitive-behavioral treatment of borderline personality disorder, 1993a. New York: Guilford.

[51] Linehan MM. Skills training manual for cognitive behavioral treatment of borderline personality disorder, 1993b. New York: Guilford.

[52] Longo LP, Johnson B. Addiction, pt 1: benzodiazepines: side effects, abuse risk and alternatives. Am Fam Physician. 2000;61(7):2121–2128.

[53] Lydiard RB, Rickels K, Herman B, et al. Comparative efficacy of pregabalin and benzodiazepines in treating the psychic and somatic symptoms of generalized anxiety disorder. Int J Neuropsychopharmacol. 2010;13(2):229–241.

[54] Mathew SJ, Amiel JM, Coplan JD, Fitterling HA, Sackeim HA, Gorman JM. Open-label trial of riluzole in generalized anxiety disorder. Am J Psychiatry 2005;162:2379-81.

[55] Mathew SJ, Garakani A, Reinhard JF, Oshana S, Donahue S. Short-term tolerability of a nonazapirone selective serotonin 1A agonist in adults with generalized anxiety disorder: a 28-day, open label study. Clin Ther 2008;30:9.

[56] Mathew SJ, Price RB, Mao X, Smith LP, Coplan JD, Charney DS, Shungu DC. Hippocampal N-acetylaspartate concentration and response to riluzole in generalized anxiety disorder. Biol Psychiatry 2008;63:891-8.

[57] Mennin DS, Heimberg RG and Turk CL. Clinical presentation and diagnostic features, 2004. In R. G. Heimberg, C. L. Turk, & D. S. Mennin (Eds.), Generalized anxiety disorder: Advances in research and practice. New York: The Guilford Press.

[58] Menza MA, Dobkin RD, Marin H. An open-label trial of aripiprazole augmentation for treatment-resistant generalized anxiety disorder. J Clin Psychopharmacol. 2007;27(2):207–210.

[59] Montgomery SA, Tobias K, Zornberg GL, et al. Efficacy and safety of pregabalin in the treatment of generalized anxiety disorder: a 6-week, multicenter, randomized, double-blind, placebo-controlled comparison of pregabalin and venlafaxine. J Clin Psychiatry. 2006;67(5):771–782.

[60] Nicolini H, Bakish D, Duenas H et al. Improvement of psychic and somatic symptoms in adult patients with generalized anxiety disorder: examination from a duloxetine, venlafaxine extended-release and placebocontrolled trial. Psychological Medicine,2009; 39, 267–276.

[61] Pande AC, Crockatt JG, Feltner DE, et al. Pregabalin in generalized anxiety disorder: a placebo-controlled trial. Am J Psychiatry. 2003;160(3):533–540.

[62] Petrovic M, Mariman A, Warie H, et al. Is there a rationale for prescription of benzodiazepines in the elderly? Review of the literature. Acta Clin Belg. 2003;58(1):27–36.

[63] Pittenger C, Coric V, Banasr M, Bloch M, Krystal JH, Sanacora G.Riluzole in the treatment of mood and anxiety disorders. CNS Drugs. 2008;22(9):761-86.

[64] Pohl RB, Feltner DE, Fieve RR, et al. Efficacy of pregabalin in the treatment of gener-
      alized anxiety disorder: double-blind, placebo-controlled comparison of BID versus
      TID dosing. J Clin Psychopharmacol. 2005;25(2):151–158.

[65] Pollack M. Levetiractam (Keppra) for anxiety. Curbside Consultant 2002; 1 (4): 4

[66] Pollack MH, Matthews J, Scott EL. Gabapentin as a potential treatment for anxiety
      disorders [letter]. Am J Psychiatry 1998;155 (7): 992-3

[67] Pollack MH, Simon NM, Zalta AK, et al. Olanzapine augmentation of fluoxetine for
      refractory generalized anxiety disorder: a placebo-controlled study. Biol Psychiatry.
      2006;59(3):211–215.

[68] Pollack MH, Tiller J, Xie F, et al. Tiagabine in adult patients with generalized anxiety
      disorder: results from 3 randomized, double-blind, placebo-controlled, parallel-
      group studies. J Clin Psychopharmacol. 2008;28(3):308–316.

[69] Pollack MH. Refractory generalized anxiety disorder. J Clin Psychiatry 2009;70
      (Suppl. 2):32-38.

[70] Power KG, Jerrom DWA, Simpson RJ. A controlled comparison of cognitive-behavio-
      ral therapy, diazepam and placebo in the management of generalized anxiety. Behav
      Psychother 1989;17: 1–14.

[71] Rapgay L, Bystritsky A, Dafter RE, Spearman M. New Strategies for Combining
      Mindfulness with Integrative Cognitive Behavioral Therapy for the Treatment of
      Generalized Anxiety Disorder. J Ration Emot Cogn Behav Ther. 2011;29(2):92-119.

[72] Rickels K, Downing R, Schweizer E, et al. Antidepressants for the treatment of gener-
      alized anxiety disorder: a placebo-controlled comparison of imipramine, trazodone,
      and diazepam. Arch Gen Psychiatry 1993; 50: 884-95

[73] Rickels K, Pollack MH, Feltner DE, et al. Pregabalin for treatment of generalized
      anxiety disorder: a 4-week, multicenter, double-blind, placebo-controlled trial of pre-
      gabalin and alprazolam. Arch Gen Psychiatry. 2005;62(9):1022–1030.

[74] Rickels K, Schweizer EE. Current pharmacotherapy of anxiety and panic. In: Meltzer
      HY, ed. Psychopharmacology: The Third Generation of Progress. New York, NY:
      Raven Press;1987:1193-1203.

[75] Roemer L, Orsillo SM, Barlow DH. Generalized anxiety disorder. In: Barlow DH, ed.
      Anxiety And Its Disorders. New York, NY: Guilford; 2002:477-515.

[76] Rynn M, Rüssell J, Erickson J. et al. Efficacy and safety of duloxeline in the treatment
      of generalized anxiety disorder: a flexible-dose, progressive-titration. placebo-con-
      trolled trial. Depress Anxiety 2008: 25 (3): 182-9

[77] Rynn M, Brawman-Mintzer O. Generalized anxiety disorder: acute and chronic treat-
      ment. CNS Spectr. 2004;9(10):716-23.

[78] Schaller JL, Thomas J, Rawlings D. Low-dose tiagabine effectiveness in anxiety disorders. MedGenMed. 2004;6(3):8.

[79] Schwartz TL, Azhar N, Husain J, et al. An open-label study of tiagabine as augmentation therapy for anxiety. Ann Clin Psychiatry. 2005;17(3):167–172.

[80] Schwartz TL. The use of tiagabine augmentation for treatment-resistant anxiety disorders: a case series. Psychopharmacol Bull. 2002;36(2):53–57.

[81] Segal ZV, Williams JMG and Teasdale JD. Mindfulness-based cognitive therapy for depression: A new approach to prevention relapse, 2002. New York: Guilford Press.

[82] Shader RI, Greenblatt DJ. Some current treatment options for symptoms of anxiety. J Clin Psychiatry. 1983;44:21-30.

[83] Simon NM, Hoge EA, Fischmann D, et al. An open-label trial of risperidone augmentation for refractory anxiety disorders. J Clin Psychiatry. 2006;67(3):381–385.

[84] Sinclair LI, Christmas DM, Hood SD, Potokar JP, Robertson A, Isaac A, Srivastava S, Nutt DJ, Davies SJ. Antidepressant-induced jitteriness/anxiety syndrome: systematic review. Br J Psychiatry. 2009;194(6):483-90.

[85] Snyderman SH, Rynn MA, Rickels K. Open-label pilot study of ziprasidone for refractory generalized anxiety disorder. J Clin Psychopharmacol. 2005;25(5):497–499.

[86] Stein DJ, Ahokas AA, de Bodinat C. Efficacy of agomelatine in generalized anxiety disorder: A randomized, double-blind, placebo-controlled study. J Clin Psychopharmacol. 2008;28, 561-566.

[87] Wittchen HU, Zhao S, Kessler RC, et al. DSM-III-R generalized anxiety disorder in the National Comorbidity Survey. Arch Gen Psychiatry 1994;51:355–364.

[88] Wittchen HU. Generalized anxiety disorder: prevalence, burden, and cost to society. Depress Anxiety 2002;16:162–171.

[89] Yonkers KA, Dyck IR, Warshaw MG and Keller MB. Factors predicting the clinical course of generalised anxiety disorder. Br J Psychiatry. 2000;176:544-49)

[90] Yonkers KA, Warshaw MG, Massion AO, Keller MB. Phenomenology and course of generalised anxiety disorder. Br J Psychiatry. 1996;168(3):308-13.

Chapter 9

New Approaches to the Psychological Treatment of Obsessive-Compulsive Disorder in Adults

Clare Rees and Rebecca Anderson

Additional information is available at the end of the chapter

1. Introduction

The key features of Obsessive-Compulsive Disorder (OCD) are the experience of recurrent, unwanted and intrusive thoughts (obsessions) and/or the completion of repetitive ritualistic behaviours (compulsions). Compulsions are frequently performed to reduce the distress associated with the obsessional thoughts [1]. The lifetime prevalence of OCD is estimated to be 2-3% in the general population, with epidemiological studies indicating consistency in rates across different countries and cultures [2,3].

OCD is a severe anxiety disorder that is associated with significant disability. In fact, the World Health Organisation has rated OCD as the tenth leading cause of disability in the world. If left untreated, OCD typically becomes a chronic problem with a pattern of frequent re-occurrence and relapse [2]. Unfortunately, many individuals will significantly delay help-seeking, due to reasons such as a fear of embarrassment, and thus suffer for years with significant symptoms and distress [4,5].

OCD is typically diagnosed according to Diagnostic and Statistical Manual of Mental Disorders criteria [1]. These stipulate that the individual must experience either obsessions, compulsions, or both, and that these must interfere with the individual's life due to the time they consume (i.e., more than one hour per day) or by causing marked distress or significant impairment. To obtain an accurate diagnosis, clinicians will often use structured diagnostic interviews such as the Mini International Neuropsychiatric Interview (MINI) [6], Anxiety Disorders Interview Schedule (ADIS-IV) [7], or Structured Clinical Interview for the Diagnostic and Statistical Manual of Mental Disorders (SCID) [8]. Furthermore, clinicians and researchers will frequently utilize a selection of measures to ascertain symptom severity and to assess for clinical outcomes. The most common of these include the Yale-Brown Obsessive Compulsive Symptom Checklist (YBOCS) [9], and the Obsessive Compulsive Inventory – Revised (OCI-R) [10].

2. Why new approaches to treatment are needed

For some time now, the dominant approach to treating this disorder is a behavioural therapy called Exposure and Response Prevention (ERP). ERP is considered the gold-standard treatment as it currently has the most convincing evidence of efficacy from several controlled trials [11] and metaanalytic studies [12] spanning a number of years. In a study examining the change scores as a result of treatment outcomes, Fisher and Wells [13] found that 50-60% of participants were likely to be classified as recovered following ERP treatment. ERP is typically delivered on an individual basis and may be implemented as a stand alone treatment, or combined with cognitive strategies under the label of Cognitive Behaviour Therapy (CBT). Despite the success of ERP in alleviating the symptoms of OCD for many individuals, there remains much scope for further improving the success of psychological treatments for the disorder. Issues such as treatment refusal, non-completion of ERP, non-response in some cases and restricted accessibility are just some problems effecting outcomes.

Presently, there are major issues with costs and limited psychological therapy resources in the public healthcare system [14]. There are very limited therapeutic services available to the public in the area of OCD, and the majority of individuals do not have access to good treatments. According to Shafran and colleagues [15], evidence suggests that even though a number of evidence-based psychological treatments have been developed, clients are not receiving them within clinical settings. Furthermore, when evidence-based psychological treatments are delivered, they are often not delivered to an optimal standard [15]. Shafran and colleagues [15] provided a number of recommendations to approach this gap in well-delivered evidence-based psychological treatments, however, it may take time to increase awareness and knowledge about evidence-based psychological treatments, as well as the implementation of them. Given the lack of available therapeutic services being provided to the public as well as the delivery of evidence-based psychological treatments, a stepped care approach could provide another solution in the meantime to this problem [14].

A stepped care approach simply refers to treatments at differing intensities [14]. Within a stepped care approach, the treatment must be the least restrictive, but still provide significant improvements to health. With this in mind, if a treatment is provided at a lower level or step, and the client is not improving post-treatment, the client's needs should be evaluated, and an appropriate step to treatment provided. The restrictiveness of a treatment generally refers to the cost and personal inconvenience. When referring to the therapist, it can also refer to the availability of the therapists time and the amount of time required by a specialist therapist [14]. Given the limited number of therapists trained in the area of OCD, a stepped care approach appears to be particularly warranted in the treatment of OCD.

The National Institute for Health and Clinical Excellence (NICE) Guidelines for Obsessive-compulsive disorder [16], a world-renowned document outlining evidence-based approaches to treating the disorder, endorses the use of a stepped-care model in the prevention and provision of treatment services to individuals with OCD. The NICE Guidelines outline six levels of intervention as follows. It should be noted that all references to CBT within this stepped care model emphasize the need to include an ERP component in therapy.

Step 1: Awareness and recognition

Step 2: Recognition and assessment (including referral to appropriate services)

Step 3: Initial treatment by guided self-help and CBT via group or individual format

Step 4: For OCD with comorbidity or a poor response to initial treatment - treatment via CBT within a multidisciplinary team, possible medication

Step 5: For OCD with significant comorbidity, severe impairment or limited treatment response - specialist treatment services with expertise in CBT, possible medication

Step 6: Inpatient or intensive treatment programs including medication and CBT to reduce the risk to life, severe self-neglect or severe distress or disability.

As can be seen, while the higher level steps within this care model indicate the need for ERP based psychotherapy, which is provided on an individual basis, there is much scope for exploring less intensive, less costly, and more widely accessible formats for the delivery of ERP based treatment programs.

Furthermore, it is important to review emerging and alternate approaches to the conceptualization and treatment of this disorder. The capacity for ERP based treatments to bring about considerable and clinically significant change for many clients is well documented. However, prior studies have noted that up to 25% of patients refuse ERP treatment due to the time commitments needed to complete the treatment, a fear that the exposure exercises will bring about overwhelming anxiety, or a fear that a dreaded outcome will occur should the individual fail to complete their rituals [17]. Within this stepped care model there are limited evidence-based alternatives for treatment other than medication-based treatment, which individuals may also refuse or be unable to tolerate. It is therefore important that we continue to explore new psychological treatment approaches for this disorder and thus offer hope to those who refuse or do not respond to the current gold-standard treatment approaches.

3. New Treatment Approaches

The following section will provide a review of a number of new approaches to the treatment of OCD. First, the use of treatment modalities that differ from standard individual based CBT or ERP will be discussed. This will explore the use of the group therapy format, and the use of modern technologies in the delivery of cognitive and behavioural therapies. Next, emerging conceptualizations and treatment approaches will be discussed. This will review the evidence for Metacognitive and Acceptance and Commitment based approaches to the management of OCD. Each approach will first be described, the proposed mechanisms of change outlined and then a critical review of the evidence for efficacy will be offered.

Group therapy for OCD

The predominant groups that have been evaluated for OCD are either cognitive, behavioural or a combination of both. Provision of therapy in groups for OCD makes intuitive sense because of the known issues relating to shame, isolation and embarrassment that have been identified amongst sufferers. Being able to meet others with a similar set of problems can allow for symptoms to be normalized and destigmatised. Participating in a group can allow the individual to develop a support network for sharing strategies, information and resources, and the process of helping others may enhance ones self-esteem, and sense of social competence and connectedness. From a clinical perspective, peer modeling of ERP exercises may provide additional opportunities for exposure and reinforce compliance with homework. In addition to these potential advantages, as already mentioned, stepped-care models emphasize the importance of providing treatment options which are less costly and intensive. Group therapy formats have the capacity to increase access to well-trained clinicians, and decrease potential waiting times.

Empirical Evidence for Group CBT for OCD

A meta-analysis by Jónsson and Hougaard [18] examined the effectiveness of group CBT and ERP as reported in thirteen prior treatment trials. This included randomized controlled trials, non-randomized controlled trials, and naturalistic trials. The meta-analysis indicated that group CBT and ERP yields a large overall pre-post effect size of 1.18. Importantly, group dropout rates of 13.5% were compared with reported individual treatment dropout rates of 12.1%. This was considered an indication that the group format seemed an acceptable method of treatment delivery to most patients. When this information is combined with the earlier findings that direct comparisons between group and individual based treatments have not demonstrated a significant difference in post treatment outcomes [19,20], group CBT and ERP certainly appear to be viable and efficacious treatment options in the management on this disorder. Furthermore, the meta-analysis indicated that compared to pharmacological treatment, the between groups effect size of 0.80 favoured group CBT/ERP.

Since this meta-analysis, Belotto-Silva and colleagues [21] compared group CBT (GCBT) with Fluoxetine, a Selective Serotonin Reuptake Inhibitor, in a controlled trial including 158 participants (GCBT N=70; Fluoxetine N=88). A total of 12 group therapy sessions of 2 hours duration were provided each week. The Fluoxetine group received 80mg/day for the same duration (12 weeks). Mean YBOCS scores decreased by 23% (GCBT) and 21% (Fluoxetine). The authors note that this level of symptom reduction, although significant, is less than has been observed in some other CBT studies. They conclude that this is most likely due to the high rate of comorbidity present in the sample. In fact the results are closer to other similar studies that have utilised less stringent exclusion criteria and therefore arguably more representative samples [19,22]. In another study since the meta-analysis [23], the effectiveness of GCBT for OCD was further evaluated in a representative, clinic sample in Norway. In this open trial, 54 patients diagnosed with OCD were provided with 12 sessions of GCBT. At post treatment and again at 3 and 12 month follow-up significant improvements in OCD symptoms as well as depression and anxiety were observed.

It could be argued that these outcomes are simply due to the non-specific effects of participating in a group, such as the increased social support that participants experience. A study by Fineberg and colleagues [24] therefore attempted to account for the role of non-specific group effects within their research design by including a relaxation placebo control group. The outcomes indicated that both those in the CBT and relaxation placebo group improved, and that there was no significant difference between the outcomes for the two groups. However, there was a significant bias towards non-uptake of the relaxation therapy condition. With more potential participants dropping out prior to the trial even beginning, this may mean that the final relaxation group participants represented individuals predisposed to believe that relaxation was a credible form of treatment for OCD and that they therefore had enhanced expectations of treatment. There was also a significant difference in drop-out rates across conditions with 35% of participants dropping out of the relaxation group compared to 4% in the CBT group. Due to the observed difficulties with finding a credible group placebo, we are not yet able to ascertain whether these results are simply due to the non-specific group factors. However, this study yielded a large treatment effect size of 1.45 for GCBT, providing further support for the further use of group CBT.

Overall, the large effect sizes noted in prior studies demonstrate that group CBT and ERP are viable treatment options for service provision, with comparable findings to individual therapy and pharmacological treatments for OCD. Although further group placebo controlled trials may go some way to separating out the effects of non-specific group factors, the consistent reports of clinically and statistically significant improvements for participants, and the potential improved access to expert services for clients and cost savings for clinicians indicate that group therapy is a worthy option in the treatment of this disorder.

Telemental Health Approaches

Telemental health is a term used to capture the broad application of telecommunication and information technology in the provision of various mental health services. There are a number of different applications that have been developed and trialed for the treatment of OCD in adults. A summary of the evidence base and key advantages and disadvantages of these applications is provided in Table 1.

Evidence	Decreases physical barriers to treatment	Improves access to expert clinicians	Impact on time required	Other potential advantages	Other potential disadvantages

				...of clinician		
Telephone-based						
No therapist (automated)	RCTs	Yes	No	Eliminates	Able to be completed at time selected by client	Isolation, lack of therapeutic alliance may impact on treatment adherence and retention
With therapist	RCTs	Yes	Yes	Decreases	Regular contact may improve treatment compliance, support for clients experiencing difficulty with program	Lack of non-verbal cues
Video-conferencing	Case series	Yes	Yes	No change	Able to be conducted on mobile devices and home computers, presence of non-verbal cues, observation of exposure exercises	Observation of non-verbal cues may be limited by screen set-up, clients may not be familiar or comfortable with technology
Internet-based						
No therapist	Open trial	Yes	No	Eliminates	Able to be completed at time selected by client	Isolation, lack of therapeutic alliance may impact on treatment adherence and retention
With therapist	Open trial	Yes	Yes	Decreases	Regular contact may improve treatment compliance, support for clients experiencing difficulty with program	Lack of non-verbal cues
Virtual Reality	Case series	Yes	No	Decreases	Technology may enable treatment to be conducted on mobile devices and home computers	Virtual environment may not extend to cater for idiosyncratic presentations

Table 1. Advantages and disadvantages of telemental health approaches

Telephone-Based Treatments

BT-Steps [25] is a well-evaluated behaviour therapy self-help program that is administered via the telephone. It does not involve direct therapist contact as clients simply access an automated system where they enter details of their progress and receive automatic suggestions and prompts from an electronic recording. Reductions in YBOCS symptoms of up to 30% have been reported in open studies of patients who completed the self-exposure phase of BT-Steps [26] however a major limitation of this approach is the unusually high dropout rate that has been observed in the studies. In attempt to investigate this further, Kenwright, Marks, Graham, Franses and Mataix-Cols [27] compared the self-administered BT-Steps to a BT-Steps with inclusion of nine sessions of therapist support. Those in the supported condition evidenced both improved compliance and outcomes.

Three trials of CBT via telephone with therapist contact have been conducted with increasingly improved methodological rigor. Lovell and colleagues [28] first conducted a case series with four participants examining the impact of eight weekly telephone contacts with a cognitive behavioural therapist, starting and ending with a face-to-face session. Three out of the four participants improved, with reductions of between 24% to 67% noted on the YBOCS. In a later trial, Taylor and colleagues [29] provided 12 weekly therapy sessions by phone and with provision of a self-help book and compared this to a waitlist control. Thirty three participants were included and results indicated significant reduction in symptoms for the telephone group. More recently, Lovell and colleagues [30] compared telephone-based treatment with face-to-face CBT in a non-inferiority trial involving 72 participants. In each condition participants received 10 therapy sessions however, the telephone sessions were half the duration of the face-to-face sessions. Equivalent improvements were found across both groups suggesting that the telephone condition may represent an effective treatment with considerable reduction in therapist's time requirements.

Videoconferencing

Videoconferencing is a computer-assisted approach that bears the closest resemblance to face-to-face therapy because both therapist and client interact in real-time. It has major advantages in terms of eliminating the issue of distance between therapist and client. It is particularly beneficial for clients who have restricted mobility for any reason or who might not otherwise be inclined to leave their homes to attend therapy sessions. To date, two studies have explored the treatment of OCD via videoconference. Himle and colleagues [31] utilised a multiple-base line design to analyse the outcomes of a 12-week manualised CBT intervention. Three participants were included in the study and significant improvements in symptoms were observed for all participants as measured by the YBOCS. Participants also reported high satisfaction with the therapy and excellent scores on therapeutic alliance were also obtained.

In a recent case series design, Vogel and colleagues [32] investigated the effectiveness of videoconferencing therapy with the addition of cell phones. Fifteen sessions of ERP was delivered via six teleconference and nine cell phone sessions. Four of the six participants made substantial gains and no longer met criteria for OCD at the end of therapy. Importantly, these gains were maintained at a three month follow-up, and all patients rated the treatment format as acceptable and that the working alliance with the therapist was high. The authors did note that these results should be interpreted with caution due to the small sample size, lack of a control comparison and blind ratings, and possible selection bias of participants where those who are more comfortable with technologies self-select into the study. However, it was also recognized that the addition of cell phones to the trial allowed for a back-up when teleconferencing equipment did not work, and allowed the clinician to monitor exposure exercises conducted away from the videoconferencing equipment. With the increasing number of cell phones allowing video calls, the potential for this portable technology to improve the capacity for in-situ exposure exercises should only improve with time.

Internet-Based CBT

Treatments that are delivered via computers enable a client to gain assistance from remote locations or from the convenience of their own homes. For some time now, less costly and intense forms of intervention such as bibliotherapy and self-directed exposure have been recognized as an effective option for provision of psychological treatment [33]. More recently, bibliotherapy has been brought into the technological age with the development of computerized versions that as per their original counterparts, do not include any therapist contact. However, on the whole, the evidence has suggested that better results are achieved with the addition of minimal therapist support [34].

A recent open trial of an 8-week CBT treatment ('The OCD Program') delivered via the Internet has been completed [35]. Twenty-two individuals with a primary diagnosis of OCD participated in the trial receiving eight online CBT lessons in addition to twice-weekly telephone contact from a Clinical Psychologist. It should be noted that the average amount of therapist contact time was only 86 minutes across the 8 weeks. Significant improvements in YBOCS total scores were found with a reported within-groups effect size of 1.28 at post-treatment. This suggests that significant improvements in symptoms may be possible with only very limited therapist input.

In another recent open trial [36], 23 patients diagnosed with OCD were provided with a 15-week Internet-Based CBT program with therapist support. Consistent with the Wootton study, therapist contact time was minimal (average of 92 minutes per patient across the entire 15 weeks) and the within-groups effect size on the YBOCS was large (1.56). Taken together, the results of these trials suggest that CBT provided over the Internet with only minimal therapist time can result in substantial symptom reduction of a similar magnitude to that seen in face-to-face studies. However, as these are only open trials randomized controlled trials with larger samples and comparisons against face-to-face CBT are required to strengthen the conclusions.

Virtual Reality

Riva and Gamberini [37] assert that "virtual reality is an application that lets users navigate and interact with a three-dimensional computer-generated environment in real time" (p. 327). Virtual reality can be conducted on a variety of different systems ranging from 3-dimension software installed on a personal computer to immersive headsets connected to a hand control [38]. Virtual reality therapies are based on the assumption that people feel "present" in the virtual environment, whereby at some level their perception fails to recognize the role of technology in their experience [39]. A particular advantage of virtual reality systems is that they have the potential to offer accurate standardization and replication of a prescribed environment [40].

Virtual reality therapies have been demonstrated to be more effective than no treatment for several specific phobias, including spider phobia, acrophobia, and a fear of flying [39]. However, head-to-head trials with gold-standard in-vivo ERP treatments are limited, and the value of this form of treatment over the current leading approach is therefore unclear at this stage. The potential cost effectiveness of exposure via a virtual reality system is most obvious for problems where stimuli for the exposure exercise may be difficult or expensive to come by (e.g., flights for exposure exercises to address a fear of flying, or spiders to address a spider phobia). Virtual reality therapies therefore remain a promising area for future directions in anxiety disorder treatment, but require further evaluation at this stage.

In the only study evaluating virtual reality for OCD to date, Clark, Kirkby, Daniels, and Marks [41] used an interactive virtual environment to provide vicarious exposure to dirt for thirteen individuals with OCD. Participants completed three 45-minute computer based treatment sessions at weekly intervals. During the session, the participants were instructed to direct a figure on the screen to engage in exposure, such as by touching dirt in a virtual garden, and encouraged to refrain from selecting that the figure wash their hands in the virtual sink. Participants were awarded points for exposing their figure to dirt, and then for refraining from washing their hands despite the figure rating their anxiety as high. Following treatment, participants showed a significant decrease on their depression scores and on one measure of OCD symptoms, the Padua Inventory. However, no significant change was noted on their YBOCS scores.

In a follow-up report on the same study, it was noted that across the three virtual reality sessions participants became faster at engaging in hand dirtying, and were less likely to engage in hand-washing in the virtual environment [42], indicating that participants were able to learn the principles of ERP via this format. Given the low dose of therapy applied in this trial (i.e., three sessions only), and capacity to provide this treatment without ongoing therapist input, this therapy format certainly warrants further investigation to ascertain whether learning from the virtual environment can generalize to real-world experiences. The main limitation to future development of virtual reality programs for OCD may be the need to create a sufficient range of virtual environments and activities to cater for the expansive variety of OCD symptom presentations beyond contamination fears and associated hand-washing.

Summary of Empirical Evidence for Telemental Health Treatment of OCD

Taken together, the field of telemental health treatment for OCD is very promising with a number of controlled trials now showing that treatments administered via computer with minimal or no therapist assistance can result in significant reductions in obsessive-compulsive symptoms. Particularly promising results are being seen in Internet-Based treatments whereby as little as ten minutes of telephone contact per week from a therapist is associated with large effect sizes on obsessive-compulsive symptoms. While some approaches may enable reductions in therapist contact hours, approaches such as video-conferencing may not reduce contact hours but instead enable individuals with OCD to receive expert treatment regardless of geographical location. It is therefore envisaged that future treatments within a stepped care model could utilize computer and internet based therapies at a lower step, with technologies such as video-conferencing being used to provide expertise for individuals with high levels of comorbidity or who have not responded to less intense treatment formats who would otherwise have difficulty accessing such services. While the use of virtual reality based programs requires further investigation, it is possible that should it be demonstrated as an effective treatment format, it could be built into current computer or internet based self-help programs as a stand-alone treatment, or as a component in an overall treatment which also includes psychoeducation and the development of a personalized ERP hierarchy.

Metacognitive Therapy

Metacognition refers to beliefs about thinking and strategies used to regulate and control thinking and was originally elaborated upon by Flavell [43]. Since then a number of theorists have incorporated aspects of metacognition into various psychological models of OCD [44-47]. Most notable amongst these theorists is Adrian Wells who, along with colleagues, has developed a comprehensive metacognitive account of OCD based on the Self Regulatory Executive (S-REF) model [48,49]. According to this model, a style of thinking called the cognitive attentional syndrome (CAS) is the main causal factor in prolonging all emotional disorders. However, Wells has gone on to specify which particular aspects of this model are most relevant to understanding OCD. Wells and Mathews [48] and Wells [46] propose that three types of metacognitive knowledge are important in the etiology and maintenance of symptoms: thought fusion beliefs, beliefs about the need to perform rituals, and criteria that signal rituals can be stopped. In this model, thought fusion beliefs are extended beyond thought action fusion (belief that having a thought increases the chance of acting on it) but also thought-event fusion (the belief that having a thought can cause an event or means that an event has happened) and thought object fusion (the belief that thoughts or feelings can be transferred into objects). According to the model the three overall types of metacognitive knowledge operate in a causal chain to explain obsessive-compulsive symptoms.

The main approach used in MCT for OCD is to help the client to become aware of their metacognitive processing and to learn to modify these higher order metacognitions such as beliefs about the importance of thoughts. MCT differs from standard CBT in that no attempts are made to modify lower order appraisals such as 'I am responsible to ensure nothing happens to my family'. Also, MCT does not include exposure exercises aimed at habituation but instead includes the use of behavioural experiments to assist in the interruption of unhelpful metacognitive processes such as attempts to suppress thoughts.

Empirical Evidence for MCT for OCD

Two small trials of MCT for adults with OCD have been conducted to date. The first case series trial included four individuals diagnosed with OCD who received 12 sessions of individual MCT [50]. Substantial reduction in obsessive-compulsive symptoms was found with all participants meeting clinical significance criteria for recovery at post-treatment and 3-month follow-up. A second open trial included 8 individuals diagnosed with OCD who received 12 sessions of group-based MCT [51]. Similar results were found in this study with seven out of eight participants achieving recovery according to the YBOCS clinical significance criteria. This result was maintained at 3-month follow-up.

Steffen Moritz and colleagues [52] developed and tested a self-help treatment called 'My Metacognitive Training for OCD' (myMCT) which contains a mixture of standard cognitive-behavioural elements plus the addition of metacognitive treatment elements. They recruited 86 individuals with OCD over the Internet and randomly assigned them to either the self-help or wait-list condition. Those in the myMCT condition were emailed an electronic version of the self-help book. Participants who received the intervention showed significantly greater reductions in obsessive-compulsive symptoms compared to the wait-list group. It should be noted that this treatment did contain traditional cognitive restructuring elements and is thus less of a 'pure' test of metacognitive treatment for OCD.

Given that all bar one participant in the earlier MCT trials achieved recovery status and had maintained this at 3-month follow-up, MCT may represent a promising way forward for clinicians and patients alike. As this therapeutic approach does not directly rely on exposure exercises, it may provide a less aversive form of therapy for those who in the past have refused to start or have initiated but then dropped out of ERP programs. The small samples sizes, lack of control conditions, and possible non-specific effects of participating in a group program do limit the conclusions of these trials. Furthermore, there has been no comparison between MCT and gold-standard ERP to date. Further research could go some way towards determining whether MCT fits within the stepped care model of treatment as an efficacious stand alone individual based treatment, an alternative to group ERP or CBT, or as a self-help based program.

Acceptance and Commitment Therapy

ACT is based on a philosophy of *functional contextualism* and the Relational Frame Theory (RFT) [53]. The basic premise of this theory is that individuals learn relationships between stimuli and responses through a number of different processes and this relationship is not necessarily contingent upon actual experience with that stimuli. For example, in the case of OCD a person may fear contamination from handrails because they are similar or grouped together with shopping trolleys which are considered 'dirty'. ACT consists of six main therapy processes that are not targeted in a linear fashion but rather are addressed within therapy when the opportunity or need arises. The six therapy processes are

1.   Acceptance,

2.   Defusion,

3.   Self as context,

4. Contact with the present moment,

5. Values, and

6. Committed Action [54].

Unlike conventional CBT, ACT does not concern itself with attempts to address the content of cognitions or behaviours in OCD but rather the processes. For example, in ACT the client with OCD is assisted to see how previous attempts to control obsessions have failed and that the focus of therapy will shift to 'accept' rather than 'struggle' to eradicate obsessional thoughts. The therapist realigns the client to consider improvement in quality of life as the goal rather than reducing or eliminating symptoms. Another major aspect of the therapy is to help the clients achieve 'cognitive defusion', in other words, to see thoughts less literally. Instead of attempting to analyse, rationally challenge or evaluate the accuracy of thoughts, clients are assisted to 'defuse' from obsessions and to alter their relationship to these experiences by treating them just as thoughts in one's head or 'relatively unimportant words' [55]. Various therapeutic exercises are used to assist the client to achieve defusion such as 'thanking' the mind for a thought. 'Self as context' simply refers to the process of helping the client to separate his or her inner experiences from self. For example, to understand that obsessional thoughts are separate from who the client is as a person. Mindfulness exercises are also used to help the client to become more aware of current experiences, such as thoughts and sensations and not to engage in avoidance but to simply observe and pay attention to those experiences. Values work in ACT focuses on helping the client to follow through on actions or behaviours that are more consistent with personally held values (e.g., being a good friend). This is in contrast to behaviours that are aimed at avoiding anxiety (e.g., completing cleaning rituals). Finally, behavioural commitment exercises are designed to ensure that the client continues to engage in behaviours that are consistent with their values. For example, making time once a week to visit friends would be a behavioural commitment.

Although ACT is described as a Behaviour Therapy and it does include exposure exercises, the difference is that ACT does not utilise these therapeutic strategies with the aim of reducing rituals or distress per se. Rather, all of the strategies are used to help the client practice acceptance and mindfulness whilst heading in valued directions. Often there will be a simultaneous reduction in frequency and distress of obsessions and compulsions as a function of other more functional behaviours taking precedence but this is not the focus of the therapy [55].

Empirical Evidence for ACT with OCD

Twohig, Hayes, and Masuda [56] conducted a multiple baseline study of ACT for OCD that included four clients with different symptom presentations (two checking, one cleaning, one hoarding). The intervention consisted of 8 hours of ACT. At the end of treatment, significant reductions in symptoms were obtained on the Obsessive Compulsive Inventory (OCI) with results maintained at 3-month follow-up. This same ACT protocol was later compared to a progressive relaxation training (PRT) control condition in the first randomized controlled trial of ACT for OCD [57]. The study included 79 adults diagnosed with OCD; with primary symptoms measured using the YBOCS. Significant improvements on the YBOCS were found for the ACT condition at post treatment and follow-up. In addition, clinically significant improvement occurred more in the ACT compared to the PRT condition. Although this study provides initial empirical support for the efficacy of ACT for OCD, further controlled trials are required as well as trials including longer follow-up periods and comparisons against other active and well established treatments such as ERP.

Summary and Conclusion

While ERP has long been established as the most effective treatment for OCD, the typical application of the treatment in an individual face-to-face format may limit client access to effective therapy and specialist clinicians. The stepped-care model suggests that lower intensity treatment formats, such as self-help and group therapy, be utilized so that only those with more complex needs are referred to the higher intensity individual format. This review has indicated that internet based CBT programs with minimal therapist support and group ERP based therapy are supported as lower intensity treatment options within a stepped care model. There is limited evidence that CBT conducted over the telephone or via videoconferencing will reduce therapist time working with patients. These formats therefore do not offer an alternative step within the stepped care model, but instead offer an additional means for delivering the higher intensity step of individual based therapy which is less susceptible to geographical or physical barriers to attending therapy. At this stage, further evaluations are required of virtual reality based programs to ascertain their effectiveness either as a stand-alone treatment or as a component within a treatment package.

Although still considered the gold-standard treatment, some patients will decline to start or complete ERP based therapy, and a proportion will not improve despite application of the treatment by expert clinicians. It is noted that the stepped care model offers limited evidence-based psychological alternatives to ERP based psychotherapy. It is therefore important that we continue to evaluate alternative approaches. Early indications from MCT and ACT trials have shown promising results. However, for both approaches the studies have involved small samples, and neither treatment has been directly compared with ERP in a clinical trial. Until such a comparison takes place, no conclusion can be made as to whether these approaches should be included as an option within the current stepped care model.

Author details

Clare Rees* and Rebecca Anderson

*Address all correspondence to: c.rees@curtin.edu.au

School of Psychology and Speech Pathology, Curtin Health Innovation Research Institute (CHIRI), Curtin University, Australia

References

[1] American Psychiatric Association. (2000). Diagnostic and statistical manual of mental disorders. *Text revision (4th ed.). Washington: Author.*

[2] Abramowitz, J., Taylor, S., & Mc Kay, D. (2009). Obsessive-Compulsive Disorder. *The Lancet*, 374(9688), 491-499.

[3] Pallanti, S. (2008). Transcultural observations of obsessive-compulsive disorder. *The American Journal of Psychiatry*, 165, 169-170.

[4] Rasmussen, S., & Tsuang, M. (1986). Clinical characteristics and family history in DSM-III obsessive-compulsive disorder. *American Journal of Psychiatry*, 143, 317-322.

[5] Steketee, G. (1993). Treatment of obsessive-compulsive disorder. *New York: Guilford Press.*

[6] Sheehan, D., Lecrubier, Y., Sheehan, K., Amorim, P., Janavs, J., Weiller, E., Hergueta, T., Baker, R., & Dunbar, G. (1998). The Mini-International Neuropsychiatric Interview (M.I.N.I): the development and validation of a structured diagnostic psychiatric interview for DSM-IV and ICD-10. *Journal of Clinical Psychiatry*, 59(20), 22-33.

[7] Brown, T., Di Nardo, P., Lehman, C., & Campbell, L. (2001). Reliability of DSM-IV anxiety and mood disorders: Implications for the classification of emotional disorders,. *Journal of Abnormal Psychology*, 110, 49-58.

[8] First, M., Spitzer, R., Gibbon, M., & Williams, J. (1996). Structured Clinical Interview for DSM-IV Axis I Disorders- Patient Edition (SCID-I/P, Version 2.0). *New York: Biometrics Research Department, New York State Psychiatric Institute.*

[9] Goodman, W., Price, L., Rasmussen, S., Mazure, C., Fleischman, R. Hill, et al. (1989). The Yale-Brown Obsessive Compulsive Scale: Development, use, and reliability. *Archives of General Psychiatry*, 46, 1006-1011.

[10] Foa, E., Kozak, M., Salkovskis, P., Coles, M., & Amir, N. (1998). The validation of a new obsessive-compulsive disorder scale: The obsessive-compulsive inventory. *Psychological Assessment*, 10, 206-214.

[11] Foa, E., Liebowitz, M., Kozak, M., Davies, S., Campeas, R., Franklin, M., Huppert, J., Kjernisted, K., Rowan, V., Schmidt, A., Simpson, H., & Tu, X. (2005). Randomized, placebo-controlled trial of exposure and ritual prevention, clomipramine, and their combination in the treatment of obsessive-compulsive disorder. *American Journal of Psychiatry*, 162, 151-161.

[12] Kobak, K., Greist, J., Jefferson, J., Katzelnick, D., & Henk, H. (1998). Behavioral versus pharmacological treatments of obsessive compulsive disorder: A meta-analysis. *Psychopharmacology*, 136, 205-216.

[13] Fisher, P., & Wells, A. (2005). How effective are cognitive and behavioural treatments for obsessive-compulsive disorder? A clinical significance analysis. *Behaviour Research and Therapy*, 43, 1543-1558.

[14] Bower, P., & Gilbody, S. (2005). Stepped care in psychological therapies: Access, effectiveness and efficiency. *British Journal of Psychiatry*, 186, 11-17.

[15] Shafran, R., Clark, D., Fairburn, C., Arntz, A., Barlow, D., Ehlers, A., et al. (2009). Mind the gap: Improving the dissemination of CBT. *Behaviour Research and Therapy*, 47, 902-909.

[16] National Collaborating Centre for Mental Health. (2005). Obsessive compulsive disorder: Core interventions in the treatment of obsessive compulsive disorder and body dysmorphic disorder. *Leicester: British Psychological Society*.

[17] Greist, J. (1998). The comparative effectiveness of treatments for obsessive-compulsive disorder. *Bulletin of the Meninger Clinic*, 62, A65-A81.

[18] Jónsson, H., & Hougaard, E. (2009). Group cognitive behavioural therapy for obsessive-compulsive disorder: A systematic review and meta-analysis. *Acta Psychiatrica Scandinavica*, 119, 98-106.

[19] Anderson, R., & Rees, C. (2007). Group versus individual cognitive-behavioural treatment for obsessive-compulsive disorder: a controlled trial. *Behaviour Research and Therapy*, 45(1), 123-137.

[20] Fals-Stewart, W., Marks, A., & Schafer, J. (1993). A comparison of behavioral group therapy and individual behavior therapy in treating obsessive-compulsive disorder. *The Journal of Nervous and Mental Disease*, 181, 189-193.

[21] Belotto-Silva, C., Belo, Diniz. J., Marino, Malavazzi. D., Valerio, C., Fossaluza, V., Borcato, S., Seixas, A., Morelli, D., Miguel, E., & Shavitt, R. (2012). Group cognitive-behavioral therapy versus selective serotonin reuptakeinhibitors for obsessive-compulsive disorder: A practical clinical trial. *Journal of Anxiety Disorders*, 26, 25-31.

[22] Tolin, D., Maltby, N., Diefenbach, G., Hannan, S., & Worhunsky, P. (2004). Cognitive behavioral therapy for medication non-responders with obsessive-compulsive disorder: a wait-list-controlled open trial. *Journal of Clinical Psychiatry*, 65(7), 922-931.

[23] Håland, A., Vogel, P., Lie, B., Launes, G., Pripp, A., & Himle, J. (2010). Behavioural group therapy for obsessive-compulsive disorder in Norway: An open community-based trial. *Behaviour Research and Therapy*, 48, 547-554.

[24] Fineberg, N., Hughes, A., Gale, T., & Roberts, A. (2005). Group cognitive behaviour therapy in obsessive-compulsive disorder (OCD): A controlled study. *International Journal of Psychiatry in Clinical Practice*, 9, 257-263.

[25] Marks, I., Baer, L., Greist, J., Park, J., Bachofen, M., Nakagawa, A., Wenzel, K., Parkin, J., Manzo, P., Dottl, S., & Mantle, J. (1998). Home self-assessment of obsessive com-

pulsive disorder. Use of a manual and a computer-conducted telephone interview: two UK-US studies. *British Journal of Psychiatry*, 172, 406-412.

[26] Herbst, N., Voderholzer, U., Stelzer, N., Knaevelsrud, C., Hertenstein, E., Schelgl, S., Nissen, C., & Kulz, A. (2012). The potential of telemental health applications for obsessive-compulsive disorder. *Clinical Psychology Review*, 32, 454-466.

[27] Kenwright, M., Marks, I., Graham, C., Frances, A., & Mataix-Cols, D. (2005). Brief scheduled phone support from a clinician to enhance computer-aided self-help for obsessive-compulsive disorder: A Randomized Controlled Trial. *Journal of Clinical Psychology*, 61, 1499-1508.

[28] Lovell, K., Fullalove, K., Garvey, R., & Brooker, C. (2000). Telephone treatment of obsessive-compulsive disorder. *Behavioural and Cognitive Psychotherapy*, 28, 87-91.

[29] Taylor, S., Thordarson, D., Spring, T., Yeh, A., Corcoran, K., Eugster, K., et al. (2003). Telephone-administered cognitive behavior therapy for obsessive compulsive disorder. *Cognitive Behaviour Therapy*, 32(1), 13-25.

[30] Lovell, K., Cox, D., Haddock, G., Jones, C., Raines, D., Garvey, R., et al. (2006). Telephone administered cognitive behaviour therapy for treatment of obsessive compulsive disorder: A randomised controlled non-inferiority trial. *BMJ: British Medical Journal*, 333, 883.

[31] Himle, J., Fischer, D., Muroff, J., Van Etten, M., Lokers, L., Abelson, J., & Hanna, G. (2006). Videoconferencing-based cognitive-behavioral therapy for obsessive-compulsive disorder. *Behaviour Research and Therapy*, 44, 1821-1829.

[32] Vogel, P., Launes, G., Moen, E., Solem, S., Hansen, B., Haland, A., & Himle, J. (2012). Videoconference- and cell phone-based cognitive behavioral therapy of obsessive-compulsive disorder: A case series. *Journal of Anxiety Disorders*, 26, 158-164.

[33] Tolin, D., Diefenbach, G., Maltby, N., & Hannan, S. (2005). Stepped care for obsessive-compulsive disorder: A pilot study. *Cognitive and Behavioral Practice*, 12(4), 403-414.

[34] Palmqvist, B., Carlbring, P., & Andersson, G. (2007). Internet-delivered treatments with or without therapist input: does the therapist factor have implications for efficacy and cost? *Expert Review of Pharmacoeconomics & Outcomes Research*, 7, 291-297.

[35] Wootton, B., Titov, N., Dear, B., Spence, J., Andrews, G., Johnston, L., & Solley, K. (2011). An internet administered treatment program for obsessive-compulsive disorder: A feasibility study. *Journal of Anxiety Disorders*, 25, 1102-1107.

[36] Andersson, E., Ljotsson, B., Hedman, E., Kaldo, V., Paxling, B., Andersson, G., Lindefors, N., & Ruck, C. (2011). Internet-based cognitive behavior therapy for obsessive compulsive disorder: a pilot study. *BMC Psychiatry*, 11, 125.

[37] Riva, G., & Gamberini, L. (2000). Virtual reality in telemedicine. *Telemedicine Journal and E-Health*, 6, 327-340.

[38] Hoffman, H., Doctor, J., Patterson, D., Carrougher, G., & Furness, T. (2000). Virtual reality as an adjunctive pain control during burn wound care in adolescent patients. *Pain*, 85, 305-309.

[39] Krijn, M., Emmelkamp, P., Olafsson, R., & Biemond, R. (2004). Virtual reality exposure therapy of anxiety disorders: A review. *Clinical Psychology Review*, 24, 259-281.

[40] Rizzo, A., Buckwalter, J., Humphrey, L., van der Zaag, C., Bowerly, T., Chua, C., Neumann, U., Kyriakakis, C., van Rooyen, A., & Sisemore, D. (2000). The virtual classroom: A virtual environment for the assessment and rehabilitation of attention deficits. *CyberPsychology and Behavior*, 3, 483-499.

[41] Clark, A., Kirkby, K., Daniels, B., & Marks, I. (1998). A pilot study of computer-aided vicarious exposure for obsessive-compulsive disorder. *Australian and New Zealand Journal of Psychiatry*, 32, 268-275.

[42] Kirkby, K., Berrios, G., Daniels, B., Menzies, R., Clark, A., & Romano, A. (2000). Process-outcome analysis in computer-aided treatment of obsessive-compulsive disorder. *Comprehensive Psychiatry*, 41(4), 259-265.

[43] Flavell, J. (1979). Meta-cognition and meta-cognitive monitoring: a new area of cognitive developmental inquiry. *American Psychologist*, 34, 906-911.

[44] Emmelkamp, P., & Aardema, A. (1999). Metacognition, specific obsessive-compulsive beliefs and obsessive-compulsive behavior. *Clinical Psychology and Psychotherapy*, 6, 139-145.

[45] Purdon, C., & Clark, D. (1999). Metacognition and obsessions. *Clinical Psychology and Psychotherapy*, 6, 102-110.

[46] Wells, A. (1997). Cognitive therapy of anxiety disorders: A practice manual and conceptual guide. *Chichester, UK: Wiley*.

[47] Wells, A. (2000). Emotional disorders and metacognition: Innovative cognitive therapy. *Chichester, UK: Wiley*.

[48] Wells, A., & Mathews, G. (1994). Attention and emotion. A clinical perspective. *Hove, UK: Lawrence Erlbaum & Associates*.

[49] Wells, A., & Matthews, G. (1996). Modeling cognition in emotional disorder: The S-REF Model. *Behavior Research and Therapy*, 34, 881-888.

[50] Fisher, P., & Wells, A. (2008). Metacognitive therapy for obsessive-compulsive disorder: A case series. *Journal of Behavior Therapy and Experimental Psychiatry*, 39, 117-132.

[51] Rees, C., & van Koesveld, K. (2008). An open trial of group metacognitive therapy for obsessive-compulsive disorder. *Journal of Behavior Therapy and Experimental Psychiatry*, 39, 451-458.

[52] Moritz, S., Jelinek, L., Hauschildt, M., & Naber, D. (2010). How to treat the untreated: effectiveness of a self-help metacognitive training program (my MCT) for obsessive-compulsive disorder. *Dialogues in Clinical Neuroscience*, 12, 209-220.

[53] Hayes, S., Barnes-Holmes, D., Roche, B. ., & Eds., . (2001). Relational Frame Theory: A Post Skinnerian account of human language and cognition. *New York: Kluwer Academic/Plenum*.

[54] Hayes, S., Strosahl, K., & Wilson, K. (1999). Acceptance and Commitment Therapy: An experiential approach to behavior change. *New York: Guilford Press*.

[55] Twohig, M. (2009). The application of acceptance and commitment therapy to the treatment of obsessive-compulsive disorder. *Cognitive and Behavioral Practice*, 16, 18-28.

[56] Twohig, M., Hayes, S., & Masuda, A. (2006). Increasing willingness to experience obsessions: Acceptance and commitment therapy as a treatment for obsessive-compulsive disorder. *Behavior Therapy*, 37, 3-13.

[57] Twohig, M., Hayes, S., Plumb, J., Pruitt, L., Collins, A., Hazlett-Stevens, H., & Woidneck, M. (2010). A randomized clinical trial of acceptance and commitment therapy versus progressive relaxation training for obsessive compulsive disorder. *Journal of Consulting and Clinical Psychology*, 78(5), 705-716.

Chapter 10

PTSD and the Attenuating Effects of Fish Oils: Results of Supplementation After the 2011 Great East Japan Earthquake

Daisuke Nishi, Yuichi Koido, Naoki Nakaya,
Toshimasa Sone, Hiroko Noguchi, Kei Hamazaki,
Tomohito Hamazaki and Yutaka Matsuoka

Additional information is available at the end of the chapter

1. Introduction

1.1. Evidence of effects of omega-3 polyunsaturated fatty acids on depression and anxiety disorder

Omega-3 polyunsaturated fatty acids (omega-3 PUFAs) such as eicosapentaenoic acid (EPA) and docosahexaenoic acid (DHA) are essential fatty acids that cannot be synthesized by humans de novo and must therefore be obtained through the diet. Omega-3 PUFAs are speculated to be beneficial against psychiatric disorders, especially depression, and an increasing growing number of randomized controlled trials (RCTs) have been carried out to verify their efficacy. In fact, a number of previous meta-analyses of RCTs support the positive effects of omega-3 PUFAs supplementation in reducing depressive symptoms [1-7]. However, a recent meta-analysis by Bloch and Hannestad in 2011 found that nearly all evidence of omega-3 PUFAs benefit was removed after adjusting for publication bias [8]. Their meta-analysis has subsequently been criticized by two papers published in quick succession [6, 7]. One of these papers, by Martins et al [6], pointed out methodological flaws with Bloch and Hannestad's analysis. For example, Bloch and Hannestad's analysis included the study examining individuals without formal psychiatric diagnosis, and 2 other studies satisfying their inclusion criteria were not included. Martins et al concluded that supplements containing EPA ≥60% of total EPA + DHA were effective against depression, a finding in agreement with a meta-analysis by Sublette et al [5]. Taken together, then, the latest evidence does suggest the efficacy of omega-3 PUFAs containing EPA ≥60% against depression.

Several biological mechanisms potentially explain the effect of omega-3 PUFAs in depression and anxiety disorder [1]. To date, however, few RCTs have been carried out to investigate whether omega-3 PUFAs are effective against anxiety disorders. While one such study suggested that omega-3 PUFAs might not be effective for patients suffering from depression with comorbid anxiety disorder [9], some RCTs found that omega-3 PUFAs decreased hostility and aggression among patients with borderline personality disorder [10].

1.2. Omega-3 polyundasurated fatty acids and inflammation

A competitive interaction exists between omega-6 polyunsaturated fatty acids (omega-6 PUFAs) such as arachidonic acid (AA) and omega-3 PUFAs in regard to their shared enzymatic pathways. Compared with the eicosanoids produced from AA, such as prostaglandin E2 (PGE2), those produced from omega-3 PUFAs, such as prostaglandin E3 (PGE3), have little pro-inflammatory activity [11]. Therefore, it is speculated that the amounts of omega-6 eicosanoids released in response to depression-associated inflammation and cell apoptosis, are determined by the fatty acid composition of the cell membrane phospholipids [12]. On this basis, it is thought that increased levels of omega-3 PUFAs in the cell membranes reduces the release of AA-derived prostaglandins, thereby reducing inflammatory activity [13].

Naturally occurring depression-related cell apoptosis may be mediated by free radicals that appear in the brain during the process of inflammatory or ischemic damage. Inflammation and ischemia are known to increase the risk for clinically defined depression [14]. Taken into account that cytokines stimulate the intrinsic pathway of apoptosis and induce depression [15, 16], it is not altogether surprising to find frequent comorbidity of inflammation and depression. The interaction between omega-6 and omega-3 PUFAs eicosanoids, therefore, partly control inflammation, apoptosis and depression as a result [14].

1.3. Omega-3 polyunsaturated fatty acids and neurogenesis

The severity of depression is known to be associated with serum brain-derived neurotrophic factor (BDNF) [17], which exerts various effects on the nervous system, including neuronal outgrowth, differentiation, synaptic connectivity, and neuronal repair and survival [18-20]. Its severity is also associated with low levels of erythrocyte omega-3 PUFAs [21]. Short-term dietary supplementation with omega-3 PUFAs has been shown to up-regulate adult neurogenesis in lobsters [22]. In rats, dietary omega-3 PUFAs increased levels of BDNF, which promotes neuronal survival and growth [23].DHA extended neurites and branches of rat hippocampal neurons in vitro [24]. DHA supplementation to rats also promoted the maturation of neurons and hippocampal neurogenesis in vivo [25].. On the basis of these findings, omega-3 PUFAs supplementation can enhance the effect of BDNF-related synaptic plasticity and neurogenesis.

Additionally, in PTSD, the pathogenesis of which is characterized by excess consolidation of fear memory and failure of extinction learning [26], it might be possible to control fear memory by regulating hippocampal neurogenesis [27]. Indeed, in mice with active hippocampal neurogenesis, the period of hippocampus-dependent fear memory was found to be shorter [28]. Given the findings of animal research conducted to date, omega-3 PUFAs seem to be the most promising candidate for dietary intervention to facilitate adult hippocampal neurogenesis following a traumatic event [25, 29]. In fact, in an open label trial in patients with physically injury, we previously found that PTSD symptoms were significantly alleviated by taking DHA-rich fish oil [30].

1.4. Background of the study

On March 11, 2011, The Great East Japan Earthquake and tsunami devastated the northeastern coast of Japan. As of July 18th, 2012, 15,867 died and 2,906 were missing arrocding to the National Police Agency. Many rescue workers, as well as survivors, were exposed to traumatic experiences. A number of studies have reported adverse psychological outcomes among rescue workers. In a study of medical care personnel sent to aid trauma victims of an airline crash, 13.5% developed PTSD within 18 months of the crash [31]. Similarly, in a study of rescue workers deployed to the site of the September 11 terrorist attack in New York in 2001, 16.7% developed PTSD and 21.7% developed depression at 13 months after the attack [32]. Moreover, peritraumatic distress (distress during and right after a traumatic experience) and TV viewing for extended periods were shown to predict PTSD symptoms in rescue workers [33, 34]. PTSD is associated with higher psychiatric comorbidity, attempted suicide, and physical illnesses [35], as well as with high medical expenses [36]. An appropriate strategy for the prevention of PTSD in rescue workers is therefore clearly required, but as yet adequate measures have not been developed.

Against this background, we carried out a study to determine whether fish oil supplementation can attenuate PTSD symptoms among rescue workers after the Great East Japan Earthquake. The main findings have been breifly reported elsewhere [37] and here we present the overall findings of the study.

2. Methods

2.1. Participants

This trial named "Attenuating posttraumatic distress with omega-3 polyunsaturated fatty acids among disaster medical assistance team members after the Great East Japan Earthquake (APOP)" was a single-blind, randomized, parallel-group field trial administered by the National Disaster Medical Center (NDMC), Tokyo, Japan. The head office of the Disaster Medical Assistance Team (DMAT) is located at NDMC. DMAT members are doctors, nurses, and operational coordination staff (medical or clerical staff who are neither doctors nor nurses) who are dispatched as a mobile medical team with specialized training that is capable of acting during the acute phase of a large-scale disaster. DMAT activities commenced on the day of the Great East Japan Earthquake, March 11, and concluded on March 22.

The DMAT members recruited to the present trial met the following inclusion criteria: 1) aged 18 years or older; 2) a native Japanese speaker or non-native speaker with Japanese conversational abilities; and 3) physically and psychologically capable of understanding and providing consent for study participation. The exclusion criterion was regular intake of warfarin for at least 3 months before deployment, because Fish oil supplementation could have provided additional anticoagulation with warfarin.

2.2. Procedures

The detailed trial procedures have been reported elsewhere [38], but briefly a written guide to the study, including an explanation of the study and informed consent, was posted to the Emergency Medical Information System by DMAT head office and a mass email was sent to all DMAT members asking for their participation. The Peritraumatic Distress Inventory (PDI) [39, 40] was used to quantify peritraumatic distress. Other detailed baseline assessment has been reported elsewhere [38].

2.3. Ethics

The study protects the rights and welfare of participants in the spirit of ethical guidelines outlined under the Declaration of Helsinki, and further respects the ethical principles of the Ministry of Health, Labour, and Welfare of Japan. The study was approved by the Ethics Committee of the NDMC on April 1, 2011. Individual participants in this study gave written informed consent.

2.4. Interventions

For participants allocated to the fish oil plus psychoeducation group, seven capsules per day, each containing 320 mg of fish oil, were provided in line with previous research [41]. The fish oil composition of each capsule was 70% DHA and 7% eicosapentaenoic acid (EPA). Each capsule was placed in a brown 500-ml polyethylene container with a wide opening. Participants were instructed to take the capsules after eating and additionally told that they might take a full day's dosage at one time. For participants of both groups, a leaflet on psychoeducation about posttraumatic distress focusing on critical incident stress was provided.

2.5. Objectives

This study aimed to determine whether fish oil supplementation can attenuate the symptoms of PTSD and other posttraumatic distress such as depression among DMAT workers who were deployed during the acute disaster phase of the Great East Japan Earthquake.

2.6. Outcomes

The primary outcome was total score on the Impact of Event Scale-Revised (IES-R) at 12 weeks after shipment of the supplements on April 19, 2011. The IES-R, developed by Weiss, is a self-reporting questionnaire about PTSD symptoms and is the most widely used measure internationally in all forms of disaster-area research [42]. The IES-R is composed of 22 items on the three largest symptoms in the diagnostic criteria of PTSD, namely re-experiencing, avoidance, and hyperarousal. Respondents rate symptoms experienced in the previous week. The validity and reliability of the Japanese version of the IES-R has been confirmed [43].

Secondary outcomes were the total scores on each of the Kessler 6 Scale, the Center for Epidemiologic Studies Depression Scale (CES-D), and the shortened 14-item version of the Resilience Scale at 12 weeks after shipment of the supplements. the Kessler 6 Scale, developed by Kessler et al. [44], is a self-reporting questionnaire designed to screen for psychiatric disorders and mood and anxiety disorders; the CES-D, developed by Radloff [45], is a self-reporting questionnaire on depression; and the shortened 14-item version of the Resilience Scale, developed by Wagnild and Young [46], is a self-reporting questionnaire for quantitative evaluation of resilience. The Japanese version of each of these three scales has been validated [47-49].

Safety of the intervention was evaluated by the presence of adverse events during the observation period, by asking the participants about the presence of such events at 2, 4, 8, and 12 weeks after the start of fish oil supplementation. Whenever inquiries were received from participants, necessary information was provided to them.

2.7. Sample size

We estimated that the mean improvement in IES-R score as the primary outcome measure would be 10 (SD 15) for the fish oil plus psychoeducation group and 0 (SD 15) for the psychoeducation alone group [30]. We set α level at.05 and β at.10. This brought us to our required sample size estimation of 48 cases per group. Because the control group in this study received psychoeducation, we allowed up to 150 cases for the intervention group and 300 cases for the control group.

2.8. Randomization

Participants were randomly assigned to either the fish oil supplementation plus psychoeducation group or psychoeducation alone group. The trial statisticians (NN and TS) independently conducted randomization by the permuted block method using a four-person block, and concealed allocation mechanism until the study was finished. The participants were stratified by sex because previous studies showed that the prevalence of PTSD and of major depressive disorder was higher in women than in men [50].

2.9. Blinding

Because placebo capsules were not provided to psychoeducation alone group, participants could not be masked. Also, the researcher who provided necessary information regarding safety management to the participants (DN) could not be masked in just a few cases when participants inadvertently stated that they took the fish oils capsules. Other researchers were masked to allocation.

2.10. Statistical methods

All analyses were conducted according to the intention-to-treat principle. A sensitivity analysis was performed using a multiple imputation procedure with SAS version 9.1 (SAS Institute Inc, Cary, North Carolina) to impute each psychological variable end point for participants who did not have a follow-up psychological variable assessed.

Analysis of covariance (ANCOVA) was used to investigate the significance of the differences in the initial values as well as those of the net changes after the intervention among the 2 groups, 95% confidence interval values, and P values. Covariates for ANCOVA were sex, age, and each psychological variable score at baseline. In addition, we examined the impact of sex difference for fish oil supplementation on posttraumatic distress. A two-tailed test was used, with the α level set at 0.05.

3. Results

3.1. Participants flow and recruitment

Figure 1 shows the trial profile. Of the 1,816 DMAT workers deployed to the disaster areas, 172 were enrolled and randomly allocated to the fish oil plus psychoeducation group or psychoeducation alone group between April 2 and 12, 2011 (Figure 1). The mean duration from baseline assessment to follow-up assessment was 14.2 weeks (SD 0.9), and from shipment of the supplements to follow-up assessment was 12.6 weeks (SD 0.8). Only 1 participant in the psychoeducation alone group was lost to follow-up.

3.2. Baseline data

The two groups were well balanced with respect to baseline characteristics, except that the IES-R total and intrusion subscale scores were relatively high in the intervention group (Table 1). The mean term of the deployment was 4.1 days (SD 2.0). Two participants (1%) were injured during deployment, 11 (6%) saved children, 24 (14%) had contact with corpses, and the median of the PDI was 12.5 (range 0-42). These variables, identified as risk factors for PTSD in previous research [31, 51], did not differ significantly between the two groups. The PDI scores were comparable to those in accident survivors (Median 15.0, range 0-40] [52, 53].

3.3. Numbers analyzed

Eighty-six participants were assigned to each group. Primary outcome data were available for all participants, except one. All participants constituted the intention-to-treat population. The imputation technique assigned changes in the effectiveness end point for the noncompleter based on the participant's baseline characteristics and baseline psychological variables.

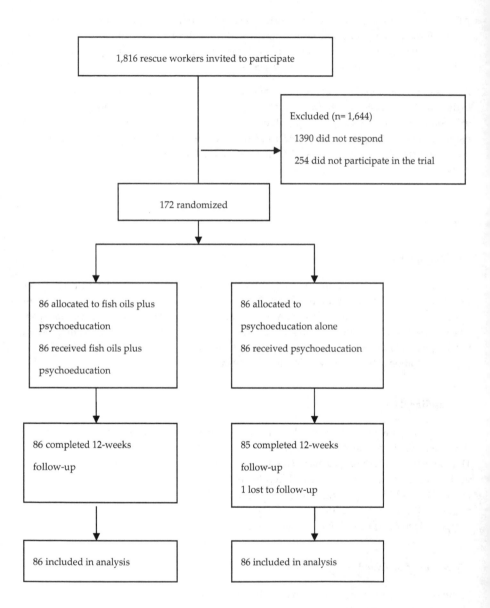

Figure 1. Flow diagram of the study

	Fish oil plus psychoeducation group (n=86)	Psychoeducation alone group (n=86)	P value[*1]
Demographic data			
Age in years (mean±S.D.)	37.9 ± 7.4	37.4 ± 7.4	0.62
Women (%)	27.9	26.7	0.86
BMI (mean±S.D.)	22.7 ± 2.8	23.0 ± 3.0	0.50
Occupation (%)			0.87
Medical Doctor	26.7	24.4	
Nurse	46.5	45.4	
Other	26.7	30.2	
Years of occupational experience (mean±S.D.)	14.5 ± 7.2	13.2 ± 7.3	0.24
Previous disaster operation experience (%)	27.9	26.7	0.86
Married (%)	67.4	72.1	0.51
Has a child (or children) (%)	57.0	61.6	0.53
Education (%)			
University or higher	47.7	53.5	0.45
Current smoker (%)	29.1	23.3	0.39
Current drinker (%)	80.2	83.7	0.55
Has past history of any physical disaeses[*2] (%)	0.0	0.0	-
Has past history of depression (%)	0.0	4.7	-
Psychological data			
IES-R (mean±S.D.)			
IES-R-Total	14.5 ± 15.1	10.7 ± 11.5	0.07
IES-R-Intrusion	6.5 ± 6.6	4.7 ± 5.1	0.05
IES-R-Avoidance	4.0 ±5.2	3.0 ± 4.2	0.16
IES-R-Hyperarousal	3.9 ± 4.6	2.9 ± 3.6	0.12
K6 (mean±S.D.)	4.5 ± 5.0	3.4 ± 4.2	0.13
CES-D (mean±S.D.)	13.6 ± 9.1	11.6 ± 8.1	0.13
RS-14 (mean±S.D.)	65.5 ± 10.3	67.1 ± 9.9	0.31

Abbreviations: IES-R, Impact of Event Scale-Revised; K6, Kessler 6 Scale; CES-D, Center for Epidemiologic Studies Depression Scale; RS-14, Resilience Scale 14-item version

*1) Student's t test or Chi-square test

*2) Physical disease defined as cancer, cardiovascular disease, stroke, chronic renal disease, chronic liver disease, and accidental injury.

Table 1. Characteristics of the study population at randomization

3.4. Outcomes and estimation

ANCOVA adjusted for sex and age showed a significant reduction in IES-R intrusion and hyperarousal subscale scores in the fish oil plus psychoeducation group. When adjusted for the scores at baseline, however, no significant difference in primary outcome was seen between the two groups when adjusted for the scores at baseline (-0.9, 95% CI, -3.0 to 1.2; P = 0.39) and no significant differences were seen in any of secondary outcomes (Table 2).

Variables	Baseline (mean±S.D.)	After 12 weeks (mean±S.D.)	Net change 1 (95% CI)	P value	Net change 2 (95% CI)	P value
IES-R-Total						
Fish oils group	14.5 ± 15.1	9.0 ± 9.5	-2.7	0.06	-0.9	0.39
Control group	10.7 ± 11.5	7.9 ± 10.0	(-5.5, 0.1)		(-3.0, 1.2)	
IES-R-Intrusion						
Fish oils group	6.5 ± 6.6	3.3 ± 3.4	-1.5	0.03	-0.5	0.28
Control group	4.7 ± 5.1	3.1 ± 3.7	(-2.8, -0.2)		(-1.3, 0.4)	
IES-R-Avoidance						
Fish oils group	4.0 ± 5.2	3.3 ± 4.4	-0.04	0.94	0.3	0.44
Control group	3.0 ± 4.2	2.4 ± 3.7	(-1.0, 0.9)		(-0.5, 1.1)	
IES-R-Hyperarousal						
Fish oils group	3.9 ± 4.6	2.3 ± 2.7	-1.1	0.03	-0.6	0.11
Control group	2.9 ± 3.6	2.5 ± 3.5	(-2.1, -0.1)		(-1.4, 0.1)	
K6						
Fish oils group	4.5 ± 5.0	2.9 ± 3.4	-0.4	0.52	0.2	0.62
Control group	3.4 ± 4.2	2.2 ± 3.7	(-1.5, 0.8)		(-0.6, 1.1)	
CES-D						
Fish oils group	13.6 ± 9.1	10.8 ± 6.3	-1.5	0.20	-0.3	0.73
Control group	11.6 ± 8.1	10.3 ± 7.2	(-3.9, 0.8)		(-2.1, 1.5)	
RS-14						
Fish oils group	65.5 ± 10.3	67.2 ± 11.3	2.7	0.09	2.2	0.15
Control group	67.1 ± 9.9	66.1 ± 13.3	(-0.4, 5.8)		(-0.8, 5.2)	

Abbreviations: IES-R, Impact of Event Scale-Revised; K6, Kessler 6 Scale; CES-D, Center for Epidemiologic Studies Depression Scale; RS-14, Resilience Scale 14-item version; CI, confidence interval

Net change 1: Analysis of covariance (ANCOVA) adjusted for sex and age

Net change 2: Analysis of covariance (ANCOVA) adjusted for sex, age and each psychological variable score at baseline

Table 2. Change in IES-R, K6, CES-D and RS-14 scores of participants in the fish oils and control groups

Because previous studies showed that the prevalence of PTSD and of major depressive disorder was higher in women than in men [50], subgroup analysis by sex was pre-specified. In women, the IES-R total mean score was reduced from 15.7 (SD 14.9) at baseline to 9.3 (SD 8.8) at follow-up in the fish oil plus psychoeducation group, compared to that from 11.2 (SD 13.0) to 10.4 (SD 12.3) in the psychoeducation alone group. In men, the IES-R total score was reduced in both groups, from 14.0 (SD 15.3) to 8.9 (SD 9.9) in the fish oil plus psychoeducation group and from 10.5 (SD 11.1) to 6.9 (SD 9.0) in the psychoeducation alone group. Remarkably, even when adjusted for age and IES-R scores at baseline, change in the IES-R score of women in the two groups from baseline to 12weeks was -3.9 (95% CI, -7.5 to -0.3; P = 0.04) (Table 3).

Regarding adherence, 7 out of 86 participants (8%; 6 male, 1 female) in the fish oil plus psychoeducation group took fish oil supplements 2 days or less per a week.

3.5. Adverse events

The occurrence rate of adverse events was not significantly different between the two groups, with 32 participants (37%) in the fish oil plus psychoeducation group reporting at least one adverse event versus 22 (26%) of the psychoeducation alone group doing so. Of these events, none were regarded as serious or led to withdrawal. The main adverse events included loose bowel (21 (24%) in the fish oil plus psychoeducation group versus 15 (17%) in the psychoedu-cation alone group) and belching (12 (14%) in the fish oil plus psychoeducation group versus 7 (8%) in the psychoeducation alone group).

4. Discussion

4.1. Interpretation

This trial regretfully did not show the superiority of fish oil supplementation plus psycho-education over psychoeducation alone for the prevention of PTSD and depressive symptoms among rescue workers. Even though a relatively good improvement was seen in IES-R score in the fish oil plus psychoeducation group, the improvement did not reach statistical signifi-cance. Furthermore, we recorded no significant differences between the two groups for the 3 secondary outcomes.

One of the possible reasons for not detecting the effectiveness of fish oil supplementation was that posttraumatic distress was reduced in both groups. A previous study of disaster workers at the September 11 terrorist attack sites showed that depressive symptoms were increased from 7 months after the disaster to 13 months after, while PTSD symptoms were reduced from 1 week to 13 months afterward [32]. In the present study, all psychological variables were reduced to some extent in both groups. Participants in both groups were contacted at 2, 4, 8, and 12 weeks for safety management and necessary information was provided to them upon request for ethical reasons: such contact might have been supportive for both groups of participants. Psychoeducation provided before the baseline assessment also might affect the results.

Variables		Net change (95% CI)	P value
IES-R-Total			
	Women	-3.9 (-7.5, -0.3)	0.04
	Men	0.2 (-2.2, 2.7)	0.86
IES-R-Intrusion			
	Women	-1.3 (-2.9, 0.4)	0.12
	Men	-0.1 (-1.1, 0.8)	0.78
IES-R-Avoidance			
	Women	-0.4 (-1.9, 1.1)	0.58
	Men	0.6 (-0.4, 1.6)	0.23
IES-R-Hyperaruosal			
	Women	-1.9 (-3.4, -0.5)	0.009
	Men	-0.1 (-1.0, 0.8)	0.77
K6			
	Women	0.1 (-1.9, 2.1)	0.90
	Men	0.2 (-0.7, 1.2)	0.61
CES-D			
	Women	-2.8 (-6.4, 0.8)	0.13
	Men	0.5 (-1.5, 2.6)	0.60
RS-14			
	Women	3.7 (-1.5, 9.0)	0.16
	Men	1.7 (-2.0, 5.4)	0.36

Abbreviations: IES-R, Impact of Event Scale-Revised; K6, Kessler 6 Scale; CES-D, Center for Epidemiologic Studies Depression Scale; RS-14, Resilience Scale 14-item version; CI, confidence interval

Net change: Analysis of covariance (ANCOVA) adjusted for age and each psychological variable score at baseline

Table 3. Change in IES-R, K6, CES-D and RS-14 scores of participants in the fish oils and control groups stratified by sex

The fish oil capsules used in this study contained 1,568 mg DHA and 157 mg EPA per day. Based on previous studies [25, 29], DHA rather than EPA appeared to facilitate adult hippocampal neurogenesis. However, there is evidence to support the effectiveness of EPA monotherapy or a combination of EPA and DHA for depressive disorders [1]. A recent review showed that a 2:1 EPA:DHA ratio might be optimal for the treatment of depressive disorders [54]. In fact, our open label trial in physically injured patients failed to alleviate depressive symptoms, while alleviating PTSD symptoms [30]. To our knowledge, no previous studies have examined the effectiveness of fish oils to prevent PTSD. The appropriate composition of fish oil capsules to prevent PTSD warrants attention.

Remarkably, fish oil supplementation plus psychoeducation significantly lowered the IES-R total and hyperarousal subscale scores in women, despite the small sample size of women. To our knowledge, this is the first randomized controlled trial to show that fish oil reduced PTSD symptoms in women. While this outcome could be caused by chance because this was a secondary analysis, our finding coincides with that of previous longitudinal studies in Finland, Spain, and the United States [55-57] showing dietary intake of fish decreased the risk of developing depression in women, but not in men. Moreover, in Japan, a very low intake of fish was found to be associated with increased risk of suicidal death in women [58]. Although the difference in depressive symptoms assessed by the CES-D did not reach statistical significance among women in the present study, further studies with a large sample size may prove the effectiveness of fish oil supplementation for attenuating depressive symptoms in women. Also, our finding that women who took the fish oil supplements had a significant reduced score on the hyperarousal subscale is also partly consistent with a previous study showing that DHA intake prevented aggression from increasing at times of mental stress [41]. It is unclear why fish oils play an important role for regulating psychological well-being only in women, but it could be explained by the fact that estrogens cause higher DHA concentrations in women than in men [59]. Future studies should determine the effect of the sex difference in the effectiveness of fish oil supplementation for PTSD and posttraumatic depressive symptoms.

In addition to the possibility that fish oils do attenuate PTSD symptoms in women, it is well known that fish oils are effective for the secondary prevention of cardiovascular disease. An ecological study revealed that the availability of omega 3 PUFAs was inversely related with disease rates in 12 risk models, such as mortality from stroke and cardiovascular disease, as well as depression [60]. Given these positive effects on physical health and low rates of severe adverse events, fish oil supplementation could be a safe and novel strategy for the prevention of PTSD in women.

4.2. Generalizability

As shown in the figure 1, 1,390 out of 1,816 rescue workers invited to participate did not respond, which could limit the external validity of the findings. This might be because many rescue workers committed themselves to important roles at their own hospitals immediately after their deployment and could hardly afford to participate in this study.

4.3. Limitations

This study has some strengths. The participants are representative of all DMAT workers in that they are based across Japan. Baseline assessments were conducted within 1 month after the earthquake, which would minimize recall bias, and the attrition rate (<1%) was extremely low.

However, the study also has some limitations. First, this study was not a placebo controlled, double-blind trial. Because this study was implemented at a time of crisis, we could not prepare placebo capsules. It might be possible that we found a placebo effect acted more strongly in women who took the fish oil supplements. We are currently implementing a double-blind, placebo control trial of fish oils for the prevention of PTSD in physically injured patients (ClinicalTrials.gov Identifier: NCT00671099]. Second, this study relied on self-reports of adherence to the protocol, rather than biomarkers. We are currently measuring fatty acid composition of red blood cell membranes in a double-blind controlled trial mentioned above. Third, the finding of efficacy for women is driven by the significant reduction in hyperarousal cluster symptoms. Hyperarousal cluster symptoms are not PTSD-specific and are similar to the symptoms of other anxiety and mood disorders. Because assessment of PTSD is a self-report screening instrument rather than a structural interview, this study could not rule out an alternative explanation of the positive finding for women that attributes that difference to changes that are not related to PTSD.

5. Conclusion

This trial did not show the effectiveness of fish oil supplementation for the prevention of PTSD and depressive symptoms in rescue workers. However, the supplements did reduce PTSD symptoms significantly in women. Due to limitations mentioned above, the result of this study is a preliminary and should be accepted cautiously, but at the same time it is an encouraging finding. Not only rescue workers but large numbers of people were traumatized by natural disasters such as the Great East Japan Earthquake, and psychiatric resources to support them have been limited. Against this background, daily life-based intervention for the prevention of PTSD is preferable. Fish oil supplementation may offer a safe strategy for preventing PTSD in women, and thus is an important topic that should be further explored in disaster mental health care.

Acknowledgements

The authors would like to thank Professor Kaoru Inokuchi for generous financial support. We also thank Dr. Hisayoshi Kondo and Mr. Masayuki Ichihara for coordination with participants, and Mss. Kyoko Akutsu and Yumiko Kamoshida for data management and Ms. Hiroko Hamatani for preparation of bottled supplements. Professors Yasuhiro Otomo and Takeshi Terao and Dr. Katsumi Ikeshita joined this study as a member of the data and safety monitoring board. All of the supplements used in the study were supplied by Kentech Co., Ltd., Toyama, Japan.

Author details

Daisuke Nishi[1,2,3], Yuichi Koido[1], Naoki Nakaya[4,5], Toshimasa Sone[6], Hiroko Noguchi[2,3], Kei Hamazaki[3,7], Tomohito Hamazaki[3,7] and Yutaka Matsuoka[1,2,3]

1 National Disaster Medical Center, Japan

2 CREST, Japan Science and Technology Agency, Japan

3 National Center of Neurology and Psychiatry, Japan

4 Kamakura Women's University, Japan

5 Tohoku University, Japan

6 Tohoku Fukushi University, Japan

7 University of Toyama, Japan

References

[1] Freeman, M. P, Hibbeln, J. R, Wisner, K. L, Davis, J. M, Mischoulon, D, Peet, M, et al. Omega-3 fatty acids: evidence basis for treatment and future research in psychiatry. J Clin Psychiatry. (2006). Dec; , 67(12), 1954-67.

[2] Ross, B. M, Seguin, J, & Sieswerda, L. E. Omega-3 fatty acids as treatments for mental illness: which disorder and which fatty acid? Lipids Health Dis. (2007).

[3] Lin, P. Y, & Su, K. P. A meta-analytic review of double-blind, placebo-controlled trials of antidepressant efficacy of omega-3 fatty acids. J Clin Psychiatry. (2007). Jul; , 68(7), 1056-61.

[4] Martins, J. G. EPA but not DHA appears to be responsible for the efficacy of omega-3 long chain polyunsaturated fatty acid supplementation in depression: evidence from a meta-analysis of randomized controlled trials. J Am Coll Nutr. (2009). Oct; , 28(5), 525-42.

[5] Sublette, M. E, Ellis, S. P, Geant, A. L, & Mann, J. J. Meta-analysis of the effects of eicosapentaenoic acid (EPA) in clinical trials in depression. J Clin Psychiatry. (2011). Sep 6.

[6] Martins, J. G, Bentsen, H, & Puri, B. K. Eicosapentaenoic acid appears to be the key omega-3 fatty acid component associated with efficacy in major depressive disorder: a critique of Bloch and Hannestad and updated meta-analysis. Mol Psychiatry. (2012). Apr 10.

[7] Lin, P. Y, Mischoulon, D, Freeman, M. P, Matsuoka, Y, Hibbeln, J. R, Belmaker, R. H, et al. Are omega-3 fatty acids anti-depressants or just mood-improving agents? The effect depends upon diagnosis, supplement preparation, and severity of depression. Mol Psychiatry. online publication (2012). July 24.

[8] Bloch, M. H, & Hannestad, J. Omega-3 fatty acids for the treatment of depression: systematic review and meta-analysis. Mol Psychiatry. online publication (2011). Sep 20.

[9] Lesperance, F, Frasure-smith, N, St-andre, E, Turecki, G, Lesperance, P, & Wisniew-ski, S. R. The efficacy of omega-3 supplementation for major depression: a randomized controlled trial. J Clin Psychiatry. (2010). Aug; , 72(8), 1054-62.

[10] Zanarini, M. C, & Frankenburg, F. R. omega-3 Fatty acid treatment of women with borderline personality disorder: a double-blind, placebo-controlled pilot study. Am J Psychiatry. (2003). Jan; , 160(1), 167-9.

[11] Calder, P. C. Polyunsaturated fatty acids and inflammatory processes: New twists in an old tale. Biochimie. (2009). Jun; , 91(6), 791-5.

[12] Su, K. P. Biological mechanism of antidepressant effect of omega-3 fatty acids: how does fish oil act as a'mind-body interface'? Neurosignals. (2009). , 17(2), 144-52.

[13] Fernandes, G, Chandrasekar, B, Luan, X, & Troyer, D. A. Modulation of antioxidant enzymes and programmed cell death by n-3 fatty acids. Lipids. (1996). Mar;31 Suppl:S , 91-6.

[14] Pascoe, M. C, Crewther, S. G, Carey, L. M, & Crewther, D. P. What you eat is what you are-- a role for polyunsaturated fatty acids in neuroinflammation induced depression? Clin Nutr. (2011). Aug; , 30(4), 407-15.

[15] Eilat, E, Mendlovic, S, Doron, A, Zakuth, V, & Spirer, Z. Increased apoptosis in patients with major depression: A preliminary study. J Immunol. (1999). Jul 1; , 163(1), 533-4.

[16] Harlan, J, Chen, Y, Gubbins, E, Mueller, R, Roch, J. M, Walter, K, et al. Variants in Apaf-1 segregating with major depression promote apoptosome function. Mol Psychiatry. (2006). Jan; , 11(1), 76-85.

[17] Shimizu, E, Hashimoto, K, Okamura, N, Koike, K, Komatsu, N, Kumakiri, C, et al. Alterations of serum levels of brain-derived neurotrophic factor (BDNF) in depressed patients with or without antidepressants. Biol Psychiatry. (2003). Jul 1; , 54(1), 70-5.

[18] Schinder, A. F, & Poo, M. The neurotrophin hypothesis for synaptic plasticity. Trends Neurosci. (2000). Dec; , 23(12), 639-45.

[19] Huang, E. J, & Reichardt, L. F. Neurotrophins: roles in neuronal development and function. Annu Rev Neurosci. (2001). , 24, 677-736.

[20] Hashimoto, K, Shimizu, E, & Iyo, M. Critical role of brain-derived neurotrophic factor in mood disorders. Brain Res Brain Res Rev. (2004). May; , 45(2), 104-14.

[21] Lin, P. Y, Huang, S. Y, & Su, K. P. A meta-analytic review of polyunsaturated fatty acid compositions in patients with depression. Biol Psychiatry. (2010). Jul 15; , 68(2), 140-7.

[22] Beltz, B. S, Tlusty, M. F, Benton, J. L, & Sandeman, D. C. Omega-3 fatty acids upregulate adult neurogenesis. Neurosci Lett. (2007). Mar 26; , 415(2), 154-8.

[23] Wu, A, Ying, Z, & Gomez-pinilla, F. Dietary omega-3 fatty acids normalize BDNF levels, reduce oxidative damage, and counteract learning disability after traumatic brain injury in rats. J Neurotrauma. (2004). Oct, , 21(10), 1457-67

[24] Calderon, F, & Kim, H. Y. Docosahexaenoic acid promotes neurite growth in hippocampal neurons. J Neurochem. (2004). Aug; , 90(4), 979-88.

[25] Kawakita, E, Hashimoto, M, & Shido, O. Docosahexaenoic acid promotes neurogenesis in vitro and in vivo. Neuroscience. (2006). , 139(3), 991-7.

[26] Ressler, K. J, & Mayberg, H. S. Targeting abnormal neural circuits in mood and anxiety disorders: from the laboratory to the clinic. Nat Neurosci. (2007). Sep; , 10(9), 1116-24.

[27] Matsuoka, Y. Clearance of fear memory from the hippocampus through neurogenesis by omega-3 fatty acids: A novel preventive strategy for posttraumatic stress disorder? Biopsychosoc Med. (2011). Feb 8;5(1):3.

[28] Kitamura, T, Saitoh, Y, Takashima, N, Murayama, A, Niibori, Y, Ageta, H, et al. Adult neurogenesis modulates the hippocampus-dependent period of associative fear memory. Cell. (2009). Nov 13; , 139(4), 814-27.

[29] Wu, A, Ying, Z, & Gomez-pinilla, F. Docosahexaenoic acid dietary supplementation enhances the effects of exercise on synaptic plasticity and cognition. Neuroscience. (2008). Aug 26; , 155(3), 751-9.

[30] Matsuoka, Y, Nishi, D, Yonemoto, N, Hamazaki, K, Hashimoto, K, & Hamazaki, T. Omega-3 fatty acids for secondary prevention of posttraumatic stress disorder after accidental injury: An open-label pilot study. Journal of Clinical Psychopharmacology (2010). , 30(2), 217-9.

[31] Epstein, R. S, Fullerton, C. S, & Ursano, R. J. Posttraumatic stress disorder following an air disaster: a prospective study. Am J Psychiatry. (1998). Jul; , 155(7), 934-8.

[32] Fullerton, C. S, Ursano, R. J, & Wang, L. Acute stress disorder, posttraumatic stress disorder, and depression in disaster or rescue workers. Am J Psychiatry. (2004). Aug; , 161(8), 1370-6.

[33] Nishi, D, Koido, Y, Nakaya, N, Sone, T, Noguchi, H, Hamazaki, K, et al. Peritraumatic Distress, Watching Television, and Posttraumatic Stress Symptoms among Rescue Workers after the Great East Japan Earthquake. PLoS One. (2012). e35248.

[34] Nishi, D, & Matsuoka, Y. Peritraumatic distress after an earthquake: a bridge between neuroimaging and epidemiology. Mol Psychiatry. online publication (2012). Jul 3.

[35] Davidson, J. R, Hughes, D, Blazer, D. G, & George, L. K. Post-traumatic stress disorder in the community: an epidemiological study. Psychol Med. (1991). Aug; , 21(3), 713-21.

[36] Walker, E. A, Katon, W, Russo, J, Ciechanowski, P, Newman, E, & Wagner, A. W. Health care costs associated with posttraumatic stress disorder symptoms in women. Arch Gen Psychiatry. (2003). Apr; , 60(4), 369-74.

[37] Nishi, D, Koido, Y, Nakaya, N, Sone, T, Noguchi, H, Hamazaki, K, et al. Fish oil for attenuating posttraumatic stress symptoms among rescue workers after the Great East Japan Earthquake: A randomized controlled trial. Psychother Psychosom. (2012). , 81, 315-317.

[38] Matsuoka, Y, Nishi, D, Nakaya, N, Sone, T, Hamazaki, K, Hamazaki, T, et al. Attenuating posttraumatic distress with omega-3 polyunsaturated fatty acids among disaster medical assistance team members after the Great East Japan Earthquake: The APOP randomized controlled trial. BMC Psychiatry. (2011). Aug 16;11(1):132.

[39] Brunet, A, Weiss, D. S, Metzler, T. J, Best, S. R, Neylan, T. C, Rogers, C, et al. The Peritraumatic Distress Inventory: a proposed measure of PTSD criterion A2. Am J Psychiatry. (2001). Sep; , 158(9), 1480-5.

[40] Nishi, D, Matsuoka, Y, Noguchi, H, Sakuma, K, Yonemoto, N, Yanagita, T, et al. Reliability and validity of the Japanese version of the Peritraumatic Distress Inventory. Gen Hosp Psychiatry. (2009). January- February; , 31(1), 75-9.

[41] Hamazaki, T, Sawazaki, S, Itomura, M, Asaoka, E, Nagao, Y, Nishimura, N, et al. The effect of docosahexaenoic acid on aggression in young adults. A placebo-controlled double-blind study. J Clin Invest. (1996). Feb 15; , 97(4), 1129-33.

[42] Weiss, D. S. The Impact of Event Scale-Revised. Second Edition ed. Wilson JP, Keane TM, editors. New York: Guilford Press; (2004).

[43] Asukai, N, Kato, H, Kawamura, N, Kim, Y, Yamamoto, K, Kishimoto, J, et al. Reliability and validity of the Japanese-language version of the impact of event scale-revised (IES-R-J): four studies of different traumatic events. J Nerv Ment Dis. (2002). Mar; , 190(3), 175-82.

[44] Kessler, R. C, Andrews, G, Colpe, L. J, Hiripi, E, Mroczek, D. K, Normand, S. L, et al. Short screening scales to monitor population prevalences and trends in non-specific psychological distress. Psychol Med. (2002). Aug; , 32(6), 959-76.

[45] Radloff, L. S. The CES-D scale: a self-report depression scale for a research in the general population. Appl Psychol Measurement. (1977). , 1, 385-401.

[46] Wagnild, G. M, & Young, H. M. Development and psychometric evaluation of the Resilience Scale. J Nurs Meas. (1993). Winter; , 1(2), 165-78.

[47] Furukawa, T. A, Kessler, R. C, Slade, T, & Andrews, G. The performance of the K6 and K10 screening scales for psychological distress in the Australian National Survey of Mental Health and Well-Being. Psychol Med. (2003). Feb; , 33(2), 357-62.

[48] Shima, S, Shikano, T, Kitamura, T, & Asai, M. A new self-report depression scale. Seishinigaku (1985). in Japanese), 27, 717-23.

[49] Nishi, D, Uehara, R, Kondo, M, & Matsuoka, Y. Reliability and validity of the Japanese version of the Resilience Scale and its short version. BMC Res Notes. (2010). Nov 17;3(1):310.

[50] Kessler, R. C, Sonnega, A, Bromet, E, Hughes, M, & Nelson, C. B. Posttraumatic stress disorder in the National Comorbidity Survey. Arch Gen Psychiatry. (1995). Dec; , 52(12), 1048-60.

[51] Schlenger, W. E, Caddell, J. M, Ebert, L, Jordan, B. K, Rourke, K. M, Wilson, D, et al. Psychological reactions to terrorist attacks: findings from the National Study of Americans' Reactions to September 11. Jama. (2002). Aug 7; , 288(5), 581-8.

[52] Nishi, D, Matsuoka, Y, Yonemoto, N, Noguchi, H, Kim, Y, & Kanba, S. Peritraumatic Distress Inventory as a predictor of post-traumatic stress disorder after a severe motor vehicle accident. Psychiatry Clin Neurosci. (2010). Apr; , 64(2), 149-56.

[53] Nishi, D, Usuki, M, & Matsuoka, Y. Peritraumatic Distress in Accident Survivors: An Indicator for Posttraumatic Stress, Depressive and Anxiety Symptoms, and Posttraumatic Growth. In: Ovuga E, editor. Post Traumatic Stress Disorders in a Global Context: InTech; (2012). , 97-112.

[54] Mcnamara, R. K. Evaluation of docosahexaenoic acid deficiency as a preventable risk factor for recurrent affective disorders: current status, future directions, and dietary recommendations. Prostaglandins Leukot Essent Fatty Acids. (2009). Aug-Sep; 81(2-3):223-31.

[55] Timonen, M, Horrobin, D, Jokelainen, J, Laitinen, J, Herva, A, & Rasanen, P. Fish consumption and depression: the Northern Finland 1966 birth cohort study. J Affect Disord. (2004). Nov 1; , 82(3), 447-52.

[56] Sanchez-villegas, A, Henriquez, P, Figueiras, A, Ortuno, F, Lahortiga, F, & Martinez-gonzalez, M. A. Long chain omega-3 fatty acids intake, fish consumption and mental disorders in the SUN cohort study. Eur J Nutr. (2007). Sep; , 46(6), 337-46.

[57] Colangelo, L. A, He, K, Whooley, M. A, Daviglus, M. L, & Liu, K. Higher dietary intake of long-chain omega-3 polyunsaturated fatty acids is inversely associated with depressive symptoms in women. Nutrition. (2009). Oct; , 25(10), 1011-9.

[58] Poudel-tandukar, K, Nanri, A, Iwasaki, M, Mizoue, T, Matsushita, Y, Takahashi, Y, et al. Long chain n-3 fatty acids intake, fish consumption and suicide in a cohort of Japanese men and women--the Japan Public Health Center-based (JPHC) prospective study. J Affect Disord. (2011). Mar;129(1-3):282-8.

[59] Giltay, E. J, Gooren, L. J, Toorians, A. W, Katan, M. B, & Zock, P. L. Docosahexaenoic acid concentrations are higher in women than in men because of estrogenic effects. Am J Clin Nutr. (2004). Nov; , 80(5), 1167-74.

[60] Hibbeln, J. R, Nieminen, L. R, Blasbalg, T. L, Riggs, J. A, & Lands, W. E. Healthy intakes of n-3 and n-6 fatty acids: estimations considering worldwide diversity. Am J Clin Nutr. (2006). Jun;83(6 Suppl):1483S-93S.

Permissions

The contributors of this book come from diverse backgrounds, making this book a truly international effort. This book will bring forth new frontiers with its revolutionizing research information and detailed analysis of the nascent developments around the world.

We would like to thank Federico Durbano, for lending his expertise to make the book truly unique. He has played a crucial role in the development of this book. Without his invaluable contribution this book wouldn't have been possible. He has made vital efforts to compile up to date information on the varied aspects of this subject to make this book a valuable addition to the collection of many professionals and students.

This book was conceptualized with the vision of imparting up-to-date information and advanced data in this field. To ensure the same, a matchless editorial board was set up. Every individual on the board went through rigorous rounds of assessment to prove their worth. After which they invested a large part of their time researching and compiling the most relevant data for our readers. Conferences and sessions were held from time to time between the editorial board and the contributing authors to present the data in the most comprehensible form. The editorial team has worked tirelessly to provide valuable and valid information to help people across the globe.

Every chapter published in this book has been scrutinized by our experts. Their significance has been extensively debated. The topics covered herein carry significant findings which will fuel the growth of the discipline. They may even be implemented as practical applications or may be referred to as a beginning point for another development. Chapters in this book were first published by InTech; hereby published with permission under the Creative Commons Attribution License or equivalent.

The editorial board has been involved in producing this book since its inception. They have spent rigorous hours researching and exploring the diverse topics which have resulted in the successful publishing of this book. They have passed on their knowledge of decades through this book. To expedite this challenging task, the publisher supported the team at every step. A small team of assistant editors was also appointed to further simplify the editing procedure and attain best results for the readers.

Our editorial team has been hand-picked from every corner of the world. Their multi-ethnicity adds dynamic inputs to the discussions which result in innovative outcomes. These outcomes are then further discussed with the researchers and contributors who give their valuable feedback and opinion regarding the same. The feedback is then collaborated with the researches and they are edited in a comprehensive manner to aid the understanding of the subject.

Apart from the editorial board, the designing team has also invested a significant amount of their time in understanding the subject and creating the most relevant covers. They scrutinized every image to scout for the most suitable representation of the subject and create an appropriate cover for the book.

The publishing team has been involved in this book since its early stages. They were actively engaged in every process, be it collecting the data, connecting with the contributors or procuring relevant information. The team has been an ardent support to the editorial, designing and production team. Their endless efforts to recruit the best for this project, has resulted in the accomplishment of this book. They are a veteran in the field of academics and their pool of knowledge is as vast as their experience in printing. Their expertise and guidance has proved useful at every step. Their uncompromising quality standards have made this book an exceptional effort. Their encouragement from time to time has been an inspiration for everyone.

The publisher and the editorial board hope that this book will prove to be a valuable piece of knowledge for researchers, students, practitioners and scholars across the globe.

List of Contributors

Jasminka Juretić and Ivanka Živčić-Bećirević
University of Rijeka, Faculty of Humanities and Social Sciences, Department of Psychology, Croatia

Maria Michail
School of Nursing, Midwifery & Physiotherapy, University of Nottingham, UK

Jorge Javier Caraveo-Anduaga, Alejandra Soriano Rodríguez and Jose Erazo Pérez
Instituto Nacional de Psiquiatría "Ramón de la Fuente Muñiz", México

Guillem Pailhez and Antonio Bulbena
Anxiety Disorders Unit – INAD, Hospital del Mar, IMIM (Hospital del Mar Medical Research Institute), Barcelona, Spain

Roberta Anniverno, Alessandra Bramante, Claudio Mencacci and Federico Durbano
Center for the prevention of depression in women – Neuroscience Department, A.O. Fatebenefratelli e Oftalmico, Milan, Italy
Neuroscience Department, A.O. Fatebenefratelli e Oftalmico, Milan, Italy

Ebru Şalcıoğlu
Institute of Psychiatry, King's College London, University of London, UK
Istanbul Centre for Behaviour Research and Therapy, Istanbul, Turkey
Department of Psychology, Haliç University, Istanbul, Turkey

Metin Başoğlu
Institute of Psychiatry, King's College London, University of London, UK
Istanbul Centre for Behaviour Research and Therapy, Istanbul, Turkey

Catherine Fredette and Veronique Palardy
University of Quebec at Montreal, Quebec, Canada
Mcgill University, Quebec, Canada

Ghassan El-Baalbaki
University of Quebec at Montreal, Quebec, Canada
Mcgill University, Quebec, Canada

Sylvain Neron
Mcgill University, Quebec, Canada

Nesrin Dilbaz and Aslı Enez Darcin
Üsküdar University, Neuropsychiatry (NP) Hospital, Istanbul, Turkey

Clare Rees and Rebecca Anderson
School of Psychology and Speech Pathology, Curtin Health Innovation Research Institute
(CHIRI), Curtin University, Australia

Daisuke Nishi and Yutaka Matsuoka
National Disaster Medical Center, Japan
CREST, Japan Science and Technology Agency, Japan
National Center of Neurology and Psychiatry, Japan

Yuichi Koido
National Disaster Medical Center, Japan

Naoki Nakaya
Kamakura Women's University, Japan
Tohoku University, Japan

Toshimasa Sone
Tohoku Fukushi University, Japan

Hiroko Noguchi
CREST, Japan Science and Technology Agency, Japan
National Center of Neurology and Psychiatry, Japan

Kei Hamazaki
National Center of Neurology and Psychiatry, Japan
University of Toyama, Japan

Tomohito Hamazaki
National Center of Neurology and Psychiatry, Japan
University of Toyama, Japan

Printed in the USA
CPSIA information can be obtained
at www.ICGtesting.com
JSHW011427221024
72173JS00004B/707